Acknowledgments

I want to express my deepest gratitude to Ajana, graphic artist and illustrator, for gracing this book with your wonderfully creative imagination and extraordinary talent. Your aesthetic spirit, wit, and creative excellence generously conveyed by the illustrations lying within these pages openly reflect a uniquely brilliant consciousness I find intrinsic to your generation…. Speaking of which, I sincerely thank you too, James Snow, for your regard and friendship. Your clever mind and discerning herbalist's eye have enhanced this herbal and spared me litters of technical chagrin. I also wish to extend my gratitude to Dave Broach for your good-natured willingness to manifest the cover photo with your patience, your Hasselblad, and the singular touch of your light, and shutter skills. And while I'm on this roll, thank you Elaine Gill and skilled staff members of The Crossing Press. Your support, your fluid spirit of co-creating, and your confidence in my work as an herbalist and writer leave little wonder in my mind why your catalog's repertoire of publications is bursting with the works of so many excellent authors. This is not to say that we didn't have to get down and dirty while tussling with a few differences of opinion, the aftermath of which found a number of Ajana's most splendid illustrations adorning the cutting room floor, alas never to be seen by the reader's eyes; and that is the tragic component of this story. However, the ending is of course a happy one, for all who enjoy entering aesthetic realms of exquisite fantasy can visit Ajana's captivating Web site at <www. ajana-art.com> and experience the beautiful sanctums of her talent and creative vision. Please note, dear reader, this is not one of those commonplace commercial plugs; this is a dad's fervent praise of his daughter's superb talent and fascinating mind…big difference, big, big difference. Go check it out…you'll come back delighted.

THE HERBAL MEDICINE-MAKER'S HANDBOOK

A HOME MANUAL

James Green, Herbalist

Illustrated by Ajana Green

Cautionary Note: The information contained within this book is in no way intended as a substitute for medical counseling. Please do not attempt self-treatment of a medical problem without consulting a qualified health practitioner.

The author and The Crossing Press expressly disclaim any and all liability for any claims, damages, losses, judgments, expenses, costs, and liabilities of any kind or injuries resulting from any products offered in this book by participating companies and their employees or agents. Nor does the inclusion of any resource group or company listed within this book constitute an endorsement or guarantee of quality by the author or The Crossing Press.

For information on bulk purchases or group discounts for this and other Crossing Press titles, please contact our Sales Manager at 800/777-1048.

Visit our Web site on the Internet: **www.crossingpress.com**

Library of Congress Cataloging-in-Publication Data

Green, James, 1940-
 The herbal medicine-maker's handbook: a home manual / by James Green.
  p. cm.
 Includes bibliographical references and index.
 ISBN 0-89594-990-3 (pbk.)
 1. Materia medica, Vegetable—Handbooks, manuals, etc. 2. Traditional medicine—Handbooks, manuals, etc. 3. Herbals—Handbooks, manuals, etc. I. Title.

RS164.G674   2000
615'.321--dc21   00-030708

For
Bre and Ajana,
my gifted daughters
and artful companions

We dance our madness;
we dance our joy.
Oh precious ones, the fun has just begun.
Wild music is in the air;
there's beauty flowing everywhere.

Table of Contents

APPENDICES

A WORD BEFORE THE MEDICINE SHOW

"The day you decide to appreciate yourself is the day you begin to dance."
— T. Elder Sachs

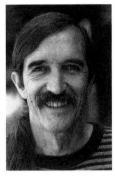

Herbal medicine-making is much like dancing; it's easy, it's natural, and it's undeniably delightful. To say the least, it is a lucid expression of one's distinct character. If you have never worked with medicinal plants or made herbal medicines for yourself, you will have to take my word for this. However, as you experiment with the procedures suggested in this manual, I promise that during some private moment, maybe when "shaking your tinctures" or while "garbling" some dreamy Mugwort, you will find yourself thinking, "Hey, that Green guy was right. This is more damn fun! I think I might even go dancing tonight!" And like dancing, once you find the rhythm of the music and begin moving your body with it, you'll never want to stop.

The ever-engaging green-melodies of herbal medicine-making are sung by the seductive voices of your neighboring leaves, roots, barks, rhizomes, flowers, and seeds, while the rhythm you move to is composed entirely within yourself, by the cadence of your creative enjoyment. You'll find yourself swinging to the pleasures of simple fun, personal independence, and a renewed connection with Earth's natural beauty and perpetual abundance. And that's feelin' good, which is the essence of health. The making is the taking of herbal medicine.

Keep in mind that herbs, the principal ingredients in homemade herbal medicines, are basically free once you learn how to correctly harvest them for yourself (which we will cover in Chapter Three). Therefore, I can assure you that herbal medicine-making performed in the home-kitchen is not only simple and fun, it is universally affordable. This makes perfect sense, for the art and empirical science of Herbalism were engendered eons ago by the wit and enduring ingenuity of some remarkably intelligent, resourceful, and visionary people—our ancestors. This is our cultural heritage.

Herbalism is one of those people's things. It is indigenous to all communities of our globe, which is why it thrives so harmoniously in our homes. To manifest high-quality, health-pumping herbal preparations, you can take this plant lore in hand, make your own preparations, and thereby liberate yourself, your family, your community, and your monetary resources from dependence on others. Why pay others to frolic in the luscious gardens of Earth, picking flowers and enjoying themselves making herbal products? You can do all that frolicking, immersing yourself in wondrous herbal beauty, and uplifting your mind and spirit. Making your own herbal medicine both enhances your happiness and boosts your immune system. And the herbal preparations you make can be every bit as excellent as those you bring home from the store. Actually they will be better, profoundly better; this I can also promise you. Ralph Waldo Emerson, another born-again herbalist, expressed similar feelings, "When I go into my garden with a spade, and dig a bed, I feel such an exhilaration and health that I discover that I have been defrauding myself all this time in letting others do for me what I should have been doing with my own hands." I always suspected that Waldo was in the garden.

Another word, if I may; then we'll get on with the medicine show. For much of my life, I have focused my attention on health, herbs, foods, gardens, and making plant medicine. They are my passion, and I feel passionately about them. As such, tendrils of my feelings and opinions will undoubtedly intertwine with the rhetoric of this manual. Knowing the inevitability of this, I want to restate (with some minor alterations) a passage from the prologue of my other book, *The Male Herbal*. I haven't evoked a better way than I did therein to say to you what I want to say here. Being the sedulous Sagittarian that I am, I'm accomplished at quoting my own thoughts, as references anyway.

So, "When an individual goes public, publishing a book discussing his experiences, beliefs, and opinions, especially in the realms of health and personal power, it is important to give the reader a self-disclosure of one's bias. Currently, in this Western culture of ours, the fact that what I have written has been published tends to display me as an authority. In light of this strange cultural phenomenon, I wish to supply the discriminating reader and herbal learner with appropriately insightful information to help him or her question this authority. Nothing that I say is presented by me as the Truth! I am merely disclosing my current truth. The printed voice of this book will share my knowledge, observations, and opinions based on my experiences, punctuated by what wisdom I have gathered. Every individual has a share of wisdom to pass around. As your mind travels through the landscape of ideas I design and construct for you in this herbal manual, please do not slip into a passive state of observation. In the light of your life experiences, measure and question my opinions and conclusions. I accept the risk of being proven wrong. If the fervor of my expression of these opinions ascends a street orator's platform for a paragraph or two, allow me the social blunder; it's just an idiosyncrasy of my particular humanness. Do not fault me for my passion. Rather, make note of any disagreements you may have, get back to me, and point out the possible errors of my current beliefs. This way we can interact and communicate as co-seekers and creators, and as co-members of a species that obviously has much to discover about itself and about the transcendent universe in which it thrives.

"We are, with one another, co-creating a most magnificent and fascinating age. And our current creation is so very splendid precisely because each of us contributes a unique perspective. The term 'expert' is derived from the verbal root per meaning to try, to risk, to press forward. All of us do that with every new thought and experience we create. Living a life qualifies each of us as an expert. We don't have to agree with each other for things to work, merely appreciate one another and enjoy our differences. I can live with the fact that some people will always think of authors as experts, as long as it is duly noted that the universal characteristic of experts is that they normally disagree with one another."

I'm almost finished here....

As we proceed through this handbook, I will not be giving you long lists of things to get. I will give you short lists of equipment and resources that will be completely adequate to get you started. I encourage you to trust your innovative cunning to guide you further in a suitable expansion of your assemblage, deciding for yourself what you will need to best support your particular style and evolving techniques. Learn the elementary principles, then unfold in your own way.

I'm not going to include innumerable, point by point, watch-me-do-it illustrations either. With a few (adroitly placed) drawings, this handbook will get you started in splendid fashion; it will give you cardinal processes as practical allies that point the way and encourage you to embark dauntlessly on your journey. Your imagination and intrinsic abilities will usher you on from there. Herbal medicine-making is more engaging this way, and you will beget astonishingly clever ideas. Remember, Herbalism is a human response to plants, and this response ever dwells alive and well within each of us. I ask you to relate to the learning of the overall process of making herbal medicine more like the way you might relate to creating art or reading a novel, rather than the way you might relate to viewing a movie or a TV program that leaves little if anything to your imagination. Like a Zen painter (don't I wish), I will create some empty space suggesting forms and ideas which your creative imagination can fill in as we proceed. This way we co-create while experiencing the ripening fruits of this medicine show. (There are some instances, however, when I will tend to go on and on; kind of like I am now.) We know that young children enjoy themselves for a significantly longer time and experience far more quality time when given simple pine cones, small rocks, colorful ribbons, and randomly shaped blocks of wood to play with than they do when given complex, perfectly molded, and fully complete toys. The opportunity to pour their own vision into the empty spaces of the unfinished picture presented by their elemental toys ignites the fertile fires of their imagination, giving them the joy of unleashed creative pleasure. The subtle suggestions stimulated by these rudimentary building units become their most entertaining playmates and beneficial teachers. Likewise, children soon become bored with toys that leave little to their innovative imagination; and so it is with adult human beings, for we are all avid creators and we all love to play.

As the medicine show proceeds from stage to stage in your home, create an herbal pharmacy that you tailor to your lifestyle; develop and refine your medicine-making techniques to suit yourself; and make notes that clearly record your experiences for future reference. Rely on the ideas in this handbook merely as starting places that will give you solid ground on which to place your feet, then leap high into your creative, innovative nature. Students become skilled in the basics under the guidance of an experienced teacher, but they become masters only after leaving the teacher and exploring areas into which the teacher had not ventured.

Have fun, don't hesitate. I appreciate your life.

CHAPTER 1
A FIELD TRIP

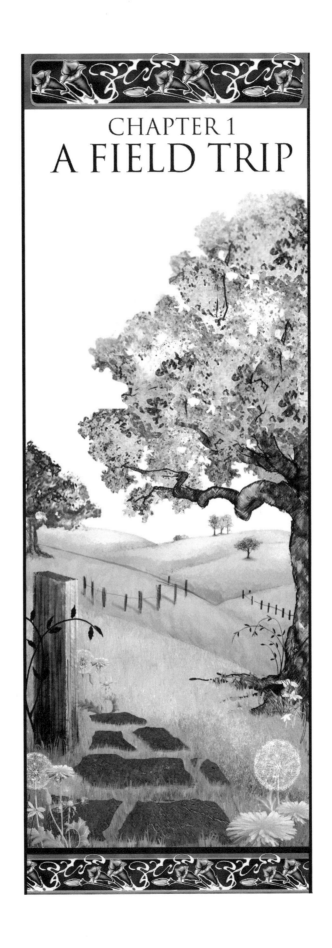

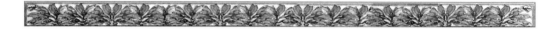

Let's begin our immersion into the mosaic of ideas and techniques that describe herbal medicine-making by first harvesting a wild plant and making an herbal extract: a Dandelion tincture.

We'll begin this green medicine journey outside your dwelling place—where the wild plants are. Herbal medicine lives outdoors, where nature spirits arouse our enchantment, and our vitality is naturally quickened. With your involvement and, I hope, a freshly awakened passion, you'll initiate your apprenticeship by experiencing the elation of harvesting a wild plant and, with it, creating a simple herbal medicine of excellent quality. So, if you are not already outdoors reading these words, please, weather permitting, step outside with me and we'll find *Taraxacum officinale*, a most notorious wild plant....

This is the plant that herbalists, children, and poets call Dandelion.

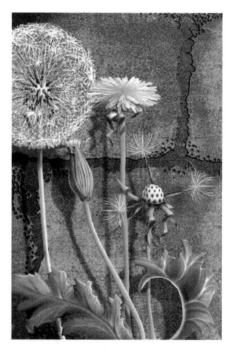

Dandelion

Many other people call it a weed and treat it rather rudely.

Let us refer to it as a wild medicinal plant and perceive the extract we're about to make with it as an herbal tonic. Our intention is to connect with a plant spirit and with its alliance create a nutritional preparation that is easy to assimilate and can be depended upon to help our digestion, our liver, and our kidneys to feel good. Then, while this first-born extract is macerating (soaking) in its menstruum (solvent), we'll proceed through the following chapters of this handbook and peruse the rest of the medicine-making ideas that await our attention.

Common Dandelion (botanical name, *Taraxacum officinale*) grows just about everywhere. It should be fairly simple for you to discover this flowering ally. It is usually denoted by one or more bright yellow floral asterisks randomly displayed in urban laws, in grazed fields, or along neighborhood footpaths.

Dandelions are one of the most common medicinal herbs that live with us in our neighborhoods. In fact, every year petrochemical companies reap additional millions from the urban community by manufacturing and marketing a myriad of designer poisons devised specifically to alienate and destroy these wily turf-gangsters. In contrast, communities in China eagerly harvest and eat young Dandelion greens to enrich their diets, along with Purslane (*Portulaca oleracea*), and Kudzu (*Pueraria lobata*), which are two more "weeds" we tend to curse in this culture. The people of our southern communities could control the rampant spread of Kudzu vine through their countrysides by eating it; it's a superb cardiac tonic, and it controls alcohol craving—if one wants to; if not, Kudzu curbs headache and hangovers.

Dandelion's species name, *officinale*, means "used in the office or the workshop." This indicates that historically Dandelion was (and of course still is) used medicinally. Dandelion's genus name, *Taraxacum*, is derived from the Greek *taraxis*, meaning disorder, and *akas*, a remedy, further echoing our ancestors' traditional esteem for this herb. Keep in mind that there are other plants that, at casual glance, look similar to a Dandelion. Fear not, though, there are no toxic or poisonous lookalikes in this country, and it is very easy to identify the official *Taraxacum*. Therefore, as I describe to you the true Dandelion, please *pay attention to detail* (the third rule of good herbal medicine-making).

The Dandelion has a single golden-yellow flower head sitting on top of each individual flower stalk. This flower head can grow up to 2 inches wide. These flowers open with the rising of the morning sun and close down in the evening. They can appear almost any time of the year, but mainly you find them from April to November in meadows, pastures, gardens, along the roadsides, and inevitably, within the rigid boundary lines of all manicured lawns. Dandelion's impetuous blossoming is Nature's never-ending reminder that diversity is favored, and therefore rules. The plant's graceful green stalks are round, smooth, brittle, and hollow. They grow from 2 to 18 inches tall, and have no other stalks branching off them. Each Dandelion stalk is straight and unjointed (no stalks branching off it), growing individually and separately out of a base having a rosette crown of numerous bright green leaves. These flower stalks often appear to be growing directly out of the ground. Dandelion never grows a central stalk. If the plant you are looking at has a tall stalk that is bearing leaves and flowers, it's not a Dandelion. However, there can be a number of flower stalks rising from the center of each Dandelion plant. Each stalk, as I have mentioned, holds up only one bright yellow flower head, or one flower bud, or possibly a single gossamer sphere of plumed seeds. The mature flower can transform into this globular seed head (faerie's afro) overnight. The lobes or edges of the long, lance-shaped Dandelion leaves have deeply serrated, unevenly pointed teeth (*Dent-de-lion*, lion's tooth in Old French). These pliable leaves are 3 to 12 inches long, 1/2 to 2 1/2 inches wide. The top surfaces, the undersides, and the midribs of Dandelion's leaves are bald and feel quite smooth to the touch. They are not hairy, warty, or prickly like some Dandelion lookalikes. When you dig a Dandelion up

There are three true Dandelion species found in the U.S.: *Taraxacum officinale*, common Dandelion, and *T. laevigatum*, a red-seeded specimen, both of which grow in disturbed soils throughout the temperate regions of the U.S. The third species, *T. ceratophorum*, is found in meadows and other moist places in the mountains throughout the boreal zone, south, and at high altitudes.

"Down with lawns; up with herbs."
— RYAN DRUM

from the ground, with profound respect and deep gratitude (the first rule of good herbal medicine-making), you'll find its root to be thick and brittle, having a thin beige skin on the outside and sap-filled, milky-white vegetable flesh within. This is commonly called a taproot. Dandelion's taproot can be branching, and it can grow up to 10 inches long. All parts of the Dandelion plant, when either broken or wounded, will bleed a bitter-tasting milky-white sap. You'll find this juice to be a little sweeter in the spring plants.

Once you have found some Dandelions, harvest an entire plant including the root, leaves, buds, blossoms, and seed heads, if there are any. If a portion of the root breaks off and remains in the ground, great! This root piece will regenerate and produce a new plant—yet another vegetable contribution to Earth's dynamic theater of perpetual abundance.

Now that you have properly identified and graciously harvested this plant, offer gratitude once again for its life. Consider leaving an offering, like a strand of your hair, a prayer, a song, a story, whatever; plant spirits are known to be deeply touched by simple gestures of appreciation. Wash all the soil off the plant, and bring it home to your kitchen. If the Dandelion plants you find are small, you might want to harvest six or seven of them.

If you are unable to locate any living Dandelions in the neighborhood, or if you suspect the plants that are there have been sprayed or are too close to the road and might be coated with odious residues of auto exhaust, the next best thing for you to do is harvest organically grown or wildcrafted, freshly dried (dehydrated) Dandelion from an herb or natural food store.

Purchase an ounce of the highest quality Dandelion root you can find and an ounce of Dandelion leaf. Make sure the dried root material is a deep rich brown color and has a full bitter flavor when you chew on a piece. Make sure the dried leaf material shows a rich green color and also has a discernible bitter flavor. This leaf, dried properly, should definitely not be brown. If it is brown, don't bother with it. It's no good; shop somewhere else.

Now, lay your fresh medicinal plant(s) on your kitchen countertop. Cut the root and other parts into small pieces. How small? As small as your patience and enthusiasm permit. The smaller the better, because more surface area is exposed. If you are using dried plant materials, crush or grind them into small pieces, using a small coffee bean grinder or a mortar and pestle (See Chapter Four, "Kitchen Pharmacy Equipment"). Place these tiny pieces in a jar with a tight-fitting lid. Use a pint- or quart-size jar depending on the amount of plant material. Pour 100-proof vodka into the jar, filling it to the top of the plant material. If you are working with fresh plant material, at this point you might pour the plant with its menstruum into a blender and liquefy it to expose more surface area to the solvent. Wipe the top ridge of the jar, cleaning off any stuff that might be clinging to it. Put a piece of wax paper over the opening as a gasket, and screw down the jar lid. Tighten it firmly. Shake your tincture energetically. Now, take a moment to look at it. Admire it for a while, because it is indeed precious. It is your plant medicine, the enchanted doorway through which you just entered the enthralling world of Herbalism. Label the container appropriately. On this label include the name of the herb, the part of the herb used, (i.e., Dandelion root and top, *Taraxacum officinale*) and the date that will arrive fourteen days from the date you are preparing this extract. This date you write on the label is the day your tincture will be ready for you to separate the saturated liquid (the tincture extract) from the then-depleted plant material (the marc). During those fourteen days, at least once, even better two or three times a day, affectionately and vigorously shake your tincture (the "sixth" rule of good medicine-making) with your mind focused on your appreciation of the plant and your intention for its use. This is an important routine to attend to, for it maintains the extraction energy of the menstruum at a more efficient rate, and it permeates the maturing medicine with your mindful attention and the healing power of your personal energy.

After a minimum of fourteen days and nights, separate the spent plant material from the liquid extract. A simple method for doing this is to line a large hand-held strainer with a square-shaped piece of cotton muslin cloth (undyed and preferably unbleached cotton muslin), large enough to hang about an inch or two over the edges of the strainer.

Place the muslin-lined strainer into a glass or stainless steel receptacle, and slowly and carefully pour your entire extract into this straining apparatus. Allow all the liquid to flow through the cloth. After the liquid has finished flowing through the cloth, join together all four corners of the cloth and hold them above the plant material. Grasp them firmly together with one hand, and with the other hand grasp the ball of plant material and twist it and squeeze it to press out the rest of the liquid thoroughly. Remove as much of the liquid as possible

from the depleted plant fiber (the marc). After doing this to your satisfaction, you can discard the marc into the compost.

Now, pour this herbal extract into a bottle that can be tightly capped (brown amber glass bottles are the most ideal) and store it in a cool, dark location. This alcohol/water extract will keep for many years. (A solution like this requires a minimum of 18–20 percent of the total volume of the liquid to be ethyl alcohol in order for the alcohol to adequately preserve it. Pure 100-proof vodka is 50 percent ethyl alcohol, and even when diluted by the juices of this fresh plant will render sufficient preservative action.)

You have handcrafted an herbal medicine; your initiation is complete—welcome to the swiftly growing community of independent lay-herbalists. To conclude this exercise, I would like to also applaud the co-creator of your handcrafted tincture by summarizing for you the personal and ecological health-promoting gifts of the wild Dandelion.

An Earth-enriching co-habitant of almost every community, Dandelion promotes healthy local turf everywhere it grows, unless it is foolishly poisoned to death. The particular design of Dandelion's root system breaks up soil in a unique manner which greatly enhances the condition of any garden soil. In fact Dandelion and its sister compositae, Chamomile, another soil-conditioning plant, have been referred to in farming cultures as "the soil doctors." Dandelion's randomly scattered flowers relieve rampant urban-lawn monotony. Its vibrant yellow blossoms are aesthetically and emotionally uplifting. For those who like to play and even giggle the way you did when you were a babe, Dandelion's mature seed heads are a joyous toy which entice bustling

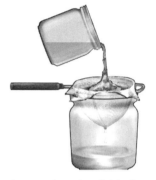

Strainer Lined with Muslin

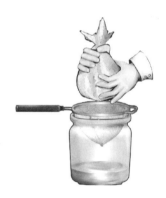

Squeezing the Liquid Out

human beings to pause, pick, and blow off its downy hairdo into passing air currents, watching the seeds eject dramatically, scattering in random directions, then parachuting serenely to the ground. I pursue this whimsical ritual as eagerly today as I did when I was a small child, and the spontaneous affair with these little blowballs remains as delightful as it always was.

When used to affect our body directly, common Dandelion is one of the finest foods and medicines found in the herbalist's materia medica. Young springtime Dandelion leaves have a pleasantly bitter aromatic flavor. They blend well with other fresh salad plants, and they carry with them a rich load of bitters and micro-nutrients, especially the minerals potassium and calcium, and vitamins A and C. Eating Dandelion greens and other bitters prior to meals is invaluable for stimulating one's appetite, digestion, and assimilation. Regular use of Dandelion extracts often relieves the uncomfortable maladies commonly experienced in the upper and lower digestive tract such as poor digestion, gas, nausea, and constipation.

In general, Dandelion carries substances that stimulate the function of many glands and organs, especially the kidneys and liver. It has a tonic affect on the kidneys and encourages kidney function with its diuretic action, while at the same time it increases the body's potassium content, rather than depleting it as other diuretics commonly do. Dandelion is an excellent substance to employ for prevention and treatment of biliary problems. It is a liver and gallbladder tonic that stimulates the healthy discharge and flow of bile. When taken over a period of 4 to 6 weeks, it can work as an efficient preventive agent for those individuals who have a constitutional disposition to form gallstones.

Following are some specific indications and an adult dosage for using the whole-plant Dandelion tincture you are presently making (see Chapter Twenty-Five, "*Dosage*," to help determine corresponding children's dosages).

For physical comfort take 30 to 50 drops of tincture 3 to 4 times daily to:

• relieve intestinal gas and poor digestion that is due to insufficient bile

• relieve constipation that is due to sluggish liver activity

• help eliminate skin eruptions that are due to sluggish liver activity

• relieve difficulty in urinating and/or water retention

• use as a blood purifier to treat chronic autotoxemia which is contributing to rheumatism, arthritis, and/or skin eruptions

The dosage I have suggested is low for this particular herb, for Dandelion is safe, gentle, and shows no toxicity. Some herbalists recommend 150 to 300 drops (approx. 5 to 10 ml) of Dandelion tincture three times a day as a basic adult dosage. However, it is prudent to begin with a low dosage regardless of the herb you consider using. Dosages can always be increased after observing your reaction to a new substance. To gain the full benefit of Dandelion when employing it as a tonic, it is often best to continue its use for at least one month up to a year, depending on the individual's response and needs. A second year of use can be beneficial and appropriate for some individuals. For the bodies of these folks, Dandelion is good food.

This act of nourishing yourself with herbs is fully affordable now that you are harvesting your own herbs and learning to make tinctures and other extracts for yourself. Remember, like the mind, the body appreciates and responds most favorably to variety (diversity). Don't take any food or herbal remedy every day. Take the remedy for 6 days a week with a random day off; do this for three to four weeks, then take a few days off, and so on. And when using Dandelion, it is quite appropriate to change the delivery vehicle by preparing this tonic herb as an herbal tea (a decoction). Drink it with the tincture, or alternate a dose (1 cup) of tea with a dose of tincture, or use Dandelion tea in place of Dandelion tincture altogether, drinking a cupful twice a day.

So, now you have an herbal tincture in the making, and you know how to store and use this specific health-supporting herbal tonic once the extraction process is completed. Meanwhile, during the following hours when you are not eating, dreaming, working, playing, or shaking your tincture, we can explore more ideas concerning the home practice of Herbalism and consider other forms of herbal extracts you can make.

CHAPTER 2

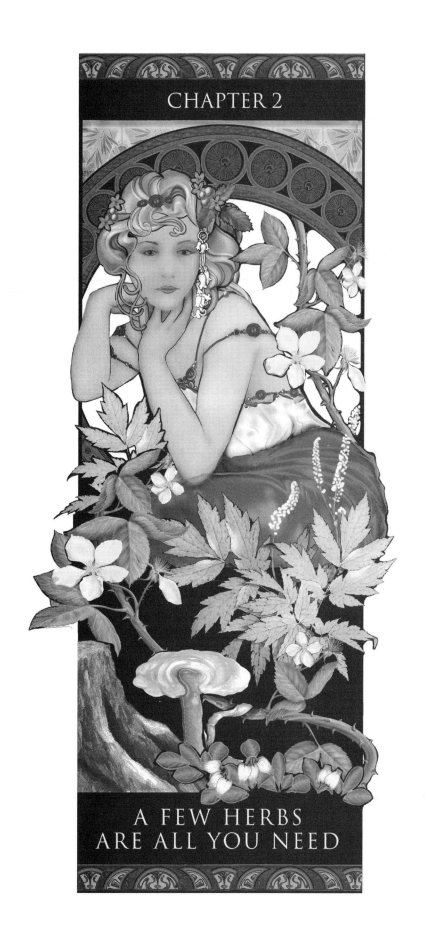

A FEW HERBS
ARE ALL YOU NEED

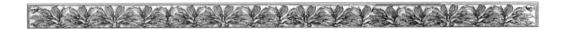

It's a jungle garden out there; roots and flowers are everywhere. That's why this leafy turquoise planet is so dear to the hearts of herbalists. Here we enjoy an unending variety of plants and animals to embrace as our allies and teachers. But for an enthusiastic student herbalist, who has just entered through some unassuming personal gate into the vast forest of Herbalism, sorting out Earth's immense herbal diversity can be somewhat bewildering.

Question: How many herbs should I know to be an effectual herbalist?

Answer: 30…well, maybe 35…and probably a fungus as well.

How's that for an assertive air of authority? Someone has to act like he or she knows the answer to that question. I'll reference the source of this authority shortly.

Certainly, most herbalists I know strongly recommend that a student limit his or her studies to "a few select herbs." Get to know them well by learning to identify them, experience growing them when possible, communicate with them, discern when, where, and how best to harvest them, make medicine with them, *touch, taste, smell,* and *use them.* The energies of thirty to thirty-five herbs will enchant you and keep you sufficiently busy for the following year or two. Distinguished individuals from the remain-

ing myriad of herbs that dwell on Earth will, one by one, as situations arise, attract your attention and attach themselves to your initial repertory.

So, the subsequent question arises: "Which few select herbs should I choose?"

Well, the most important principle to guide you in this very personal selection is to embrace any and all plants that you are intuitively attracted to: those that touch your spirit in an exceptionally deep and personal way. These are relationships that you never want to ignore. A second reliable criterion is to select herbs that grow near you and can be found thriving in the bioregion you inhabit, or in closely neighboring bio-regions. The plants you select should be fairly easy to acquire and always of excellent quality. Flirt with the currently fashionable and exotic imports, by all means, but don't become dependent on their availability.

Most herb students commence their studies by gleaning information found in popular herb books, and the number of herbs discussed in today's herbal literature can be overwhelming. At least, I have found this to be the experience of many students before they connected with a teacher or attended an herb school. So, if I may assist you with some specific suggestions, I will give you an historic and authoritative list of plants that you might consider as you orchestrate your first line of green allies, or you can at least refer to this list as a model for choosing a comparable group of plants that live in your area.

The authoritative history: In the late 1980s the California School of Herbal Studies (CSHS) was co-directed by six herbalists: Tim Blakley, David Hoffmann, Amanda McQuade Crawford, Mindy Green, Gina Banghart, and myself. We decided that, in order to align our individual classes throughout the year, it would be helpful for all of us to focus on the personalities, actions, and indications of a central core of tonic and therapeutic plants. As an initial step to develop this group of medicinals, each of us agreed to provide a list of thirty favored plants that we felt could be relied upon to supply an herbalist with pretty much any and all the herbal actions and uplifting virtues required to provide good health care in a home and community. The succeeding task of grafting our lists together and then pruning the aggregation back to thirty plants proved to be an interesting journey of forbearance and compromise; the results of that saga attest to the fact that, on a rare occasion, even experts can come to an agreement, or at least cross-pollinate their opinions. The hybrid list we ultimately compiled and felt reasonably good about included the following thirty plants.

CSHS List of 30 Herbs

Blackberry (*Rubus villosus*)

★**Black Cohosh** (*Cimicifuga racemosa*)

Calendula (*Calendula officinalis*)

Cayenne (*Capsicum annuum*)

Chamomile, German
  (*Matricaria recutita*)

Cleavers (*Galium aperine*)

Comfrey (*Symphytum officinale*)

Crampbark (*Viburnum opulus*)

Dandelion (*Taraxacum officinale*)

★**Echinacea** (*Echinacea purpurea*)

Elder (*Sambucus nigra*)

Fennel (*Foeniculum vulgare*)

Ginger (*Zingiber officinale*)

★**Goldenseal** (*Hydrastis canadensis*)

Gumweed (*Grindelia spp.*)

Hawthorn (*Crataegus oxyacanthus*)

Marshmallow (*Althaea officinalis*)

Mugwort (*Artemisia vulgaris*)

Mullein (*Verbascum spp.*)

Nettle (*Urtica spp.*)

Peppermint (*Mentha piperita*)

★**Pipsissewa** (*Chimaphilla umbellata*)

Plantain (*Plantago lanceolata* or *P. major*)

St. John's Wort (*Hypericum perforatum*)

Scullcap (*Scutellaria spp.*)

Valerian (*Valeriana officinalis*)

Vitex (*Vitex agnus-castus*)

Willow (*Salix alba*)

Yarrow (*Achillea millefolium*)

Yellow Dock (*Rumex crispus*)

I have asterisked the plants which are broadly used in commerce and which, due to over-harvest, loss of habitat, or by the nature of their innate rareness or sensitivity are either at risk or have significantly declined in numbers within their current range. Use substitute plants when possible (see the discussion on page 24).

Yes, I know; where's Milk Thistle, where's Sage, where's Usnea, where's….Undeniably, this list screams out the names of countless time-honored herbs that have not been included, and I must say (using this opportunity to get in a "last word"), the herbs that would be at the top of the list of thirty (if anybody would have listened to me) are listed below.

GREEN'S LONG-AWAITED EMBELLISHMENTS

Burdock (*Arctium lappa*)

Ginkgo (*Ginkgo biloba*)

Oat (wild: *Avena fatua*, cultivated: *Avena sativa*)

Saw Palmetto (*Serenoa serrulata*)

Siberian Ginseng (*Eleuthrococcus senticosus*)

And then there's **Reishi** mushroom (*Ganoderma lucidum*), a fungus, and….Well, you can appreciate the problem we faced.

Please note that most of the thirty plants on the CSHS list grow in abundance in the northern California region where our school is located, but as you may also notice, love transcends all rules and common sense, and some of our most favored plants that made it onto the list don't normally grow here. Ginger thrives in moist tropical regions; Goldenseal and Black Cohosh live in moist and shady Eastern hardwood forests; Echinacea lives in the open plains of the Midwest; and Pipsissewa, although it lives in Pacific Northwest forests, grows very slowly,

and therefore, even if harvested correctly does not recover rapidly. With the recently ballooning popularity of herbal medicine in this country, these five plants have all become highly sought-after medicinals, and while Ginger is abundantly cultivated and therefore not threatened by its popularity, the other four plants are not yet being adequately cultivated and are being plucked from their relatively small native stands at far too rapid a rate. They are simply being overharvested from their native environment in order to supply the soaring commercial demands of people living in the other bioregions of the U.S. as well as in Canada and many countries overseas.

The survival of these four plants is currently at great risk, and therefore humans need to find substitutes whenever possible (preferably plants that grow in our own backyard bio-regions) until these plants can be cultivated adequately to supply our commercial demands. As you can see, since the time we developed our CSHS list of thirty herbs, herbalists and other plant people have become quite alert to the fact that a number of important medicinal plants (in addition to the four on our list) are currently extremely harvest-sensitive. So, with deep regard for all these plants, I offer the following suggestions and ask you to heed them:

In general, regarding the four at-risk plants that appear on the above list of thirty:

• Please become familiar with United Plant Savers' (UpS) list of "at-risk" medicinal plants and avoid using them until we can escort them back to their natural state of abundance. (See Appendix A for this list as well as an introduction to the work of UpS.)

• Use Black Cohosh sparingly, *only* when it

is specifically indicated (see indications, page 30) and when there is no substitute available. In this regard, for those living in the Pacific Northwest region, there is our Baneberry (*Actea rubra*), a close relative of Black Cohosh, that can be harvested and prepared as a reliable substitute. The root of Baneberry offers nearly all the same actions as Black Cohosh root. Yes, the berries of Baneberry are toxic, but its root is not (that's why we don't call it Baneroot). In fact, in the early 1900s batches of Black Cohosh were often adulterated by mixing Baneberry root with the Cohosh. When taken as a tincture, Baneberry root bestows the same anti-inflammatory, sedative, and anti-spasmodic action for relieving the vast array of dull aching pains as does Black Cohosh. For a multitude of reasons, but specifically for invaluable insight into the use of this plant as an important substitute for the endangered Black Cohosh, I suggest and highly recommend that you consult *Medicinal Plants of the Pacific West*, researched and written by herbalist Michael Moore.

• In place of Pipsissewa when treating urinary tract inflammation, substitute Uva Ursi (*Arctostaphylos uva-ursi*) for its excellent diuretic, antiseptic, and astringent properties. Prepare it as a cold infusion to eliminate the extraction of most of its condensed tannins that can be irritating to some folks, and combine this with Marshmallow root to help soothe and protect any irritated tissue.

• When utilizing Goldenseal to employ its berberine alkaloid component, use it only when the plant's overall specific indications are absolutely required (see indications, page 30); otherwise use other berberine-containing plants such as Barberry (*Berberis vulgaris*), or Oregon Grape (*Mahonia aquifolium*), or at least dilute Goldenseal whenever using it: mixing 1 part Goldenseal to 4 parts Barberry or Oregon Grape root. When you feel you must use Goldenseal undiluted, use a reduced dosage, for, when it is truly the specific plant to use, a small dose is wholly adequate.

• Use only *organically cultivated* Echinacea. Avoid using wild Echinacea or any commercial products that use wildcrafted or wild-harvested Echinacea in their ingredients. Three species of Echinacea are used commercially: *E. purpurea*, *E. angustifolia*, and *E. pallida*. Echinacea purpurea is easily and presently cultivated, whereas the other two species are more difficult to grow and therefore not so widely cultivated. Due to over-aggressive wildcrafting, the native stands of all three of these species of Echinacea are disappearing rapidly.

In addition to the drama of innumerable heartbreaking revelations of personal love affairs with certain herbs, there was a rational method to the madness that was conjured up as we six herbalists compiled the above CSHS list of thirty herbs. Along with seeking plants that grow well in our climatic zone, we looked very closely at the *actions* (also referred to as therapeutic or medicinal *properties*) of these plants, and we made sure our final group of herbs embraced all the actions that we know are essential and therefore necessary in a well-endowed herbal pharmacy.

Pertaining to these actions, the science of Herbalism, like all therapeutic sciences, has its particular language. The nutritional and medicinal actions of each herb in our materia medica constitute the fundamental vocabulary of the language of Herbalism. Knowledge of the actions (the biochemical energetics) of each plant and the plant's

Goldenseal, Black Cohosh, Echinacea, and Pipsissewa are four plant allies that are due a collective show of human appreciation and currently require our concerted acts of tender loving care. Discontinuing the wild harvesting of these plants while using other herbs as appropriate substitutes will give these generous medicinals time to repopulate their natural habitats and will give herb growers time and resources to develop their skills in cultivating these herbs for commercial use. *Merci.*

spontaneous affinity for various systems of the body is basic to successfully employing herbs in health maintenance, disease prevention, and curative self-care.

Understanding the inherent energetics of each plant that one uses gives insight and increased autonomy in personal and family health care. It is too limiting to think or ask, "What herb do I take for…" or "What herb will cure my…." This approach stems from the "magic bullet" (one drug for one disease) myth conjured by pharmaceutical drug marketing. Herbs are more clever and practical than that. Each herb can do many things and have more than one effect on the human body and mind. The therapeutic actions and the unique blend of organic nutrients of each herb have a *natural affinity* for a variety of tissues, organs, and systems of the body. Supervised by the body's cellular intelligence which attracts to itself whatever is needed for toning and healing, these actions are contributed by the herb to the appropriate systems for preventing and/or curing a wide variety of conditions.

The art of herbal therapeutics is brought into play as one blends single nutritional and medicinal plants together into a *compound formula*, creating a uniquely synergistic quality that can support health, and when necessary stimulate or modify the body's self-healing vital energy.

Therefore, it is exceedingly useful to understand the terms and concepts that describe these herbal actions. There are hundreds of different actions that have been defined through the ages. However, for our purposes, only about 40 of these need be considered. It's important to recognize these terms and learn their definitions; I assure you it is time well spent. Reading through

the upcoming list of herbs will prove the practicality of this suggestion and afford you ample practice.

Using this "herbal actions" measure is a reliable technique to help you select your own group of core plants with which to work. When one applies it to the group of herbs selected for our CSHS list of thirty herbs, it can be seen that the actions we felt were essential are well represented. I will review this for you in the following section. Along with this, I will include a brief discussion of the actions of each of the thirty (+5) herbs and the fungus; I will also suggest the most effective vehicles for administering them by using infusion, decoction, tincture (and glycerite), oil infusion, salve, syrup, lotion, poultice, fomentation, and bolus/suppository.

As we progress through this handbook, exploring diverse techniques of medicine-making, I will use this list of thirty-five medicinal plants and a medicinal fungus as a reference and focus on specific information for extracting them in the various menstra we discuss.

I offer these lists and accompanying notations to you as a practical foundation for your personal home pharmacy, but I encourage you to modify the group of herbs to align with your intuitive preferences and, depending on where you live, to better fit the native medicinal plant population of your particular bio-region. Observe the actions and specific indications of the plants in this group and match them as best you can.

40 Herbal Actions to Know

Adaptogen—An action concept unique to herbal therapeutics. Adaptogenic or hormonal modulating action increases the body's resistance and endurance to a wide variety of adverse influences from physical, chemical, and biological stressors, assisting the body's ability to cope and adapt.

Alterative—Gradually restores health and vitality to the body by helping the body assimilate nutrients, eliminate waste, and restore proper function.

Anodyne, analgesic—Relieves pain when administered orally or externally.

Antacid—Neutralizes excess acid in the stomach and intestinal tract.

Anticatarrhal—Counteracts the build-up of excess mucus and inflammation in sinus or other upper respiratory parts.

Antidepressant—Helps relieve or prevent depressed states of mind.

Anti-emetic—Relieves nausea and vomiting.

Anti-inflammatory—Combats extensive or too-painful occurrence of inflammation. A degree of inflammation is a necessary process in healing.

Anti-microbial (anti-bacterial, anti-viral)—Helps the body's immune system destroy or resist the proliferation of pathogenic micro-organisms.

Anti-oxidant—Protects the body against free radical damage (free radicals are highly reactive compounds that bind to and destroy other molecules).

Antiseptic—Prevents or eliminates sepsis (infectious destructive condition of tissue).

Antispasmodic—Prevents or eases spasms or cramping in the body.

Aperient—A gentle stimulant to digestion, having a *very mild* laxative action.

Aphrodisiac—Increases sexual excitement and desire (libido).

Astringent—Contracts, firms, and strengthens body tissues by precipitating proteins, and can reduce excess secretions and discharge.

Bitter—Stimulates the normal secretion of digestive juices, benefiting digestion. This stimulating action helps counteract physical and, to a certain extent, emotional depression.

Carminative—Rich in aromatic volatile oils having a sweet, spicy or fragrant aroma which can lend a pleasant flavor to other herbs, excite peristalsis, promote the expulsion of gas, and soothe the stomach, supporting healthy digestion.

It is most useful to recognize and understand the terms that describe herbal actions. These simple concepts constitute a major portion of the vocabulary of herbal knowledge.

Cholagogue—Promotes the discharge and flow of bile from the gallbladder (*gogue* = to flow).

Counter-irritant (revulsive)—Induces local irritation of skin, drawing blood and other materials to the surface from deeper tissues, relieving congestion and inflammation.

Demulcent—Mucilaginous herbs which relax, soothe, and protect tissue.

Derivative—Draws blood and other fluids from one part of the body to relieve congestion in another.

Diaphoretic—Induces increased perspiration, dilates capillaries, increasing elimination through the skin.

Diuretic—Increases the flow of urine.

Emmenagogue—Increases menstrual flow.

Emollient—Applied to the skin to soften, soothe, and protect.

Expectorant—Supports the respiratory system by assisting it to remove excess mucus.

Febrifuge—Assists the body to reduce fever.

Galactagogue—Increases the flow of mother's milk.

Hemostatic—Arrests bleeding.

Hepatic—Strengthens and tones the liver, stimulating its secretory function.

Hypnotic—Has a powerful relaxant and sedative action and helps to induce sleep.

Hypotensive—Reduces elevated blood pressure.

Immune stimulant—Helps stimulate immune response and deal with infections.

Laxative—Promotes evacuation of the bowels.

Lymphatic—Support the health and activity of the lymphatic system.

Nervine—Affects the nervous system; having either a relaxing, stimulating, and/or tonic effect, depending on the herb used.

Refrigerant—Cooling agents which lower body temperature and relieve thirst.

Rubefacient—Generates a localized increase in blood flow when applied to the skin. Often used to warm the skin and ease the pain and swelling of joints.

Sedative—Calms the nervous system by reducing stress and nervous irritation throughout the body.

Sialagogue—Promotes the flow of saliva.

Stimulant—Warms the body, quickens circulation, and breaks up obstructions and congestion.

Stomachic—Stimulative tonic to the stomach.

Styptic—Reduces or stops external bleeding by astringent action.

Tonic—Stimulates nutrition by improving assimilation which improves systemic tone, giving increased vigor and strength to the tissues of body organs.

Vasodilator—Expands blood vessels, allowing increased circulation.

Vulnerary—Assists the body to heal wounds. This action is used externally.

ACTIONS AND INDICATIONS FOR THE CSHS LIST OF 30 HERBS

Blackberry (Bramble) is astringent, especially for the gastrointestinal tract. It allays excessive fluid loss from diarrhea, and when medical intervention is not available may save lives. Hemostatic—it stops bleeding of the gastrointestinal tract.

Black Cohosh (an at-risk plant, seek organically cultivated or employ substitutes when possible) is antispasmodic, anti-inflammatory, and analgesic and is most useful for its ability to reduce dull aching pain just about anywhere in the body. Along with this generalized effect, Black Cohosh has a specific affinity for the reproductive organs. It relieves the aching pains in the reproductive tract of males, but is most often used as a regulator of female imbalances. As an emmenagogue, it is used for relief of painful menstruation, but is also very effective for relieving suppressed menstruation. This, along with the fact that its effects are often long-lasting, suggests that it has a generalized tonic effect on the uterus and most likely on the male reproductive organs as well. This plant is widely used for the treatment of rheumatism and neuralgia and all cases characterized by that kind of pain known as rheumatic, dull, tensive, and intermittent. Black Cohosh is nervine, hypotensive, having a powerful influence over the nervous system as it appears to have a sedating effect on the perception of pain.

When using Baneberry root (*Actea rubra*), which is recommended as a substitute for Black Cohosh for relieving pain, use a reduced dosage, as noted in the latter part of Chapter Twelve, "Tincturing by Maceration."

Calendula (Marigold) is anti-inflammatory, vulnerary, lymphatic, anti-microbial, and anti-fungal. It is unsurpassed for treating local skin problems that are due to infection, and for treating wounds, burns, bruises, or strains due to physical damage. It is excellent for internal digestive inflammation and ulceration. Calendula is antispasmodic, lymphatic, and emmenagogue for normalizing the menstrual process, and cholagogue for aiding in the relief of a gallbladder problem and its accompanying digestive complaints; hepatic.

Cayenne (Capsicum) is a general tonic, but it's also quite specific to the circulatory and digestive systems. It is the most useful of the systemic stimulants, strengthening the heart, arteries, capillaries, blood flow, peripheral circulation, and nerves. It helps in conditions of debility, especially of the elderly, and wards off colds and catarrh. It is also carminative, and sialagogue. Applied externally, it is rubefacient and is most useful for cold hands and feet (sprinkled in socks), and problems like rheumatic pains and lumbago, and for hoarseness as a gargle; anti-microbial and an ouchful! but very effective styptic (s & m variety).

Chamomile is anti-inflammatory and pain-relieving for a wide range of conditions along the entire digestive tract; antispasmodic for easing muscle cramps; nervine. Chamomile is probably the most widely used relaxing nervine tonic. It is also used to relieve mental stress and tension. It is carminative and a mild bitter.

Cleavers is lymphatic; a lymphatic cleanser which relieves lymphatic swelling, particularly where there is an acute "hot" inflammation; it is a cooling diuretic that soothes an irritable urinary tract; tonic, and alterative.

Comfrey (Knitbone) is vulnerary and demulcent, having unparalleled wound, ulcer, and fracture healing action. It is anti-inflammatory and soothing to dry inflamed digestive tract; astringent, able to allay hemorrhaging wherever it occurs; and expectorant as an age-old remedy for dry irritable coughs, especially when accompanied by blood streaked mucus.

Comfrey has been praised throughout history as a premier healing plant used extensively in folkloric Herbalism internally and externally for the repair of innumerable body wounds and illnesses. However, in the past few years reductionist science has proclaimed Comfrey (in particular, the root and the early spring leaves) to be the possessor and conveyer of certain toxic components called pyrrolizidine alkaloids which are said to cause damage to the liver of human beings. Many herbalists have accepted this as truth and a number of us have not. Therefore, in order to provide full disclosure in this printed manual concerning the use of Comfrey, I feel it prudent to inform the reader of this debate and give current standard precautions: It is recommended that pregnant women, young children, and persons with manifest liver disease avoid the consumption of Comfrey (external use is no problem). Others are advised to use Comfrey root and leaf on a short-term basis and preferably avoid the use of the spring leaf, but instead use the leaf that appears on the latter (second) growth of the year. There are available in the marketplace pyrrolizidine-free Comfrey tinctures in which the suspect alkaloids have been removed.

Crampbark is an antispasmodic that relieves voluntary and involuntary muscular spasm of the entire pelvic viscera, bladder, womb (anti-abortive), ovaries, and the limbs; it allays convulsions, asthma, thigh and back pain, and it's an anti-inflammatory and nervine, helping to restore sympathetic/parasympathetic balance. Its astringent action helps allay excessive blood loss in menstruation and especially in menopause; emmenagogue.

Dandelion (also see Chapter One, "A Field Trip") has many healing actions. The root is a general tonic and an effective liver tonic, hepatic, which acts to "cool" (detoxify) the liver; its cholagogue action decongests the gallbladder by increasing bile flow; and its choleretic action promotes bile production. It is anti-rheumatic, as it stimulates cell metabolism in the body, assisting the body to dump metabolic waste into the blood to be cleansed by the liver. It is alterative, relieving skin disorders and degenerative joint disorders, lowering blood cholesterol. It is a mild laxative, bitter. The leaf is a safe, highly effective diuretic, the best natural source of potassium which avoids potassium depletion, so common with the use of other diuretics; bitter. Young leaves can be eaten raw in salads; they are best mixed with other salad greens and tossed with a favorite salad dressing.

Echinacea (an at-risk plant, use only organically cultivated) is an immune stimulant, assisting the body to resist infection more efficiently; it is anti-microbial and increases cellular resistance to virus, and activates the macrophages that destroy both cancerous cells and pathogens; it is anti-catarrhal and alterative.

Elder, Black, if I recall correctly, stood at the top of each of our CSHS lists, being nearly a complete pharmacy by itself. Elder's leaves used externally are vulnerary and emollient. When used internally the leaves are purgative, expectorant, diuretic, and diaphoretic. Its flowers prepared as a cold infusion are diuretic, alterative, and cooling; as a warm infusion the flowers are diaphoretic and gently stimulating. Its berries are diaphoretic, diuretic, aperient, and when fresh they make good juice and jam. Elder is the reliable home remedy for cold, flu, fever, skin eruptions, sprains, bruises, wounds, hayfever, sinusitis, tension, constipation, rheumatic discomfort, and so on. Look this plant up in a variety of sources; probably no single herbal tells Elder's complete story.

Fennel is carminative, relieving flatulence and colic, and stimulating digestion and appetite. It is very helpful in improving the flavor of other herbs. Combined with Catnip (*Nepeta cataria*), it makes the best child's remedy for fever, colic, and general restlessness; it is anti-spasmodic, having a calming effect on coughs and bronchial disorders, and anti-inflammatory as a compress and eye wash for infected eyes and inflamed eyelids, and galactogogue.

Ginger is a diffusive stimulant that is warming by increasing peripheral circulation; an emergency remedy whenever immediate stimulation is needed, a master herb for relieving nausea and motion sickness; an anodyne in gastric and intestinal pain; a carminative and anti-spasmodic in the digestive tract; diaphoretic for promoting perspiration in feverish conditions; anti-inflammatory particularly useful in rheu-

matic conditions that benefit from heat; anti-microbial; rubefacient; and a reliable emmenagogue.

Goldenseal (an at-risk plant; use cultivated Goldenseal or substitute with other berberine-containing plants or other plants that offer similar actions) is hepatic, cholagogue, a bitter digestive stimulant, and a primary anti-microbial for acute infection. It is an invaluable tonic stimulant for over-relaxed, profusely secreting mucous membranes having a wide effect on the respiratory, digestive, and genito-urinary systems, and it has an anti-catarrhal effect, especially in sinus conditions. It is astringent and emmenagogue.

Gumweed is a relaxing expectorant, which relaxes the smooth muscles. It is antispasmodic and hypotensive, useful for treatment of asthmatic and bronchial conditions, especially when accompanied by rapid heartbeat and nervous response.

Hawthorn is a heart tonic of the first order which maintains the heart in a healthy condition. It directly effects the cells of the heart muscle, enhancing both activity and nutrition. It is a specific remedy in most cardiac disease and facilitates a gentle but long-term sustained effect on degenerative, age-related changes in the entire cardiovascular system; astringent. It is hypotensive and diuretic.

Marshmallow, due to its abundance of mucilage, is emollient when used in salves for external use. Used internally, it is a soothing demulcent indicated for inflamed and irritated states of mucous membranes. The root is used to treat all inflammatory conditions of the gastrointestinal tract, including the mouth, gastritis, peptic ulcers, colitis, etc. The leaves are diuretic, expectorant, and anti-inflammatory, and are used to relieve dryness of lungs and a burning or irritated urinary tract; its abundant mucopolysaccharides mildly stimulate the body's immune function.

Mugwort is a bitter tonic and foremost digestive stimulant. It is anti-oxidant, which helps in the metabolism of rancid fats and protects the liver from damage from free radicals. It is cholagogue, giving a general stimulating effect on bile flow, helping to remove liver congestion, especially for those who have eaten (rancid) oily food. As a nervine tonic, it eases tension, and is anti-depressant, as it aids in depression, particularly when this is due to liver congestion, a virus, and/or a sedentary lifestyle; it is emmenagogue.

Mullein is expectorant, an extremely beneficial respiratory remedy that tones the mucous membranes, reduces inflammation, and stimulates fluid production, thus facilitating expectoration. It is also demulcent, diuretic, nervine, anti-spasmodic, alterative, astringent, anodyne, vulnerary, and anti-inflammatory. The oil infusion of the fresh flowers is particularly effective for soothing and healing any inflamed surface and easing ear problems (pain). As a fomentation of leaves it is excellent for local application to any inflamed parts.

Nettle leaf is a spring tonic and a general alterative detoxifying agent which clears out waste products, strengthens the mucosa of the urinary, digestive, and respiratory systems, and when taken fresh works against the allergic response to hayfever. It prevents uric acid build-up in joints and is extremely helpful in cases of gout, rheumatism, and arthritis. It is an astringent, which is useful for relieving excessive discharge and bleeding, and is diuretic and hypotensive. Nettle root is tonic for the genito-urinary system. It is a good prostate tonic and quite helpful for benign prostatic enlargement. It is an excellent potherb cooked like spinach or any other fresh greens.

Peppermint is one of humanity's favorite and most uplifting flavors. It is carminative and anti-spasmodic, having a relaxing effect on the muscles of the digestive system; it combats flatulence and stimulates bile and the flow of digestive juices. It is carminative, diaphoretic, and anti-emetic. As a mild anesthetic to the stomach lining, it often allays feelings of nausea. It is nervine, and anti-microbial. This plant (combined with Elder and Yarrow) is a traditional treatment for fevers, colds, and influenza and thereby has saved countless lives throughout the ages.

Pipsissewa (an at-risk plant, well substituted for by using an Uva Ursi and Marshmallow combination) Therefore, **Uva Ursi** (Bearberry) is diuretic; it has a specific antiseptic and astringent effect upon the membranes of the urinary system, which it can be relied upon to soothe and tone. With its anti-microbial action, it is wonderfully effective for treating bladder infection, gravel, or a stone in the kidney. It is helpful to blend this plant with Marshmallow root to increase the soothing and protectant demulcent action.

Plantain is a magnificent weed that grows everywhere and is readily available throughout the year. It is vulnerary, expectorant, demulcent, anti-inflammatory, astringent, diuretic, and anti-microbial, having excellent healing properties. It is a gentle expectorant that will soothe inflamed and painful membranes, ideal for coughs and bronchitis. Its astringency aids in diarrhea, hemorrhoids, and bladder inflammation where there is bleeding. It relieves inflammation of the skin and intestinal tract. It is a valuable treatment for diseases of the blood and glandular conditions. It is a traditional cure taken internally, and as a poultice for treating the stings and bites of snakes, spiders, and insects, and as a dressing for cuts, wounds, and bruises.

St. John's Wort is nervine. Taken internally, it has a sedative and pain-relieving effect appropriate for treating neuralgia, anxiety, and tension, and any irritable and anxious effects of menopausal changes. As an anti-depressant, it is highly recommended for treatment of melancholia or "the blues." As an astringent, it is used externally as an oil or salve. It is a valuable healing vulnerary and anti-inflammatory remedy for nerve injuries, muscular bruises, painful wounds, swelling, varicose veins, and mild burns.

Scullcap is a nerve tonic, having a mild sedative, anti-spasmodic edge. It is especially appropriate as a primary nervous system tonic and relaxant for stalwart individuals who have fiery emotions that promote nerve and muscle tension. This plant is also used specifically in the treatment of seizure, hysterical states, and epilepsy, as well as for general muscular and nervous irritability and tension. It is also well used where there

is nervous disorder that develops twitching, tremors, restlessness, or irregular muscular action. As a cardiac relaxant, it is useful in sedating heart imbalances caused by overactive nerves; bitter.

Valerian is primarily a nervine tonic. It is helpful to know Valerian has a stimulating, warming nature which does not work well for those who tend to have too great a blood flow to the brain, and too great a nerve force already. Rather, Valerian, having a warming and stimulating effect on the body, is a remedy used better for a nervousness and irritability that comes secondarily to deficiency. It is best used in people with poor blood circulation in general, but particularly poor circulation to the brain and nervous centers. It is well used for anxiety, despondency, and nervousness in individuals whose face and skin look pale and lifeless, and the skin and body is cool. It is a particularly useful remedy when there is intestinal tension leading to gas, cramps, constipation, or irritable bowel type conditions. For a tonic effect, it should be taken as a fresh plant extract. This plant is also hypotensive and is used as a relaxing remedy in hypertension and stress-related heart problems. As a hypnotic it is well known to improve sleep quality, especially amongst those who consider themselves to be poor sleepers. Besides its wonderful relaxing effects, Valerian is also anti-spasmodic and emmenagogue. It is a suitable remedy for excessive caffeine intake.

Vitex (Chasteberry) is a uterine tonic which stimulates and normalizes pituitary gland functions, especially its progesterone-stimulating function, and therefore acts to normalize the activity of female sex hormones. This is the basis for its use in everything from PMS and recovery from taking birth control pills, to dysmenorrhea and menopause. It is used to stabilize the ovulation cycle. It is well used to help reduce the undesirable symptoms of menopause and is helpful in irregular menstruation, especially if accompanied by endometriosis. It helps relieve hormonally related constipation, and can assist in the control of acne in teenagers.

Willow is an ancient analgesic remedy used for its pain-relieving, anti-inflammatory effects. In various forms, it has been employed to relieve the discomforts of headache, cold, flu, fever, gout, and the aches and pains of all description.

Yarrow is one of the best of the diaphoretic herbs, making it a standard remedy for reducing fever. It is used for treating hypertension. This action is attributed to its vaso-dilating and diuretic properties. As a tonic, this herb's main uses are as an astringent, anti-septic, anti-inflammatory, anti-spasmodic, and a diuretic remedy for the genito-urinary system. It is used as an astringent, anti-inflammatory, and bitter tonic in the gastrointestinal system, where it can help normalize irritated and inflamed states of the digestive tract, as its volatile oils contain similar anti-inflammatory constituents as Chamomile. Its astringent, hemostatic, and anti-inflammatory properties also make this plant useful for intestinal bleeding, hemorrhoids with bloody discharge, uterine hemorrhage, profuse, protracted menstruation, and leucorrhea. It is also quite effective in relieving menstrual cramps. Used externally, it is styptic and a wound-healing vulnerary.

Yellow Dock is a hepatic liver stimulant and laxative. As a laxative, its activity lies somewhere between the bile stimulants (Dandelion, Oregon Grape) and the more strongly laxative anthraquinone group (Bitter Aloe, Senna, Buckthorn). Its combination of liver-cleansing properties and laxative effect seems to assist the body in dealing with the metabolic wastes often associated with a low-fiber, high-fat, and meat diet. As a cholagogue, it stimulates the flow of bile and has a therapeutic effect on jaundice when this is due to congestion. Yellow Dock is a wonderful alterative for treating oily and exudative skin conditions. It seems to work through the liver and bowel to help remove metabolic wastes from the blood. By improving the liver's ability to metabolize wastes and fats it takes the burden off of secondary pathways of elimination, such as the skin.

GREEN'S 5 ADDITIONAL HERBS AND THE FUNGUS

Burdock is a "deep food" and alterative that moves the body to a state of well-nourished health, promotes the healing of wounds, and removes the indicators of system imbalance such as low energy, ulcers, skin conditions, and dandruff. As a diuretic and alterative, it works through the liver and kidneys to protect against the build-up of waste products and is considered to be one of the best tonic correctives of skin disorders. Burdock is a classic remedy for skin conditions which result in dry, scaly skin and cutaneous eruptions (eczema, psoriasis, dermatitis, boils, carbuncles, sties), as well as also being helpful in relieving rheumatism and gout. As a mild bitter that stimulates digestive juices and bile secretion, it aids appetite and digestion and is well used in anorexia. Externally,

Gobo is a young and tender Burdock root commonly used in Japanese cuisine and available in many local produce sections.

Oat spirit is the commuter's green angel. She graciously feeds the nervous system of those who overwork themselves, function on nervous energy (and caffeine), are chronically under stress, simply burned out, and possibly a bit depressed by it all.

it is an exceptional fomentation or poultice to promote the healing of wounds and ulcers, especially when also taken internally on a regular basis.

Ginkgo is first and foremost a vasodilator. It improves circulation to the brain and periphery and has a normalizing action on the vascular system, making it important in all conditions stemming from poor circulation. It improves circulation to all poorly nourished areas. It enhances memory by improving nerve cell transmission and brain metabolism by increasing the utilization of oxygen and glucose. As a brain tonic, free-radical scavenger, and anti-oxidant, it helps prevent cardiovascular damage and counters the general effects of aging.

Oat is one of the best nerve tonics for feeding the depleted nervous system of those who overwork and undernourish themselves, or for those who function on nervous energy (or caffeine) for too long without replenishing their reserves. Oat is specific for the individual who is chronically under stress and is simply burned out. Its anti-depressive activity is specific for nervous exhaustion and debility when associated with depression. It is a nutritive that is well used for convalescence following any prostrating disease and/or nervous breakdown. Externally, it is demulcent and vulnerary, making a soothing bath for use in neuralgia and irritated skin conditions.

Saw Palmetto is a nutritive tonic whose influence is directed toward the entire reproductive apparatus. It works cleverly as a remedial tonic that stimulates the nutrition of the nerve centers upon and through which it operates. For the male, this action

focuses particularly on the prostate gland, which it keeps in a state of wellness. For an enlarged prostate gland and accompanying diminished sexual drive, it is remarkably therapeutic, as it reduces the size of the gland and quickly relieves the other disorders that commonly occur with this condition's symptoms (i.e., dribbling urine, slow initiation of urination, incomplete bladder evacuation). In females, this plant is beneficial for treating ovarian enlargement, weakened sexual drive, and with continual use its nourishing components can help develop small underdeveloped mammary glands. As a diuretic, antiseptic, and tonic it is a valuable remedy in treating any infection of the genito-urinary system. As a nutritive endocrine agent, it is safely used to give a boost to the male sex hormones and has been reported to reverse sterility in woman where there is no organic disease or injured tissue. This berry tastes to me like rancid soap, so I find it is most palatable when taken in capsule form. For those whose nature will do well with the actions and flavor of Licorice, this herb does a decent job of covering Saw Palmetto's controversial flavor.

Siberian Ginseng is a classic adaptogen in that when taken consistently it produces a state of non-specific stress resistance. It helps modify the underlying imbalance caused by stressors, regardless of the specific nature of the stressor (chemical, physical, psychological, etc.). In order for an herb to be classified as an adaptogen, not only must it help one deal with "stress," but it cannot cause an imbalance in physiological functions; it must basically be harmless and should help normalize functions, regardless of whether they are underactive or overactive.

Siberian Ginseng's adaptogenic qualities have been shown to improve generalized resistance to infectious diseases, to lessen muscular fatigue, to help balance hypertension, and to reduce damage from radiation. Although its effect on the adrenal cortex gives it wide-ranging uses, it seems to have a special affinity for the circulatory system. It has been shown to balance both high and low blood pressure, reduce serum cholesterol levels, and relieve anginal pain.

The wide-ranging effects of Siberian Ginseng can be traced largely to its ability to have positive effect on the general adaptation syndrome. When confronted with long-term stress, the original response known as the "alarm reaction" is less severe; the resistance phase (i.e., when you are coping with a stress) is prolonged, and the exhaustive stage that can follow long-term stress is better handled. All in all, Siberian Ginseng allows one to better handle a tougher work load, emotional and chemical stressors, living in congested cities, and the general frazzle of living in our twenty-first century civilization.

Reishi (*Ganoderma lucidum*) is a remarkably beneficial fungus for the human body. First of all, it is a primary supporter of the immune system, as it is believed to enhance white blood cell production, stimulate macrophage (scavenger cells of the immune system) activity, help protect against cancer, and work against viruses. It is shown to modify the body's allergic response. Reishi also provides cardiovascular protection by helping to lower excessively high blood pressure. It helps lower cholesterol while it increases the ratio of HDL (good cholesterol) to the LDL (not so good) cholesterol. At the same time, it inhibits platelet dysfunction (platelets are components of blood that promote clotting). In addition to all this, Reishi is a liver protective against damaging agents, and it seems to have a calming and strengthening effect on the nervous system, as it is mildly adaptogenic and antioxidant by protecting the body against free radicals. That's an herbal ally, my friends!

HERBS TO AVOID IN PREGNANCY

Barberry (which I suggested using as a substitute for Goldenseal)

Black Cohosh (except for the last month of pregnancy) and its substitute Baneberry (see page 30)

Cayenne (use sparingly)

Comfrey

Ginger (use very sparingly)

Goldenseal

Mugwort

Oregon Grape (which I suggested using as a substitute for Goldenseal)

Yarrow

Suggested Methods of Extraction

	Bolus/ Suppository	Decoction	Fomentation	Infusion	Lotion	Oil	Poultice	Salve	Syrup	Tincture
Blackberry		●							●	●
Black Cohosh		●							●	●
Burdock (root and/or seed)		●	●				●		●	●
Calendula	●		●	●	●	●	●	●		●
Cayenne				●		●		●	●	●
Chamomile				●					●	●
Cleavers				●						● fresh plant
Comfrey	●	●	●	●	●	●	●	●	●	●
Crampbark		●								●
Dandelion		● root		● leaf					●	● root, leaf
Echinacea	●	●					●			●
Elder				● leaf, flower		● leaf		● leaf	●	● flower
Fennel				● crushed seed					●	●
Ginger		●		●					●	●
Ginkgo				●						●
Goldenseal				●		●		●		●
Gumweed				●						●
Hawthorn		● berry		● leaf, flower					● berry	● berry, leaf, flower
Marshmallow				● root, leaf cold infusion		●		●	●	●
Mugwort				●						●
Mullein				●		● flower			●	● leaf, flower

	BOLUS/ SUPPOSITORY	DECOCTION	FOMENTATION	INFUSION	LOTION	OIL	POULTICE	SALVE	SYRUP	TINCTURE
Nettle				●		●			●	●
Oat				●			●			●
Peppermint				●					●	●
Plantain				●		●	●	●	●	●
Reishi		● decoct 45 min.								●
Saw Palmetto		●								●
Siberian Ginseng		●								●
St. John's Wort				●		●		●	●	●
Scullcap				●						●
Uva Ursi				● cold infusion						
Valerian				● cold infusion					●	●
Vitex				●						●
Willow				●						●
Yarrow			●	●			●	●		●
Yellow Dock		●					●		●	

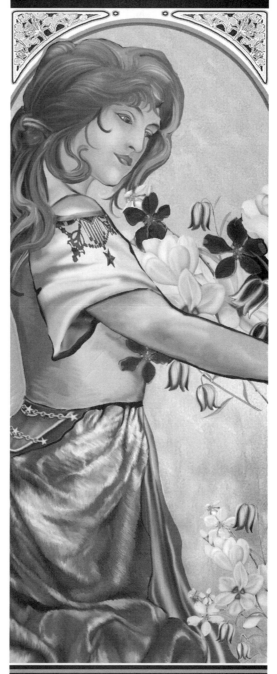

CHAPTER 3

GARDENING AND HARVESTING, DRYING, GARBLING, AND STORING

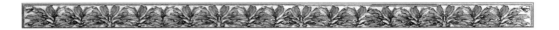

I find gardening to be the most companionable and fulfilling of all my herbal experiences. I am wholly, entirely, and utterly convinced that the power of gardening to promote healing and sustain wellness goes far beyond that of any other form of medicine, herbal or otherwise. In fact, with certain individuals I've noted that gardening is the only herbal remedy whose antidepressant action truly uplifts their spirit and successfully relieves their depression. Having discovered it, gardening has become the only medicine path they steadfastly rely on.

Collecting and planting seeds, touching the Earth, relating to plants, and caring for them as you attune to the flow of the seasons, simply feels good. All phases of gardening touch my being in a spiritual, mental, emotional, and physical way. It always fills my heart and mind with delicious anticipation, which stimulates the vital flow of any human being's life force.

In the concluding chapter of *The Male Herbal*, I asked these questions regarding Western culture: "Where are all the old men? Where have they gone? What are they doing? Where have the seeds of male maturity fallen?" A few years have passed since then, and during that time I've located a vast number of these male elders; they're in the garden (with Waldo). That's why we don't

hear much from them. They've withdrawn from much of society's commotion and chatter, and they're busy talking with plants. They've become active greenmen, and their primary dialogue has transcended to one of quiet words, the language fulfilled human beings use to commune with plant spirit. These elders are well and doing fine, living their wisdom. I've been noticing these days an ever-increasing number of younger men hanging out in gardens, as well.

But I don't figure that you picked up this book in search of a gardening manual, so I will get on with other information—even though my gardening manual would simply say: "Just put your hands, some roots, and some seeds into the receptive earth and grow something." I will, however, place some medicine gardening documents in the back of this book as Appendix B, and they'll be there for you when you seek them.

The innate joy of being with plants is reflected in the spontaneous uplifting of our human spirit as we commingle with our vegetable allies. Conscientious herbal medicine-making is a transformative process that materializes this communion, expressing it in the forms of nourishing plant concoctions and subtle energetic elixirs, and most importantly as sustained, thriving plant communities.

In my travels as an herbalist, the experience of harvesting medicinal plants has become the most intimate and compassionate portion of this communion. As I harvest a plant being, I put forth my desire to make medicine, and in turn plant spirits acquiesce to my request for the aid of their embodied nutrients and aesthetic healing vibration. I strive to receive these gifts with gratitude, and feel the sacred circle of giving sanction our union. That is a very good feeling, a feeling of health. In my practice as an herbalist, I deeply revere this mutually conscious act of alliance.

It is my belief that plants have manifested as one of this planet's foremost expressions of love. The clear vibration of love that radiates from plants is one of the fullest expressions of unconditional love that I witness. Harvesting is a way of calling forth and receiving this love. It has become a sacred act in my practice, one that I try to participate in wholeheartedly with grateful consciousness and clear communication of my intent.

I recommend herbal medicine-makers involve themselves in this segment of medicine-making with clear purpose in mind and inner commemoration in heart. Plant spirits will respond likewise. They are highly conscious. They are of the same spiritual essence we are. They adore us, and they communicate this to us with every vibration of their pure positive energy. Plants are responsive allies and trustworthy companions, and when we ask them to make medicine with us, we will do well to approach them with mutual regard, care, and intelligence.

Herbal medicine-making is the dynamic synapse that lays the roadway between harvesting plants and consuming plant preparations. Therefore, the ritual-process of harvesting is the very foundation of preparing and potentizing these medicines for our use. Intimate attention to the details of our harvest process is the rite that allows the medicine-maker to contact and communicate with the spirit of the plant and imbue this plant spirit in his or her food and medicine. If we choose to devalue this act by ignoring or disregarding the presence of plant spirit, we carry off the physical remnants of the plant, but lose access to the most vital healing power of the herb. And with this same heedless thrust, we can damage the sustaining stability and beauty of our environment. I try to bear this in mind whenever I participate in the circle of giving as the harvester of another being. This holds for all Earthly harvests—plant, animal, and mineral.

Certainly, the science and technology we employ to prepare our herbal preparations are important factors in bringing forth high-quality herbal medicines, and the main body of this handbook offers guidelines for these techniques. But as author of this work I must allege, as I repeat, these are not the most crucial factors. *The harvest is.* Therein lies the art and soul of excellent medicine-making.

A clear compassionate intent for one's use of a harvest, coupled with an animated connection with the plant (one that embraces a sincere regard for the continual welfare of the plant's community), is what draws forth the spirit of plants to accompany one's medicine. This "plant spirit" is the "active ingredient" in herbal preparations that medical pharmaceutical science and many commercial herbal industries are so desperately

In my opinion the harvesting of a plant is the most critical element in the process of making truly fine herbal medicine.

seeking. The active ingredient of herbal medicine, the one that truly supports human health and healing, is not scientifically captured in high-tech wonder-labs, mysteriously contained and transformed by stainless steel vessels and bubbling glass beakers. It is simply embraced in the woodlands, meadows, seashores, and in the domestic gardens where plants and plant communities live. It is conveyed by a green spirit, whoever she or he might be, wherever she or he might work.

TWO RITUALS

Following are two focusing rituals you might find useful.

These rituals are clearly not intended to impress the plants, and they are not ordained to flip on some sort of magic switch; plants are already our allies, and the magic Nature surrounds us with all the time, where everything imaginable is possible, is always on. These rituals are for you. To receive what you want, you merely have to tap into natural enchantment in a nonresistant fashion. Ritual helps you allow yourself to function at an altered state of knowing and receptivity. In ritual you focus precisely on what you want and hold your attention on the vibrations you choose to harmonize with—at present, the vibration of plant spirit.

The first procedure is a ritualized method for allowing yourself to communicate with plants and receive them as personal allies. The second is a ritual that aligns the pace of your physical and mental energy with the energy of the plant entities you wish to harvest. Both rituals can help you focus on your intent and align your spirit in a relationship with a plant, a relationship that allows you to carry the spirit of the plant along with your harvest of its physical being. If either one or both rituals appeal to you, adopt them, or modify them to suit your nature. If they're not your style, create your own way. These are merely my means to an end; there are innumerable other ways to woo plant spirit. Seduction is a highly personal adventure. Ritual is a partner helping create the energy of a dance; you are the drummer.

I'd like to slip a note in here to readers who live in cities' densely populated neighborhoods or other areas where intentional gardens are not apparent and open spaces are often inaccessible. Plant spirit resides in each and every plant. Regardless of the size of the metropolis you inhabit or the thickness of its concrete complexion, you can spot wild plants growing throughout its brittle surface. There's simply no holding them down. Walk the streets and check it out; healthy plants are rising through the city grid. You'll see them standing in anonymous cement cracks and poking out of the narrow seams where building walls reach down and touch adjoining sidewalks. You can find plants growing all along streetside curbs and down adjacent alleyways; and, their green spirit lounges as communities of weeds at the edges of asphalt parking lots. Arriving with the wind, the seeds of diverse plants abound in pretty much every patch of city dirt. When you start looking, you find Earth's plants hanging out all over town. Even the most plant-resistant environments host their bands of outlaw weeds. Actually plant spirit, in one form or another, envelops the entire city—every city. Boundless numbers of fertile seeds lie under city streets and beneath each metropolitan structure. The precious seeds and spores of

Earth's ancient forests, jungles, grasslands, and wetlands reside peacefully in the soils below the urban hubbub, patiently biding their time, prepared to reemerge whenever opportunities arise. Left unattended, as our current civilizations move on to other things, cities will quickly become wild gardens again—it's inevitable. Humanity in its expansive exuberance has mowed down the forests for the time being but certainly has not eliminated them from Earth's timeless demeanor. We tend to credit ourselves with abilities on this orbiting garden we do not truly possess. We are Earth's hyperactive children; she loves us and lets us play, but we're not running her show. Not really. So for now, there may not be a sufficient amount of plants growing on urban turf to harvest, but there are always plenty to relate to and commune with, and, like other plants, they respond to us. Acknowledge plant spirit that greets you on the street. Respond to its communication. It's a silent language, remember; other humans won't hear you. Reach out and touch plants too, rubbing their leaves between your fingers and smelling their green aromas. Other folks won't pay much attention to this gesture either. And if I might add a P.S. to this note, the plants you encounter on your streets are noteworthy candidates to adopt as urban allies. Their vibrations are as clear and uplifting as those of plants growing in gardens and country wilds. If you feel a green companion touch your spirit, plant its image in your mind and heart. Let it grow in there too and enjoy the connection; the plant's companionable spirit will always be there for you to access. Cities are rarely lonely places for those who speak with the plants.

We are Earth's hyperactive children; she loves us and lets us play, but we're not running her show.

A Ritual of Communion

"The greatest gift of the garden is the restoration of the five senses."

—Hanna Rion

To begin with, let me suggest that there are plants out there fully prepared and eager to communicate with you. They offer no resistance whatsoever to the adventure of communicating with a receptive human being. Over 99 percent of our (human) being is a vibrational communicator. Under 1 percent is a verbal communicator even with other human beings, so plants and animals being virtually 100 percent vibrational communicators are very similar to you and me in their vibrational offering. They are quite able and entirely compatible to communicate with us, and vice versa.

Go outside and look around in the garden or wander through the forest, the hillsides, the seashore, or along a country roadway. Note the plants that attract you most (vibrational communication). Note the ones that you have always enjoyed looking at, the plant entities that whenever you are near them you can't (and never want to) keep your eyes off. You feel pleasantly uplifted whenever you are near them (vibrational communication). These are the plants that are already your visual lovers; and believe me, if you're that attracted to them, they are appreciating you just as much (vibrational communication). So, these are the vegetable folks to start intentionally communicating with. A mutual, vibrational connection has already been established without a word having been spoken. You have entered the green.

At a time when your insides are smiling, like one of my friends once said, "At a time when you're just feeling happy for no particular reason," go sit with one of these plants; initiate enchantment. You will feel a mutual attraction touching some undomesticated, wild part of yourself. Be still and take the opportunity to listen to the sounds of Nature that surround you. Be still for as long as it takes to reunite with your deep sense of well-being. In this mutual state of consciousness plants will further respond to you. Smell the scents that are flowing around and into you. Feel everything breathing in rhythm, connecting you with Nature's intelligent beauty. Feel your absolute freedom and that of all other beings present. Touch the plant. It is vibrating in its place of absolute well-being, as are you. Feel the plant's leaf. Let your sight drink its colors. Touch the ethereal softness of its flower's petals. Let it experience your vitality and gentleness. These are the "initial words" of your communication.

Be open to all possibilities. Be open to your feelings and your visions. Dissolve any sensual separation you might feel with the plant by letting all intellectual objectivity flow away with the breeze. Instead, focus on yourself sitting with the plant, and within this subjective passion let your spirit mingle and blend with the plant's spirit.

Ask the plant to give you its name. Dismiss all you think you know or might have been taught about the plant; instead, allow *its* name to come to you. Keep the name silent within you, like the name of a clandestine lover.

Ask the plant for its song. Every plant has a song. It may give it to you to sing or to recite as poetry (or for the time being it may give you a portion of its song as a simple word for use as a mantra to focus on in meditation for later realization of the plant's power). You may also receive an image or a nature symbol to draw or paint or weave or sculpt. Songs and visual images are given to you for your personal medicine-use of the plant. Keep them intimate; hold their energy and knowledge in your heart and mind. These gifts are the ultimate harvest.

After giving you its name and song, the plant may give you other gifts by telling you what it will do for you as a medicine ally. Later, share these gifts with others if you wish, but don't exclaim them as universal truth. These are truths shared between you and the plant; they have been given specifically to you. It is your medicine.

Extend visions of well-being to the plant and to its community. They are your allies and you can always speak to them of that which you want.

Once you have communicated with a plant entity, briefly or at length, having received its name and any gifts it extends to you, continue through the succeeding days and nights to visualize and meditate on the plant's image and energy. You may be given more during these meditative states or during sleep in a dream. Expect this. It has been a long time since most of us have made ourselves available for intentional conversation with plant spirits. There is much to be communicated between plant and human species, and it is a joy for both to do so.

Later, go dancing. Dance to the rhythm of the drummers and the shakers; close your eyes and visualize and feel the energy of this plant. Dance this energy; like attracts like. In this state of consciousness, other nature spirits can come to you as you dance, or later that evening.

Remember, plants participate in very active night lives. Enter your garden during the evening hours and hang out with them in the quiet moonlight. Experience the magnificent nocturnal energy that the garden residents emanate…a very good time to exchange a few silent "words" and frolic in your garden's lunacy.

Summer Serenade for Carolyn

"Night cricket can sing you through a lonely eve; night cricket will sing you to the morning light."

—T. ELDER SACHS

A Simple Harvest Ritual

Harvest at ease, in rhythm and focus.

Sit for a while with the plants you want to harvest. Treat yourself to the splendor of their beauty; enjoy the well-being you share.

Seek out the grandmother plant, the elder of the community. Focus on this plant and yourself together. Place intimate energy around the two of you by visualizing warm light surrounding you or by shaking a rattle and feeling a field of cohesive energy encircle you (nature spirits and human babies love the sound vibrations of rattles…remember?).

Be still in body and energy. Slow down your pace of thought and action with a ceremonial offering to the grandmother and her clan. This adjusts your normal human pace to better align your energy with the energy of the plants. Just sit with the stillness and empty your mind. Meditate. Tune to your inner hearing. Plant spirit speaks to these ears.

Communicate clearly your harvest intent and clarify to the plant and again to yourself the purpose of the medicine you wish to prepare.

Ask permission to harvest, asking when to harvest, where, how, and how much. Plants, when listened to, inform you how best to harvest and receive their gifts.

At this point, it is possible that you might sense a "no" answer. Honor this. Not all of a plant's medicine energy is contained or accessed merely in its physical body. Be content for the moment to harvest plant communion and companionship. Come back again later or visit another community and extend another request.

When you feel permission to harvest, harvest softly. Impact the plant community and the ecosystem minimally. You only need enough herb for the year. Upon feeling a sense of permission, you will have strongly connected with the plant and infused your harvest with its spirit. As you work through the harvesting action, maintain communication with the individual plants you are taking, and sustain focus on your intended uses. Genius is focus.

As a conclusion to your harvest, express your gratitude to the plant community. Grandmother will be smiling and you will know it.

As you are leaving, pause for a moment and look back at the plant community. Ask yourself if you harvested softly. Does it show that you were there? How much does it show? Be with your feelings about this. Learn from them; they are your truth. A novice's mistake of effecting an over-enthusiastic harvest is always forgivable; but it is a teaching to be valued and taken to heart. Visualize the healing energy of the medicines you are about to make with the plants given to you by this community and bid farewell.

Return to your home and process your harvest immediately.

Go dancing that evening. Dance the energy and character of the plant spirit you harvested. Dance with your plant allies. Dance your happiness and your gratitude. A plant person's life is an expression of joy and companionship.

HARVESTING EQUIPMENT

There is paraphernalia necessary for the harvester. The minimum equipment required for an impassioned harvester is merely a pair of hands and some means for getting them to the plants; a healthy pair of feet is adequate for that job. But I am a stickler for taking meticulous care of all tools and equipment; therefore, I strongly recommend protective coverings for your hands and feet. Sandals and bare fingers are a pleasure to use for harvesting Red Clover or Calendula blossoms on a warm summer day, but high-top gumboots (a.k.a. duck boots, galoshes, Wellingtons) and gloves will be deeply appreciated when harvesting Stinging Nettles on a soggy river bank in early spring, or for trekking across a sloshy forest floor in search of Skunk Cabbage. A tough canvas jacket will keep you snug and protect your arms and torso from spiny stalks as you walk through forests and pull roots like those of *Oplopanax horridum* from the ground, or when you dig Blackberry roots from the earth in the spring or fall. A lightweight, long-sleeved cotton shirt worn during hot sunny days of harvesting will greatly assist your body to retain water and avoid dehydration. A variety of favorite hats protect harvesters from a hot sun, as well as from cold, rain, and the end products of bird peristalsis.

I suggest you purchase the best-quality equipment you can possibly afford. High-quality tools serve you better, are safer to use, and if taken care of will last significantly longer. The key phrase here is, if taken care of. Attention to details like keeping hands, feet, head, and torso protected and healthy; keeping blades sharp, not pushing any tool past its limits, wiping tools dry after use, cleaning and oiling them regularly, and stor-

ing them in dry places out of direct sunlight will assure you a functional, co-independent relationship with your harvesting equipment. It appears to me that inanimate objects have sensitive spirits too, and like animate objects they respond positively to any regard and attention you give them. All in all, pampered, high-quality equipment ends up being less expensive, safer, and more enjoyable to use.

In addition to body-protecting paraphernalia, you will need equipment and tools with which to cut, whittle, scrape, dig, and carry stuff in. Pruning shears, a knife, a trowel, and paper bags will do.

In my experience, the best pruning shears are Felco® brand. The makers of these cutters offer a gratifying variety of ergonomic styles for both left-handers and right-handers, and for hand sizes of men and women. Be keenly aware when using shears that they are known to bite the hand not holding them.

I also retain the services of a qualified pocketknife at all times, one whose blade will *lock* open during use. (It's a painful slice of life when a foldable knife blade suddenly closes down on one's fingers.) I carry this little tool to help me deal with those spontaneous odd jobs that inevitably arise during harvesting and gardening and for innumerable supplementary tasks such as removing soil from under fingernails, cutting large bars of chocolate, fending off bears, unwrapping Valentine gifts, and so forth. A companion pocketknife is an essential tool for an independent being. I'm not talking about a clunky foreign army version that includes fold-out dishware and a car port, just a slim, little, pocket-friendly, one- or two-blade item. I guarantee you will use it throughout your medicine-making (and other) journeys—repeatedly. When someone asks me what gift to get for someone else, man or woman, I suggest buying him or her a cool little pocketknife (they're trippy to shop for). But of course the superb suggestion is usually ignored and wanders off unappreciated.

My best trowel is made of beefy aluminum; its handle and blade are molded as a single piece, having a very sturdy shaft that doesn't bend no matter how high the fervor of my determination escalates while digging. I also rely on a hori hori, which is a brilliantly designed Japanese root digging tool that is virtually indestructible. No one said digging roots was effortless, even with the plant's permission, so be equipped.

The best paper bags to use are large, heavy-duty, recycled ones. Avoid using plastic bags; they retain heat and moisture and *quickly* compost (before you can get them home) the fresh herbs they contain.

A basket is also practical, especially one designed with a large stiff handle that arches over the top of the basket. You can stick your arm through the handle and retain the use of both hands for picking and placing the plant parts into the conveniently positioned basket hanging on your arm. This is most practical when you need to reach up to harvest Hawthorn berries or Elder blossoms or when you are perched in a tree reaching out precariously to collect other precious arboreal pickings.

In order to take good care of yourself, you will also need a full water bottle. Get a quart-size bottle, maybe two of them, as a pint of water is seldom enough. Put a fresh sprig of Mint, Lemon Balm, Lemon Verbena, or a slice of Lime in the drinking water. Never go harvesting without taking water. The arid shadow of dehydration lurks in nearly every ecosystem. Drink lots of water while harvesting and gardening. It's the medicine-maker's field tonic, and plants are indulgent water-drinking buddies.

Amidst your enchanted wonderings, you will happen upon many intriguing plants in the field. If you are a person who likes to give a name to them, carry a plant identification guide with you. Search bookstores for pocket guides that speak clearly to your intellect, ones that focus on the locations you frequent. However, when the sight of a particular plant stops you in your tracks, I suggest first sitting and asking the plant itself for its name. Then, following this private conversation, consult your identification guide, key out the plant, and note the names others have given it. Practice plant communion first, then practice using your plant key. You also have the botanical-poet's inalienable right to give the plant any "common" name you choose. I strongly suggest you revel in exercising this right. It's fun, intimate, and highly creative. Utilize all opportunities to beckon and inspire your inner poet.

Some individuals like to keep a record of their harvesting experiences. In Appendix E, I have given you a sample of the Harvesting Information Chart we recommend using at the California School of Herbal Studies for documenting the details of harvest that pertain to plants we process for our use. This form is offered merely as a sample guide. Format your own design to suit your particular interests.

First aid equipment obligatory for the harvesting tasks that await you can be summarized in three words—Lavender essential oil. I mean, you shouldn't be jeopardizing your life and limb out there in herb-land, but frequently you do put your skin at risk. What with biting and sucking critters, abrading surfaces, scraping and puncturing stickers and thorns, bumps, nicks, cuts, pruning shear bites, I tell you, it can be itchy and irritating out there. And what one needs most when a cutaneous crisis occurs is an inexpensive, soothing (anti-inflammatory), cleansing (disinfectant) accessory, that smells great. This would be a 15 ml bottle of pure Lavender essential oil. Slather it on any and all offended skin.

ECOLOGICAL HARVESTING PROTOCOL

Ecological harvesting protocol is founded on the knowledge, experience, intent, and actions of human beings who hold in their hearts and minds a deep respect for plant communities. These people I recognize as "plant persons," the green herbalists. When in the field, a green herbalist realizes that he or she is a visitor, a guest in quest of great gifts. This field persona emits respect and gratitude, and monitors one's harvesting technique in such manner that the plant community is honored and can continue to thrive. Because the relationship between the green herbalist and the plant community is such that, season to season, the number and health of the plants will have been sustained or increased, the herbalist will be welcomed back for the next harvest and the one following that, as will his or her children, apprentices, companions, and so on for generations to follow.

Please peruse the "Eight Principles of Excellent Medicine-Making" found in Appendix C offered for your contemplation.

The primary principles of gathering wild medicinal plants are discussed below.

HARVEST ABUNDANCE ONLY

Gather solely in those prime areas that you find abounding with plants of the same species. Try not to harvest the same stand year after year. Never harvest or disturb threatened or endangered plants. Plant them instead. Seek them out and sing to them. You don't have to sing out loud. If you have a singing voice like mine it's probably better that you don't. Plants hear a silent song (and often prefer it). I know this sounds a bit corny, but I find it true in my experience. Let your songs tell the plants (and wild animals) how beautiful they are and how deeply you appreciate them. Communicate to them how much you want them to remain here with us on Earth. Visualize their well-being and focus on that vision. Let the wild beings hear what's in your heart, the heart of their ally. The positive vision and songs of a singer whose passion is connected to the source of abundance can singleheartedly turn any tide from depletion to plenty.

As you gather plants, please assume the responsibility to learn which plants, if any, are currently on threatened and endangered lists in the areas you harvest. Keep in mind that a plant can be abundant in one state and at the same time rare and in great need of protection and assistance in the next state. Check with your local herbarium, botanical garden, wildflower groups, native plant society, or the United Plant Savers (UpS) list of "at-risk" plants (see Appendix A).

When digging roots, refill the holes, whether deep or shallow. Whenever possible, replant a section of any budding rhizomes or any root crowns that you can separate from the roots you harvest. Scatter the mature seeds of these root-medicine plants around the area whenever you can. Attempt to leave the area looking as undisturbed as it did upon your arrival. If possible, make the area look even better. Often

You don't need a lot of plant material to make enough herbal medicine for the year.

you will find someone's discarded trash lying around (they probably figure their high school janitor will get it later); please pick it up and cart it out. You certainly have my sincere gratitude for doing this. And please keep in mind at all times that wild (and frequently garden) plant stands also provide food for the local wildlife. Human debris left lying around can entrap and injure or kill wild fauna in the most unimaginably torturous ways.

PRACTICE AND PROMOTE DAMAGE CONTROL

Be aware of your impact on the plant communities that you are making contact with; make it negligible. Notice the impact of your footwear and your passage on the terrain. Be aware of simple erosion factors.

Hard-soled shoes are the most damaging to delicate hillside ecosystems. It is easy to damage the fragile environment of a rocky hillside or a wet stream bed by treading on them thoughtlessly.

When harvesting the foliage of bushes or trees, pick from the borders of the plants, leaving the central core of the plant to regenerate itself outward.

When harvesting a hillside, begin at the bottom and work your way up the slope. Leave all the plants growing at the top of the hill. These are the community members, often referred to as the grandparent plants, that send their replenishing seed downhill and also protect young plants. You have to love grandparents of all species. An annual Grandparents' Day would do well in this country; it could be our first interspecies holiday.

GATHER ONLY FROM HEALTHY PLANTS AND COMMUNITIES

Plants that appear to be in poor health or are being successfully harassed by gnawing and sucking insects are probably growing on the extreme peripheral border of their preferred growing conditions and are struggling to survive. These are not appropriate individuals to harvest. However, they may be harbingers of a thriving community lying nearby. Or they may be the only specimen in that area. Regardless, nod to them appreciatively and continue on.

As a general rule, don't harvest the first plants of any species you find in an area, whether weak or strong. Let these pioneering individuals alone to stake their claim and proliferate as they can. Even when you do come upon an appropriate size community of healthy plants pick from the more central portions and let the plants living on outer borders remain undiminished to tend to their venture to extend the community outward. This is especially essential when harvesting plants like St. John's Wort, which propagates itself primarily by casting its seeds and experiences a massively increased harvest due to a sudden rush of popularity. This has transformed its commercial reputation from one of a "noxious weed" to that of a "quick antidote" for human depression—foolish notions as those are.

Remove no more than 10 percent of a native plant community or 20 percent of a naturalized plant community; better yet, leave no particularly noticeable evidence you were there. Leave enough leaves, fruit, seeds, and/or flowers on the plants for them to continue to prosper healthy and strong. I repeat, you don't need a lot of plant material to make enough herbal medicine for the year. And you don't want more than a year's supply, because like gardening the act of going out into the fields and forests of nature each year and harvesting is itself one of the most healthful active ingredients in herbal medicine.

HARVEST IN UNPOLLUTED AREAS

It is best not to harvest downwind from any pollution, or on or near roadsides coated with auto exhaust residue, or any place that has been sprayed with herbicides or pesticides. In other words, harvest 50–100 yards away from public roads. I suggest not harvesting downstream from any mining or chemically laden agricultural business. The chemical runoff there is often vicious. Seriously reconsider any impulse to harvest around parking lots, public parks, fertilized lawns, and any other potentially sprayed or fumigated areas.

Avoid harvesting beneath high voltage power lines. These high-tension electric wires must trigger mutations. Yes, it's possible these mutations might prove superior to the normal plants of the species, but the deranging agitation my car radio broadcasts when I drive it near high voltage lines makes me wonder about the organic static occurring within the tissues of those hapless plants growing beneath them. No need to stress these plant communities further by harvesting them. Human nervous systems (those similar to mine anyway) don't do well beneath high-voltage lines either.

Consider initiating your own privately unpolluted growing areas. May I suggest if you have a lawn, that you quit chemicalizing it (if you have been), then quit mowing it for a while. About the time your neighbors start hassling you to cut the weeds, you will discover a volunteer pharmacy of plant medicines growing right outside your house. Tell your neighbors you're participating in a science project. That'll stall them for a couple weeks. Then place neat little rock borders around the medicinal plants you identify and tell your neighbors you're landscaping. That'll give you a few more weeks before they notify the county officials. You might consider altering your landscape design to include cultivated medicinal plants that harmonize with the wild volunteers. There is a myriad of wild and cultivated herbal alternatives to standardized urban lawns. (See Appendix B.)

GET PERMISSION

Private landowners in the U.S. and Canada love to fence themselves in and become resident ogres. North America is pregnant with chain link fences, rails, and real estate boundaries. If you are seeking to harvest "noxious weeds" such as Stinging Nettles, Dandelions, or St. John's Wort, I have found that, when asked, land owners often say, "Hell yah, take all you want; get those damn things out of here!" So you do them the favor and they love you for it. They think you're a little odd and a bit eccentric, but there is no problem. Indulge yourself in being odd now and then; it stirs the pot. However, when you seek to harvest someone's Eucalyptus, Black Walnut, or Hawthorn trees, then you might have to be a little more persuasive. But get permission. It improves the vibe. If you seek to harvest plants on Bureau of Land Management (BLM) land, you are required to obtain a free-use permit, which is obtainable, for a small fee of course. This is a permit to collect only small amounts of vegetation. (If you're a lumber company, for about the same fee you can log the entire forest.) The U.S. Forest Service and the BLM also enforce the following regulations: no picking in or near campgrounds or picnic areas; no picking any plants closer than 200 feet from trails; and no picking any plants on roadsides.

It becomes a win-win situation once we learn to harvest in a style that allows the ecology to recover. If you see that someone else, whether human or animal, has already harvested a plant community, leave it alone and move on. When you dig a root, in most cases you take the life of the plant. This is appropriate, life eats life; it is part of the circle of giving; but give sacred honor to the giver. Cultivate gratefulness in your heart for the plant's offering to your life. Prepare and dispense root medicines with this heightened appreciation. With the above acts of regard you perpetuate abundance. *The EcoHerbalist's Fieldbook*, written by Gregory Tilford, is an extraordinary work that will help you harvest with mindful heart. (See Resources.)

WHAT TO HARVEST AND WHEN

A seasoned herbalist does not gather the various parts of plants used to make herbal medicines randomly, or at just any time of the year. There is a specific time in Earth's solar and lunar cycles when an herb will yield its best "medicine." Herbalists for thousands of years have recorded information concerning the proper time to pick various herbs. And of course, being experts, they don't always agree with each other. However, most do agree that during specific periods of the plant's yearly growth and daily life cycle the medicinal constituents are more fully developed and abundant in certain parts of the plant than they are in others.

Plants are conveniently divided, for the purposes of the herbalist, into the roots (and/or rhizomes), stem, inner and outer bark, leaves, buds, flowers, saps and pitches, fruits, and seeds. These different parts require different procedures for collection, drying, and preservation.

Roots

Roots of biennial plants should be dug in the fall of the first year or in the very early spring of the second year (they die in the fall of the second year as the plant goes to seed). Perennial plants should be dug late in the fall after the aerial parts have died back and the sap has returned underground, or dig them very early in the spring when the energy of the plant is still most active in the root. If you dig them in the spring, do so immediately after the plant first appears above the ground, before too much of the sap and vital focus of the plant ascend from the root to manifest stem and leaf. In general, perennial roots should not be gathered until after two or three years' growth, and in some cases the root should be allowed three to seven years to develop full maturity. Roots of annual plants are best dug immediately before the time of flowering. However, annual plant roots are seldom used as medicines. For herbal medicine-makers who are attentive to lunar as well as solar influences, dig roots on the new moon.

Fleshy or succulent roots should be cut previous to drying to expose a large surface area to the air. Cutting roots transversely or longitudinally is more a matter of which you enjoy doing more; however, I find that if before dehydrating them you cut roots transversely in small sections, they are easier to grind into powder later, especially those roots which are quite woody or fibrous.

Root-rhizomes like Oregon Grape become very hard and woody when dry, so they are best cut into very short sections while undried. Smaller, more fibrous roots are best left whole.

If you are not using a root immediately to prepare a fresh, undried plant extract, it is important that the root or other parts of the plant be thoroughly dried. Whereas it is normally adequate to dry most plants in a heat of about 100° F., in the case of Dandelion, Burdock, and other succulent roots, apply a heat of about 150°, and thoroughly dry them in order to destroy the eggs that may have been deposited by insects. Neglecting this precaution may lead to the rapid deterioration of the root by some very contented critters to the dismay of a very discontented herbalist—not a pretty sight.

The smaller and more fibrous roots like those found with some species of Echinacea and Valerian do better with less heat in drying. As soon as these roots are dry, they should be placed in airtight containers (especially roots which contain aromatic essential oils, in order to best preserve these volatile components). It is best to use these roots within a year, for their components, unlike those of other roots, don't survive storage for long periods of time.

Stems
Stems of herbaceous plants are best gathered after leaves appear prior to flowering, unless the flowers are to be used along with the stem as one does with Hyssop and California Poppy. Harvest any aerial parts of a plant on or near a full moon.

Barks
Whenever possible, take any bark you wish to harvest from small branches or from pruned branches. Some authorities recommend gathering the bark of trees in the spring when the inner bark is transferring the heaviest concentration of water, nutrients, and medicinal components from the roots to the leaves, but I have mixed feelings about this. I feel better harvesting the bark in the fall. The mellow autumn return of the plant's sap to the roots doesn't seem to bleed out of a wound so copiously as it does during the spring when the sap bursts forth from its winter hibernation and rises fervently to feed new leaves and flowers. Ask the tree. Barks of shrubs are best harvested in the spring. At this time, the bark can be more easily separated from the wood. Of course, never ring a plant by stripping the bark completely around its girth. This will kill it. Incisions should be limited to one-quarter or less of the limb's circumference. It is generally the inner bark that is used for making medicine, so the epidermal outer bark is removed and the inner bark dried. With some plants such as Devil's Club (*Oplopanax horridus*), the whole bark of the root and lower portion of the stalk is used for medicine. This is an example of a plant that is very aromatic and high in essential oil, and its root bark must be dried and stored immediately to retain these volatile components. For some plants like Oregon Grape (*Berberis aquifolium*), the whole bark of the underground rhizome is harvested. Lunar-observant harvesters usually take plant bark during the three-quarter waning moon. If you ask, "Does that include root barks?" I'd have to say, "That's a good question; you'll have to get the answer from the plant."

Leaves
Leaves should be gathered when fully

We create win-win experiences when we learn to harvest in a style that allows plant communities to recover and thrive…our hearts and herbal pharmacies thrive as well.

developed before the flower blossoms develop, and certainly before the leaves have begun to wither and fall. Ginkgo (*Ginkgo biloba*) and Artichoke (*Cynara scolymus*) leaves are exceptions. Ginkgo leaves are best picked as they are turning yellow, while they are still on the tree and predominantly green (at least that is what the experts currently believe). Artichoke leaves are picked in both the spring and the fall, then blended, each season's leaves presenting a little different action than the other. These work well in combination.

Harvest leaves after the morning dew has dissipated and prior to the more intense heat of the day. The heat of the midday sun temporarily wilts the energy of many plants. If you notice that the leaves of plants you wish to harvest are flagging from the heat, refrain from harvesting them until the early evening when they perk up again.

Herbs high in essential oils or resins such as Rosemary, Eucalyptus, Peppermint, and Calendula should be picked in the morning after the dew dries, during the hottest part of the year when their oils and resins are most prominently developed.

Leaves of biennial plants are best picked in the spring of the second year. In the first year biennials develop their root system most extensively; in the spring of the second year, the juice shoots up into the stalks and leaves on its way to ultimately create the plant's flowers and seeds. So, gather the leaves as the sap is transiting through them. After the appearance of flowers, the leaves begin to lose their activity. The juices are now preoccupied with the development of the fruit and seeds.

The leaves of plants in the *Labiaceae* (mint) family (currently called *Lamiaceae* by professional botanists) are more aromatic as they approach the flowering tops, and the upper ones are frequently gathered with the tops.

Flowers

Flowers are gathered just before they are fully developed. The scent is more lively at this seductive stage and the color more vivid than when the blossom is fully expanded. Once the blossom is fully open and has successfully attracted a pollinating insect or has been brushed by a pollen-laden breeze, the recently fertilized ovary continues to grow at the expense of the accessory flower organs. Choose a clear, dry morning after the dew has dissipated to harvest flowers. Don't wash flowers and buds. Shake them to remove insects or debris. If you plan to dry tender, delicate blossoms, it is preferable to dry them in the shade without artificial heat.

Saps and Pitches

Take these plant secretions in late winter or early spring. They are usually flowing from a recent wound or have dried on the plant after seeping from a past wound; so before, during, and on completion of this harvest, give the tree a hug, as it can probably use it.

Fruits

Fleshy fruits which are to be used to make exquisite juices, flavoring syrups, cordials and elixirs are best plucked when they are close to, but not quite ripe. Blackberries, Mulberries, Raspberries, and Strawberries express a less glutinous and therefore more agreeable juice when not perfectly ripe. The vegetable acids at this stage are not yet completely transformed into sugar, rendering their aroma fresher and stronger.

Seeds

Seeds are the least perishable portion of the plant. Therefore, they can be and should be collected when they are perfectly ripe. They require very little, if any, drying. One just needs to make sure the seeds are not wet from dew or rain or any other external watering when they are put into storage.

The Herb

This term generally refers to the whole plant, including the leaves, stems, foliage, and sometimes the root, and all the parts of the plant are used together (i.e., Scullcap, California Poppy, Cleaver, Chickweed). The herb should be gathered when it is freshly in flower. If the flower is not to be included, the herb should be collected before the flowers appear, but after the foliage has appeared. Most plants that have thick and branching stalks or stems should be deprived of these before drying them or before using them fresh undried.

DRYING HERBS

After you harvest an herb, the next task is to prolong its potency. The most efficient way to accomplish this is to eat it on the spot, or soon thereafter, in which case the fresh plant's potency will merge with your own. This is a choice technique to indulge when harvesting palatable plants like Miner's Lettuce, Chickweed, Mullein flowers, and Nasturtium blossoms, or wild berries. You can also choose to brew a fresh plant tea. However, if you intend to postpone consumption until a later date, you must select other procedures for preserving and storing your harvest. Dehydrating (drying) plants, when done correctly, is a simple, excellent method for maintaining plant part potencies.

Your goal and the mark of success in drying plants is to end up with herbs that closely resemble the living plant in color, aroma, taste, and texture. But, in order to achieve this, the drying procedure must follow as soon after harvesting as possible. Trust me, procrastination quickly teaches the wisdom of this counsel. But go ahead, catch a movie that evening instead of tending to the St. John's Wort you spent the afternoon harvesting. Go canoeing and leave your bag of fresh Nettles sitting around for a couple days. I have. That's how I learned what I know (of course the movie was yet another Hollywood travesty, but the canoeing was an excellent adventure and the local Nettle community most forgiving of my negligence—it even showed me a slew of its other luscious patches along the river's banks).

There are a couple things to keep in mind when drying herbs. If herbs are dried too quickly by using too much heat, they roast and lose their potency. When herbs are dried too slowly, they can mold and/or self-destruct by enzymatic actions, which also seriously impoverishes their quality.

Overheating is the reason you often see commercial grade Red Clover blossoms looking pale or brown in natural food store jars, and Lavender blossoms, normally brilliant blue-violet on the stalk, looking languid and gray within this same community of jars. Dried properly, Red Clover blossoms are vibrant, pinkish red; Lavender blossoms are a deep velvety lavender.

Careless mishandling, in addition to improper heating, is another reason you find numerous specimens of brownish green and hay-colored dried leaves and stems in stores instead of the diversity of vivid green colors you see in wild and domestic herb gardens. As I mentioned above, a collection

Once succulent herbs are fully dried there is no longer enough water available in the vegetable tissues to support microorganism lifestyles; therefore the potency of one's precious harvest is greatly prolonged and herbalists are very happy.

of properly handled and correctly dried herbs will elicit the same diversity and sensual inspiration as the garden's collection of juicy green hues. Excessive age (even though almost any herb will "lose it" over time in storage) is usually the reason commercial grade Calendula blossoms often resemble leftover pieces of used Kleenex tissue you pull from the pocket of an overcoat not worn since the previous winter. Freshly dehydrated Calendula blossoms dried properly display the same bright yellows and intense oranges that they radiate while standing fresh in the garden. I could go on and on describing more examples of the inferior quality of commercial-grade bulk herbs found on many (though not all) store shelves, but I'll spare you the tedium; I get miffed thinking about it anyway. Ailing folks buy these exhausted plant materials, and of course, eventually conclude that herbs don't work. What can you expect? It's like giving wilted flowers to a friend to say you're sorry. Got to do better than that. The abundance of these examples prompts me to say, "Once you properly harvest and dry your own herbs and experience their rich color, aroma, taste, and vitality, you will seldom be satisfied with any dried herbs you find in a store." How many restaurants have you found that truly serve scrumptious "home-cooked meals?" It doesn't happen.

So, I have a few suggestions that will help you successfully preserve your freshly harvested medicinal herbs and savory spices:

• Herbs dry excellently in warm, shaded, well-ventilated areas. Circulating dry air is essential. Never dry them in sunlight. With tender, sensitive plants that you have harvested, the searing intensity of direct sunlight takes degenerating liberties often too hideous to describe. Suffice it to say, direct sunlight rapidly depreciates good herb.

• Prior to drying them, handle fresh green plants with a gentle touch and process them as soon as possible. Many freshly picked green-plant parts (Plantain leaves being a prime example) need to be handled like fragile glass, for any bruising of these leaves will make the plant turn brownish green upon drying due to the stimulation (by bruising) and quickening (by heating) of enzyme activity.

• Protect your drying herbs at night from the evening's moist air. The water in this air can rehydrate the drying herb and ignite enzymatic action and can soon transform your harvest into that brownish green vegetable carrion color I spoke of earlier. The positive side of this experience is that these herbs are still suitable for composting. And compost is good, just less heartbreaking when made with kitchen waste and grass clippings.

• Stuffing a paper bag full with fresh herb greens and/or blossoms will often in a short time ignite the composting syndrome. So, while transporting, place collections of freshly picked plant parts in a cool and shady location and get them back out of the bag and arranged in bundles for hanging or placed onto drying racks as soon as possible. Don't put this off. Don't even think of "processing" (washing, garbling, slicing) as a next step after "harvesting." It is not the next step; it is the second half—the completion—of the harvesting act. The two experiences are one. Allow as minimal a time interval as possible to occur between accomplishing both halves.

Keep in mind that, with most herbs, it is quick and easy to harvest a large quantity, but it usually takes considerably longer to process these pickings. Profuse picking followed by procrastination (or processing fatigue) is a notorious terminator of vast quantities of potentially good-quality dried herb. For the sake of the plant communities and to prevent your own disappointment, try not to over-harvest, and be determined to complete your day's work. The reward is great.

• Plants are dry enough to be placed in storage only when all of the parts are brittle. All parts must snap crisply when bent. So, in most cases, when the stem and all thicker portions of plant pieces are crisp and brittle, the herb is dry enough to be placed into a storage container. Cut large roots to see if the centers are completely dry. If any moisture remains in any portion of a plant, mold, rot, and enzyme attacks will have their way with it during storage.

• Stored herbs should be re-inspected occasionally. Dried herbs are immensely efficient at finding and absorbing any moisture that is lingering in storage containers. Check your stashes monthly, and if the herbs don't feel as crisp as they did before, dry them again. It doesn't take much time or effort to give them a desiccating booster.

HANGING BUNDLES AND DRYING RACKS

Shaded, dry heat with good air circulation creates the optimal condition for dehydrating fresh herbs. Any and all ingenious devises that create these conditions are encouraged, and if successful, applauded. The optimal air temperature to use for drying ranges from 85 to a 100° F. (30 to 40° C.), depending on the plant and the part being dried. When us-

ing drying-rack type contrivances, it is best that the warm air circulates below as well as above the drying plant parts. If you choose to bundle or string your herbs and hang them to dry, the air needs to circulate freely around them. This circulating heat carries away the plant's moisture. If the warm air that comes in contact with the moist plant parts can't move on, but instead lingers around the plant (incubating and stimulating trouble), the plant parts will either mold, have an enzyme attack, or rot, none of which leaves you with pleasant memories. Woodland bare-bottom encounters with poison oak and poison ivy and desiccating mishaps are notorious villains in herbal horror stories.

Bundling herbs and hanging them in a shaded location amidst circulating warm air is a simple, inexpensive method to dry plants. Use rubber bands for bindings; as plants dehydrate, they shrink and often fall out of twine bindings. Don't make the bundles too large, because the plants located in the center of the bundle might be cut off from the air flow, leading to mold, enzyme attack, rot. Dry or drying flower heads that are laden with seed can be bundled together, the heads stuck in a paper bag and secured, and the bundles hung up or shaken, letting the seeds dislodge from the heads and collect at the bottom of the bag.

Stringing herbs on a twine or heavy thread (clothesline-like) works for drying smaller harvests or when drying more delicate plants that are relatively light in weight. This bundling method allows each plant to adequately touch the passing air currents.

Laying plants out on sheets in the shade is another method for drying. I have never been too thrilled by this experience, because

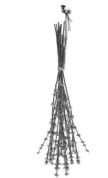

Bundling Herbs for Drying

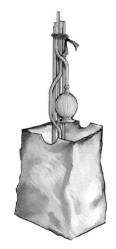

Bundling Technique for Collecting Herb Seed

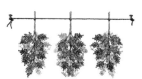

Stringing Technique for Drying Herbs

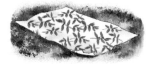

Sheet Technique for Drying Herbs

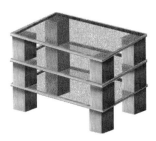

Stacked Screens for
Drying Herbs

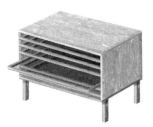

Dehydrator Used for
Drying Herbs

you have to find tall grass to lay the sheet on so air can circulate below as much as possible, or you need to find four corner posts to tie the sheet corners to, and all in all it has always been kind of a pain to contrive. So I haven't used this method very often, only as a last resort. Therefore, I am obviously not an expert in this process. But I am sure there are many folks out there who love to dry plants using a sheet, dish towel, scarf, or tablecloth; the possibilities are endless. Avoid using sheets of newspaper, however. Save these for toilet training puppies and for nesting gerbils. The printer's ink on newspapers can pollute the drying plants. It has polluted many fine minds as well.

Drying racks are my preferred contraption for dehydrating herbs. These are a series of shelves of screen network (old window screens work well) stacked in layers at suitable distances from each other, and placed in large, well-ventilated housings. Upon these racks the herbs are carefully arranged so as to overlap as little as possible, and allowed to remain subject to the desiccating action of the air circulating below as well as above until completely dried. Avoid using wire screens. The metal tends to react with certain components of fresh plants. Use nylon screen instead. Actually, we use stainless steel screen on some of our drying racks. What can I say, give 'em a little time and "experts" will disagree with their own selves too.

Commercial (or homemade) dehydrators are readily available. At one time I owned and used three wooden ones, one large one that stood on our kitchen pantry floor, and two small ones that hung out on our countertops. I'm a high energy enthusiast ("excessive" is probably a more accurate term) and often require more drying space

than others normally do. Ordinarily one dehydrator is sufficient for home use.

If you choose to use a dehydrator, I strongly suggest you locate it in or near the kitchen (lab). Make it a convenient and ready-to-use tool. Don't store it under a bunch of stuff in a cluttered hall closet that defies even the most courageous family member to enter. Relate to your dehydrator as an essential, active appliance, like the refrigerator, the stove, or the espresso maker. Give it a permanent location in the active zone of the kitchen. This will be quite practical and inspiring, encouraging you to become a prolific lay herbalist. Each time you locate a medicinal plant near your home (a Dandelion here, a Plantain there, a California Poppy, a cutting or two of your neighbor's neglected Rosemary bush, a Mullein leaf, some fresh garden Thyme, autumn leaves from the Ginkgo tree that stands down the road, and so on), you can readily harvest and dry it, and place it in a storage jar for future use. In a short time you can accumulate a year's supply of medicines and spices derived from neighborhood flora. You can do the same, of course, with any garden plants and fruits that come your way. I've even dehydrated leftover soup (soup leathers), an interesting challenge for the creative "excessive."

It's best not to use ovens or microwaves to dry your plants. You court disaster. There are too many gut-wrenching stories of people's impulsive cravings for chocolate chip cookies and preheating ovens to 375° F. just after someone else in the household had carefully laid his or her herbs in the oven to dry by the gentle heat of the pilot light. And drying fresh herb in a microwave oven is about as compatible as tank maneuvers on a golf green.

As soon as they are thoroughly dry, herbs should be processed and prepared for storage. Dried herb that is ignored and left lying or hanging around uncovered collects dust and cobwebs, and loses its vital luster. Break down bundles, garble with timely fervor, strip leaves, flowers, needles and/or berries from stems; do in general what you need to do in order to separate out the usable parts of the herb at hand. That's what "garbling" is all about. Discard the discolored, dead leaves and extraneous twigs, etc., as compost. It is best to wait until after the herb has been dried to do all this stripping and cutting. Mauling fresh herb, even gently, prior to drying, frequently leads to discoloration due to damaging of plant tissue. After the plant tissues are dehydrated, however, this no longer poses a problem.

PLANT PRESS DRYING

Pressing a plant for no other reason than that it is irresistibly beautiful, or for preserving a specimen to be identified later, can be facilitated by using a field press book. This tool is simple to construct and well worth the effort. Take time to make a good-quality one. It will serve you well for many years, and can someday transform itself into a prized and practical heirloom. Grandchildren seldom ever forget the joy of collecting wildflowers with grandma and grandpa and putting them in the press book. Your grandchildren will probably want to keep your old press book after you decide to move on to the Elysian fields to pick more flowers.

The plant pressings that you make are suitable to arrange and display in a home herbarium, a herbal scrapbook, a seasonal plant diary (call it what you will), or mounted on handcrafted greeting cards,

arranged as inspired flower pictures, or used to embellish lampshades, whatever. I find that herbal medicine is equally as effective when gazed upon as art, or walked through in a garden, or taken as a tea. Healing plant spirit can reside happily in all three.

A simple plant press is composed of three things: rigid wooden board, absorbent paper, and maintained pressure.

To construct a field press book, first place on the floor a 3/8-inch thick piece of 10-inch x 16-inch plywood (1/4-inch thick plywood is too flimsy and 1/2-inch plywood is unnecessarily heavy and bulky). Upon the plywood, stack three pieces of folded newspaper (this can be a piece of corrugated cardboard instead), two layers of paper towel or other white paper, three more pieces of newspaper or cardboard, two more pieces of paper towel and so on, until you have created a significant little pile. On top of this place a second piece of 3/8-inch plywood (cut to the same dimensions as the piece on the bottom). The plant specimen you collect are placed in between each two pieces of paper towel.

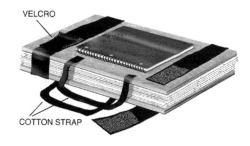

Homemade Plant Press Book

After inserting your plants in this pile, lay three bricks or heavy rocks on the pile to supply the pressure. In a short time the plants will flatten out, the paper towels will absorb moisture, and the warm location you keep this press in will assist the drying process. Give it a couple of weeks. Then check the plants, but very carefully. They are now a thin, fragile commodity. Nine out of ten times, you will be totally delighted by the results. However, things do happen that are often hard to talk about, but you'll cope, and it will all translate into meaningful experiences that you will learn from. That's Herbalism. Jot down some timely memoirs in the spiral notebook that I will soon be discussing. These notes will remind you what to do differently next time. It's good to make a mistake; it means you're courageously pushing your limits by pursuing creative new adventures, but it's dumb to make the same mistake twice. I can attest to that; I can even attest to doing it three times.

To streamline this press book, so you can carry it with you on hikes and plants walks, you can trade in the bricks for 4 feet of Velcro® and 34 inches of 1-inch wide cotton strap. You can see how and where to affix them in the illustration on page 61. The Velcro binds tightly together the two boards (and everything in between). Place your plants in between the paper towels as described above, but this time instead of laying bricks on the pile, kneel on the pile using your body weight to supply the pressure, and while kneeling wrap the bristly part of both Velcro straps around and affix them to the furry parts. You can get up now. The Velcro will sustain the memory of your body weight (could the space age exist without duct tape and Velcro?).

I suggest embellishing this basic field press book with cotton strap handgrips affixed to the boards (as illustrated) and a spiral bound notebook that has been stapled to one of the rigid boards which gives you a field desktop on which to write in the notebook. The pages of this notebook are useful for scribbling field notes and writing plant spirit-inspired lines of poetry. The 1-inch cotton straps stapled to the outside of both boards form handles with which to carry the whole works—a curious woodland briefcase for carting leaves and flowers.

GARBLING HERBS

Garbling is an exercise in the high art of paying attention to detail. Alertness to the details of harvesting and medicine-making is one of a herbalist's most creative and prosperity-promoting allies. Garbling (the word can be found the dictionary; I didn't make it up), when done correctly, is a meticulous, self-satisfying chore (a Virgo turn-on), the object of which is to remove all excess stems and twigs, impurities and adulterants, and decayed and deteriorated portions of the plant, which not only mar appearance but are apt to contaminate the usable portions. One also removes any small fauna found crawling on the goods. They were probably minding their own business, harvesting the plant for their personal agenda before you muscled in. Be kind by setting them free; they were also most likely participating in the plant's pollination conspiracy.

Garbling is an unsung backstage activity akin to the kneading of bread, the curing of firewood, proofreading manuscripts, and the arduous pulling of taffy. Mindful garbling transforms good-quality herb into great-quality herb and great-quality herb into primo herb. All superior-quality herb, by definition, is always meticulously garbled. Garbling makes herbal things better. It is appropriately undertaken anytime before, during, and after the drying process. Garbling herb is well performed in solitude, where it provides a prime opportunity to simultaneously garble one's attitude and beliefs about life. Yet I find it equally pleasant when performed in an intimate community atmosphere, wherein it attracts uplifting companionship and leisurely conversation. Its pace is similar to that of quilting and whittling, walking with little children, basket weaving, and chopping the fruits and vegetables at a potluck dinner.

STORING HERBS

Light, heat, moisture, and exposure to air deteriorate dried botanicals. Store your dried herbs in airtight, light-shielding, dry containers that will keep out insects and rodents. I prefer to use canning jars or clean recycled jars (especially the amber brown jars) that have wide mouths and tight-fitting lids. Coffee cans also make good containers, and, in some short-term situations, paper or plastic bags are appropriate containers. Do whatever you have to do to store these herb-filled containers in a cool, dark place.

Labeling Herbs for Storage
Label each container clearly including the name you use for the plant, the location of the harvest, and the date. (As I mentioned elsewhere, stored herbs can reabsorb moisture in time. Inspect your dried herb stashes routinely and re-dry them as necessary.) It is a reasonable idea to also note the general uses and dosage of the ingredients. This is a good method to refresh not only your memory of the herb's virtues but also a subtle way to pique the interest of casual on-lookers. They in turn go out and buy books like this.

When using jars as containers, it is prudent to secure the labels to the jars instead of to the lids. Jar lids are openly polygamous and have no qualms whatsoever about being affixed to any fitting jar that comes along.

I've been shocked by this conduct a number of times. If this simple precaution is taken, mislabeling jar contents can be almost entirely prevented.

Like fresh plants, dried herbs are organic entities that have various and differing tenures of stability. You seldom find a plant that retains its full potency indefinitely. Therefore, although there are exceptions, the generally accepted rules for storage time of herbs are as follows:

• Leaves, green parts, and flowers, up to one year

• Roots, seeds, and barks, two to three years

• Broken, crushed, or powdered herbs lose their value more rapidly than whole, uncut herbs.

BUYING HERBS

First of all, ask to speak to the herbalist on staff. If there is no herbalist working at the store, act astonished (they'll get the message); then do your own sleuthing. Ask where the herbs came from. Are they organically cultivated or wildcrafted, who grew them or who harvested them? Are any of the species they offer for sale threatened, and if so were they harvested consciously, etc., etc. You get the idea (refer to Rule #1 in *"Rules (Proposed) of Medicine Making,"* Chapter Twenty-Five). Encourage the herb merchant to buy from green-conscious suppliers. You'll probably find that many do, and they'll appreciate and respect you for inquiring. Those that don't buy from green-conscious sources may learn something from you.

Now check the store's herb stock. If the dried herbs displayed on the shelves are contained in clear glass jars sitting in direct sunlight, shop elsewhere; that's inexcusable.

Enjoy your garden pharmacy; garble passionately; keep an eye on those jar lids.

If the herbs on the shelves all look about the same color, they're probably "commercial grade" herb and not good quality. Shop elsewhere (refer to Rule #2 in *"Rules (Proposed) of Medicine Making,"* Chapter Twenty-Five). Varieties of herbs as they are growing and co-mingling in the garden or in the wilds naturally show a diverse array of colors and shades of green. They will continue to show a similar diversity of color when properly harvested, dried, and displayed in jars.

If the herb store passes the above examination, proceed to the taste and smell tests. Upon removing the lid from a jar of herb, you should smell a fine herbal aroma, and when a tiniest pinch of the dried herb is placed upon your tongue and slowly chewed and/or sucked on, it should provide a distinct flavor. Not necessary a yummy one, but a significant one. Good herb has color, aroma, and flavor. If all seems harmonious to your senses and to your inquiry, shop in this store. They probably have good herb to sell you; settle for nothing less (remember Rule #2).

CHAPTER 4
KITCHEN PHARMACY EQUIPMENT

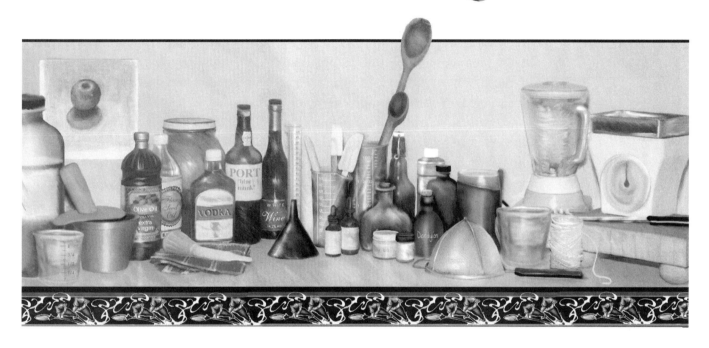

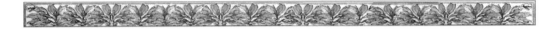

The Western symbols of medical power, knowledge, and competency standardized in mass consciousness by nineteenth and twentieth century "scientific" fanfare are the images used extensively by marketers in today's medical/pharmaceutical industry to communicate their perspective that all things are made better by the science and the high-tech industry. These same nouveau-archetype symbols are being adopted by much of today's herbal products industry to suggest that they also produce (herbal) commodities that the common person— who does not have access to the company's advanced technology and special (scientific) knowledge—can't match. During the past five years, my mailbox has found itself stuffed with full-color, high-gloss, printed literature picturing multi-story, sprawling "modern facilities," full of towering stainless steel vats sitting on polished linoleum floors, peopled by white-coated lab technicians peering through microscopes, operating computerized analysis equipment, and holding intricately designed lab-ware, testing and analyzing sterile beakers filled with colored herbal liquids and aseptic herbal powders. This attempt to impress "the mailing list" with the company's mysteriously advanced ability to produce herbal medicine is all about herbal *marketing*.

Mind you, there are some excellent herb companies active in the marketplace run by skilled herbalists whose intent is to make high-quality herbal products and a good living while also empowering their customers. These folks provide premium-quality products while evoking a marketing atmosphere of integrity and sound herbal education. I praise and honor these folks. However, the rising trend for many competing companies is to rampantly display medical cliché symbols accompanied by comparative charts that applaud their brand's self-extolled "superior delivery systems," their "clinically tested," "fast-active," "full-spectrum" this and "power-herb," "doctor-approved," "standardized" that. Please realize that the commercially correct terms and symbols being used reflect marketing strategies employed in general to overawe consumers and specifically to enhance sales; they are "business as usual." So, in face of all this, I'm strongly suggesting you not allow yourself to become overwhelmed or disempowered by the marketers' razzle dazzle. None of this glossy-slick corporate propaganda really has anything to do with you, your health, or Herbalism.

The home-tech environment of your cottage kitchen is where Herbalism lives. Herbalism thrives in the lay communities and hand-tended gardens of self-reliant plant people who cherish and practice their independence. Let the herbal marketers rave on, but know it is in your home that you can access and create for yourself the finest, most effective herbal products. In the simple environment of your domestic dwelling, you can fully empower yourself with experiences of functional herbal knowledge and competency; and all you need to help you do this is some basic knowledge and your own juicy kitchen-lab, supplied with the following equipment.

JARS AND BOTTLES

Jars are used to hold, blend, shake, seal, and store herbal stuff. Quart-size and pint-size canning jars are excellent, especially because their lids are easily renewed. Acquire a couple gallon-size glass jars, along with a diversity of miscellaneous-sized jars that reside and function in your kitchen-lab's container tribe.

Bottles are used for holding dried herbs and finished extracts. Amber glass bottles are the best to use, for they provide a shade-like shield to filter out damaging light that can deteriorate herbal material during storage.

If I may interject a suggestion here: Herbalism at its best embraces theater, and I recommend that, whenever possible, you consider doing things a little differently when you package and present your herbal wares. As a budding herbalist, don't accept false limitations. To do so only betrays your human potential. Break from the ordinary; as you collect common bottles for practical use, seek wild, colorful, whimsically shaped bottles and other types of bizarre containers as well. Use these to house and transport your herbal preparations. Render your herbal craft unique and fascinating. Why

not? It's all part of the enthusiasm and charisma of an herbal medicine show. Remember, when you make medicines at home and distribute your own herbal products to family and friends, you don't have the FDA (forever dull administration) editing your labels, monitoring your moves, or standardizing your panache. Herbalism thrives freely in the home — you can be as elaborate, outrageous, and nonconforming as you want. Package as you will. Have fun, give your herbal medicines a magical air. They will entertain and entice, manifesting ancillary wonders in a special way.

RUBBER SPATULAS

Wide ones and narrow ones to help get every bit of herbal material out of any and all sized containers. It's akin to garbling and a gesture of respect. These healing, nourishing substances are too precious to waste.

ELECTRIC COFFEE GRINDER

These post-Edison mortar and pestles provide a high-rpm pulverizing blade. Electric coffee grinders are relatively inexpensive tools that are excellent to use for powdering small portions of dried herb. Keep in mind that these are designed to be coffee bean grinding machines. They powder most herbs in good fashion, but they are not built to grind exceptionally hard materials, and they burn out when pushed too far. One has to be discriminating, somewhat gentle, and patient while using them; hardly as patient, however, as one has to be when using a pre-Edison mortar and pestle to grind and powder herbs.

MORTAR AND PESTLE

These are used more for creating atmosphere now that herbalists have electric grinders to do their pulverizing and powdering deeds. The most useful mortars and pestles are those that an herbalist can use to help prepare materials for further grinding in their electric grinder; these are the mortar and pestles designed specifically for contusion. They are made of brass, iron, or bell-metal which ideally has been molded into a deep, slender design. These tools can be used to pulverize roots, barks, and other tough woody materials by smashing down on them with the metal pestle. The narrow diameter and exaggerated depth of these devices help prevent the plant materials from flying out of the container when impacted by the pestle. A cover of stiff leather a little larger in diameter than the rim of the mortar is a further deterrent. This leather collar allows the pestle's free movement in the process of contusion.

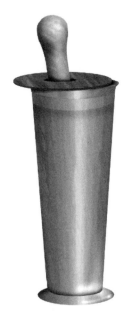

Deep contusion mortar and pestle with the leather collar

I recommend that you attain an archetypal, white porcelain Wedgwood mortar and pestle to display on a prominent shelf or countertop. These were designed for the more gentle act of trituration, which you will perform at times (see *"Trituration,"* Chapter Twenty-Five), rather than contusion. This classic symbol visually connects an herbalist's spirit to the grand heritage of the Galenic art and science of herbal medicine-making.

MEASURING CUPS AND/OR GRADUATED CYLINDERS

I find it practical to rely on plastic graduated cylinders. If you have any klutziness in you at all, or if you suspect you might have some questionable glass karma, the glass ones are too risky to use on a daily basis. I possess some beautiful Pyrex® glass cylinders that sit handsomely in my lab. They're an inspiration to behold; but I do most of my work using three plastic measuring cylinders (100 ml, 250 ml, and 500 ml sizes). In my case, it's definitely the klutz factor. And in the herb school lab we use plastic exclusively. Our lab floor is made of cement; and glass measuring devices disappear faster than Kleenex in a hayfever ward.

LID GRIPS

You'll need three of these to help you loosen jar lids that you previously tightened and allowed to sit around for a while. Inevitably, you will find it extremely difficult to remove the lid when you want to get back inside the jar. (This doesn't seem to occur as often when one employs a small kitchen-witch to reside inside or nearby the pharmacy area of the home.) When this situation does occur, however, what you do is put one lid grip on each side of the jar and place this between your thighs (I'm being serious here), and use the third grip to take hold of the lid. Squeeze your legs tightly against the jar sides and grimace as you firmly grasp and twist the obstinate lid counterclockwise. The lid will loosen. If it doesn't, repeat the above and add some light profanity. You might want to make the grimace a little more intense too. This always works for me. Using this ritual, I've never been denied entry into a jar of macerating herb.

STIRRING DEVICES

I recommend acquiring a 12- to 14-inch long by 1/2-inch diameter piece of wooden dowel, some 12-inch long wooden spoons, strong wooden chopsticks, and other stirring things that have some heft and can work well to mix and blend dense, mushy concoctions. In a short time, you will discover and adopt a favorite stick as your stirring companion. This relationship will thrive for years in a sea of activity and mutual appreciation.

STRAINERS

These are absolutely necessary to help separate depleted marcs from saturated menstruums. Acquire a variety of sizes and meshes. I use 4-inch diameter and 6-inch diameter strainers most often, but I often find that both smaller and larger ones are more helpful for specific jobs. At some point release the funds for one of those svelte, stainless steel, probably European-made, overpriced strainers that you can find in gourmet kitchen supply stores. The very fine mesh they provide is most useful for specific filtering tasks that will arise. The equally overpriced gold mesh coffee filters are useful too. You'll enjoy acquiring these tools, one by one, as you need them. Sieves and flour sifters of various-sized mesh also assist one to produce uniform-grade powders when powdering dried herb (see "*Powdering*," Chapter Twenty-Five).

DOUBLE BOILER AND A FLAME SPREADER

These are most useful for creating gentle-heat water baths and for modifying the heat coming off a stove-top burner. This equipment is useful for low heat extraction processes (i.e., preparing an oil infusion by using the digestion method).

FUNNELS

These are obviously used to get liquids (or dried herbs) into a container through a small opening without also scattering the material around the floor and countertop. I keep a variety of different sized—very small to quite large—standard funnels available for use, along with a wide-throated funnel device designed to help fill canning jars. I also bought a large plastic gasoline funnel at an auto supply store. It has a deep holding basket which is about 12 inches in diameter and a long funnel tube which I cut off about 1 1/2 inches from where it attaches to the basket. This now gives me a 3-inch diameter opening coming out of the basket. This modified device serves as a perfect funnel for transferring large amounts of dried bulk herb from paper or plastic bags into storage jars, which is also what I use the canning funnel for when relocating smaller quantities of dried herb.

MIXING BOWLS

These will be useful for a wide variety of purposes. I hold passionate affection for a 20-inch diameter wooden bowl that I found at a yard sale. I use it predominantly, even when it is obviously too big, just because it is so big—and wooden. I also recommend thin-gauge stainless steel bowls (they usually sell as sets of three concentric, differing diameters). They are available at just about every hardware store and kitchen supply section in town. Large bowls are useful for garbling fresh and dried herbs, for blending and rubbing dried herb compounds, for devising water baths, and for making adequate amounts of chocolate chip cookie dough when needed. I avoid putting oily stuff, like a cube of butter and chocolate chips, in my (great big) wooden bowl—it makes the wood permanently sticky, which complicates things when working with dry, powdery plant materials.

SCALES

Get yourself a metric scale. You can buy cheap, funky ones at kitchen supply and department stores, but the problem with these is that they normally don't register very accurately on the light end of the scale (where you will probably be doing much of your work), and they usually come with an absurdly small holding container that is not very practical when one is attempting to weigh unruly, bulky botanicals. So, I suggest that in time you buy a triple beam scale that is accurate down to a gram weight and can counterbalance a substantially sized holding basket. You'll appreciate this expenditure, and you'll enjoy your affluence. Pottery and ceramic supply stores sell triple beam scales. There are electric (battery-powered) scales also available in kitchen supply stores. They are accurate, cheaper than triple beams, and useful when working on the road.

Celebrate the New Age—go metric.

POURING DEVICES

Glass percolator coffee pot bottoms are my favorite and most sought after device to use for pouring herbal liquids. I get pushier than the teens in line for fake IDs when I see one of these well-spouted containers sitting as yet unclaimed in a yard sale or at a flea market. These glass sculptures were obviously designed by folks who knew what is required to pour blissfully with carefree confidence. The vast majority of spouted measuring cups and other spouted apparatus sold in stores today are obviously designed by the same folks who put together computer software manuals; they (the manuals and the pouring spouts) are ineffectual, having virtually nothing whatsoever to do with anyone else's reality. I suggest you hunt around for containers that have functional pouring spouts; shun and discard those that don't. Herbal extracts are too precious to squander as spillage and drippage, and one's temper is too painful to lose on a routine basis.

TURKEY BASTER

These are useful for decanting fresh-plant oil infusions and will be discussed further in the oil infusion chapter (vegan basting syringes are available at health food stores).

FILTER PAPERS

Purchase the unbleached basket style that are used for making coffee. Place these in a wire mesh strainer to hold them while you pour your extract through to filter out any unwanted particulate. You may want to strengthen these filters by using two at a time. Avoid the "cone style" filter papers, which are glued on the bottom and side. The glue might be soluble in certain solutions.

COTTON MUSLIN CLOTH

Locate a tough, unbleached cotton muslin in a fabric store. Be sure to launder it before using to rid it of the sizing found in most new cloth fabric. Muslin is used for pressing out the marc either by hand or with a mechanical press.

CALCULATOR

This is useful for doing the math when formulating a menstruum for weight/volume extraction. Pencil and paper work quite well for this too.

YOGURT THERMOMETER

This is used to monitor the temperature during the digesting process of extraction. Yogurt thermometers hover comfortably around the 100° F. zone, which is ideal for preparing oil infusions.

LABELING MATERIALS

Use whatever materials you require to create and affix labels that conform to your personal standards of aesthetics and whimsy, and the instruments to write essential information upon these engaging tags. Indelible inks are recommended.

PAPER TOWELS

The immediate availability of paper towels on demand is essential in order to maintain any semblance of sanity while making oil infusions and while pouring salves. In spite of what I said in the Prologue, this is a truth.

SPONGES AND RAGS

Have on hand a large collection of sponges and rags for spill control and general cleanup. A natal moon in the constellation of Virgo dictated this suggestion; and this is merely a suggestion. Impetuous, disorderly, hang-loose, rumpled herbal medicine-making is good too.

And at some point along your acquisition journey, you may want to acquire the following.

DEHYDRATOR

In the long run, this is probably the most important tool a domestic herbalist will obtain, and it is worth the expense to buy one that has a fine-tuned temperature control. I recommend that once you acquire a dehydrator, you give it a prominent place in the active area of your kitchen-lab. Each time you come across a wild plant that is harvestable, you can take it home and place it in the dehydrator, dry it, and in a hassle-free, short time add it to your annual stash of that particular plant-medicine. Dandelion, Chickweed, Plantain, Calendula blossoms, Red Clover blossoms, Cornsilk,

and so forth can be accumulated relatively effortlessly this way, and by autumn you will have acquired a substantial, high-quality herbal pharmacy in your home. Inevitably, within a couple of solar cycles, buying herbs from a store will have become merely a vaguely disturbing memory.

BLENDER/JUICER

Get the original Vita-Mix® 3600 Plus stainless steel model which has a 72-ounce stainless steel container (some containers come with a spigot, some don't; they both work). I have found these in yard sales, used-stuff stores, and flea markets; and some folks have acquired theirs by putting up wanted signs at large health food stores. These machines will probably be showing up more frequently now that the Vita-Mix corporation is marketing its newly designed polycarbonate container. The previous 3600 Plus Vita-Mix model, which is all stainless steel except for the plastic "two-piece Action Dome" that attaches to the top of the container, costs about $300 to $400 when purchased new. I've found them used and in excellent shape for $20, $60, and $150 Canadian in British Columbia; however, for the work this tool does, it is worth the $300. This is the best domestic designed machine I've found for powdering herbs and for blending fresh-plant extracts. It is a powerful, versatile, and very durable product that is well worth its cost to an inspired medicine-maker. We use these machines in the California School of Herbal Studies lab, where they have served many productive, but not always gentle, herb students over the past 20 years. The new model juicers that Vita-Mix now manufactures have "space-age material" plastic containers (which I'm told will also fit the older 3600 model motor base); I don't know, however, how well these will hold up to the beating of grinding herbs. The all-stainless steel machines used to come with a five-year warranty. (Actually, way back, they used to have a lifetime warranty.) But this most recent model comes with only a one-year warranty. I guess the space-age material is still in its experimental stage.

YOGURT MAKER

This is well designed for macerating small quantities of oil infusions at a low heat.

CROCK POT

This would be a superb warming (digestion) vessel for making oil infusions if it would maintain a heat of 100° F. But in my experience these cooking devices do not go lower than 150° F., which in my opinion (others will disagree) is too high a temperature for making good oil infusions. Perhaps one could employ a clever electrician to somehow derange a crock pot's rheostat, so it will consent to remain around 100° F.; this would then be a superb tool for this purpose.

FOOD PROCESSOR

This is not a priority, but if you have one or can easily acquire one, it is an excellent tool for mincing fresh garlic and other non-woody, fresh plant parts in preparation for extraction.

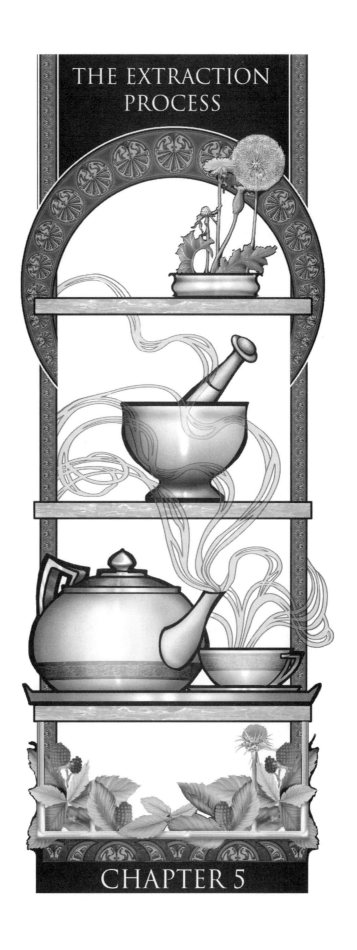

THE EXTRACTION
PROCESS

CHAPTER 5

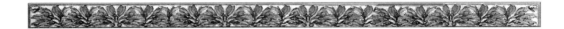

One can imagine how the first sparks of our vast herbal heritage were ignited. The inaugural attempts at the extraction of herbal properties were probably made soon after our deep ancestors discovered that certain plant materials were useful as food for nourishment, agents for altering consciousness, and medicines to alleviate physical and mental discomfort. Herbs collected for these purposes soon dried out, and it is logical to assume that our ancestral foreherbalists made attempts to restore the succulent qualities of these plants by steeping them in water. From this act, it was a simple step to discover that soaking plants in certain liquids dissolved the therapeutic powers of the plants and allowed their use in a more convenient, less cumbersome, and often more palatable form.

Applying heat was probably the subsequent step in the evolution of more specialized methods of soaking (macerating) with water. Therein the fundamental extraction processes of warm infusion, decoction, and digestion were devised. Later, the superior preservative properties and in some circumstances the superior solvent properties of vinegar and wine were recognized. Thus followed in natural progression the rudimental development of herbal extraction and medicine-making by human beings on this planet. It all germinated and evolved within the domestic arena of our common ancestors.

Concentrated ethyl alcohol was not available to the ancient herbalists as a solvent/preservative for maceration until after the twelfth century, when it was derived by the distillation of wine. It is not clear exactly when this happened, but by the sixteenth century alcohol-based tinctures and "quintessences" were attaining widespread use.

With the inflation of western reductionist science in the eighteenth and nineteenth century, paralleled by the pursuit of "rational" drug therapy in the allopathic medical arena, the processes of extraction and the isolation of plants' so-called "active ingredients" commanded the focus of a burgeoning pharmaceutical industry. The herbalist's inclination to summon and commune with the spiritual essence of a plant conjoined with a ceremony of appreciating the full array of the plant's physical and non-physical nature receded, along with the sightings of faeries and unicorns, into myth, magic, and "folkloric fancy."

Concurrently, the common practice of medicine-making in the home and the layman's practice of self-medicating with simple plant preparations declined to near extinction. As commercialized pharmaceutical technology evolved through this era in concert with allopathic medical theory and practice, the development of ever more technologically complex methods of extraction such as percolation, diacolation, mulcolation, and evacolation were devised.

This development of ever more complex systems of extraction has been a highly creative adventure in the world of pharmacy, and this has served the purpose of many. But all and all, for those individuals who are once again inclined to focus on the profound subtle energy of the plant more than on the technologies of physical extraction, no advancement beyond the fundamental rituals that derive infusions, decoctions, concentrates, and tinctures is required. Undeniably, extraction techniques that are more technologically elaborate or complex than these have provided many an adventurous herbalist with inspired enjoyment and the pleasure of satisfying their technological curiosity. Obviously, these laboratory furtherances have also allowed medical industries to produce plant-derived pharmaceutical drugs and herbal industries to manufacture standardized quasi-drugs. However, the potent simplicities of the fundamental extraction processes we will pursue in this home manual require no further complexity to serve the purposes of a conscientious lay herbalist. The simple alchemical acts of infusing, decocting, digesting, tincturing, and compounding medicinal plants are as sublime, complete, and transformative today as they were when our ancestors originally devised them.

Regardless of the technology employed, the *intent* and *joy* of the medicine-maker coupled with the consciousness of the harvester's *relationship* with the plant remains the truly empowering heart and the salient spirit of Herbalism and herbal medicine-making. Uncomplicated, ardent medicine-making is as fundamental to the art and science of Herbalism as simple passionate cooking is to the art and science of nutrition. High technology has never increased the nutritional power of good food, simply prepared.

EXTRACTION

The purpose for extraction is to draw out an herb's unique organization of chemical components along with its distinctive energetic virtues, and render these organic idiosyncrasies into a form that is more easily absorbable, possibly more concentrated, more palatable, and more convenient to administer than the original unprocessed form of the plant.

Maceration, or soaking a plant in a solvent, is performed to draw into a liquid solution the soluble constituents of the plant and to separate this solution from the insoluble residue or the marc. This liquid extract can be dispensed directly as is, or it can be readily incorporated into other delivery vehicles by mixing it with honeys, syrups, waxes, foods, and so on.

Alcohol, water-alcohol, and to some extent glycerin extracts offer the lay herbalist an added benefit of a greatly prolonged preservative action.

WHAT GOES ON DURING THE EXTRACTION PROCESS

When a freshly harvested plant is dried, the moisture present in the tissues evaporates. The walls of the cells and the ducts shrink, and at the same time the substances inside the cells previously held in solution by the water crystallize or dry to a solid amorphous mass. Later, when this dehydrated

Extraction allows us to have our herbs for a long time and makes it easier for us to eat them too.

plant is immersed in a water (aqueous) or water-alcohol (hydro-alcoholic) menstruum, the above process is reversed. In this instance, the menstruum is absorbed, causing the cells to swell and break, leading to direct contact with the menstruum and the soluble materials inside the cells go back into solution.

In the case of dried plants whose tissues are relatively soft or spongy, such as Burdock root or Nettle root, this process takes place comparatively fast; however, when a plant material is hard or callous, such as dried Wild Yam, Stone Root, Oregon Grape root, or Turmeric, much more time is required. Before the tissues of these plants can absorb a sufficient amount of menstruum, they must be broken up into fine pieces in order to expose their softer internal tissues to the action of the solvent. This is also required when extracting many seeds and leaves. Designed to shed water in nature, the walls of the outer (ectodermal) layers of these particular plant parts are impervious to water, but the walls of their inner (mesodermal and endodermal) cells are permeable and readily permit a solvent to diffuse through them and to dissolve the soluble portion of their contents. Therefore, the outer layer of cells of most leaves and seeds must be broken down like the hard tissues of plants mentioned above.

Regardless of the materials of which the cell walls of any plant part are constructed, the passing of the soluble constituents through the walls can be a slow process, but it can be quickened by increasing the surface area of the plant before extraction is begun. Again, this is accomplished (sometimes easily, sometimes not) by powdering the dried plant. This not only greatly increases the area that can be exposed to the

solvent, but also causes many of the ectodermal surface cells to be broken, so that the menstruum can come in direct contact with the cells' contents. The application of heat will also hasten the process of passing a plant's soluble constituents through the cell walls, and this is what the specialized maceration processes of hot infusion, decoction, and digestion are all about (we'll discuss those soon). It may be necessary in some circumstances, however, to avoid high temperatures during an extraction process. Heat will destroy enzymes which are sometimes desired; it will drive off volatile components, such as essential oils; it will coagulate plant proteins which can impede the extraction process; and it can dissolve out too much of the gums and proteins.

In extraction of dehydrated plant material by maceration, the dried plant material is normally powdered before applying a menstruum. The powdered plant is then allowed to remain in contact with a relatively large volume of menstruum until the extractive matter is distributed uniformly throughout the liquid. The saturated liquid is then poured off (decanted) and the marc (insoluble pulp) pressed or squeezed to procure any remaining liquid.

When percolation is used as the extraction process, a column of menstruum is allowed to flow down through a body of uniformly packed powdered herb carrying the extractant along with it as it exits the percolator cone, leaving behind the fully exhausted marc.

If instead, fresh undried plant material is being extracted by maceration, the menstruum is poured onto the plant and the entire mixture is pulverized in a blending machine (like an herbal smoothie) for an adequate time to break down the cell walls and expose them to the solvent action of the menstruum, or the fresh plant material can be simply chopped and macerated in pure ethyl alcohol, which acts to dehydrate the plant, drawing the plant juices and their chemical constituents into solution (more about these techniques later).

Before we get into a discussion of plant constituents and their main solvents, I would like to circumvent those details and give you an overview of what I consider the most efficient extraction technique for making superlative herbal medicine.

THE SENSUAL APPROACH TO SUCCESSFUL TINCTURING AND OTHER METHODS OF HERBAL EXTRACTION

1. The most important step. Acquire organically cultivated or ethically wildcrafted, meticulously garbled, high-quality herb that flaunts rich color, a deep aroma, and vivid flavor, because, please take out your stone notebook and etch the following: "My herbal extracts can never be any better than the quality of the herbs I begin with." (the 2nd rule of good herbal medicine-making).

2. Prepare the most suitable and efficient menstruum you can based on your previous experience and your knowledge of the plant properties. This information will be discussed in the following chapter. Remember to make detailed notes about the menstruums you formulate (the 4th rule of good medicine-making).

3. Make your tincture or other form of extract. (Refer to Chapters Eight through Seventeen.)

4. Now, use your common senses. Smell your finished extract, draw some of it into a glass dropper (pipette) and observe closely its color, put a drop or two of it on your tongue and taste it...Mmm! Or maybe, Yuck! ("Yuck!" is not necessarily bad, but merely intense or surprisingly unusual.) If your settled extract does not remain cloudy (at first most extracts appear cloudy before suspended sediment settles out), and it smells and tastes like the plant it was derived from, you've formulated a good menstruum for the herb at hand.

5. Dispense your herbal preparation. If it performs as you want it to, you've made a good extract; you have your herbal tonic/medicine. If you're not totally pleased, next time (and maybe the time after that) modify your menstruum until you are pleased; we've all done this many times; experience is the story of one's venture into the unknown.

Again I stress, make detailed notes for yourself. Refer to the sample Extract Information Form for medicine-making notes found in Appendix D. Modify this sample form to suit your own unique style and method of experimentation. Making herbal medicine is a very personal and sensual art and craft; don't hesitate to be adventurous and possibly blow it on occasion, just be sure you make notes. Ultimately, your experience, which is a creative integration of your successes and your mistakes, is your best teacher and finest trainer. Enjoy the plants, savor your extracts, and prize your notes.

SOLVENTS

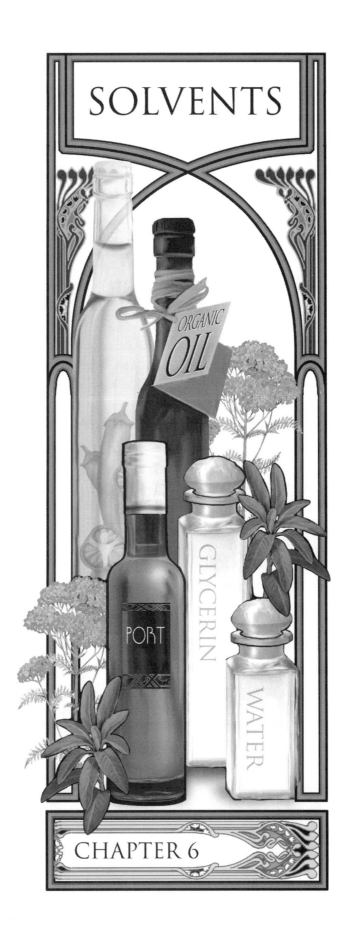

ORGANIC OIL

GLYCERIN

PORT

WATER

CHAPTER 6

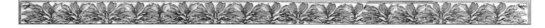

MENSTRUUM MENU— 7 LIQUIDS TO USE AS SOLVENTS

There are seven liquids readily available to us which we will discuss for use as menstrua in this manual. They are water, wine, vinegar, ethyl alcohol, alcohol-water mixture, oil, and glycerin, your basic community "potluck" components.

These seven menstrua are common kitchen supplies (except maybe the glycerin) that are abundant, easy to acquire, safe to use, and for our purposes, excellent solvents for making liquid extracts and herbal medicine in a home lab. In fact, most of these seven liquids are the principal solvents the pharmaceutical and herb industry professionals use as their primary menstrua (so much for that proprietary "scientific" mystery). There are many other menstrua used by these industries also, such as acetone, chloroform, methyl alcohol, denatured alcohol, amylic alcohol, acetic ether, sulfuric ether, hexane, and carbon disulfide. In my belief system, bodily contact with these particular solvents is neither safe nor pleasant. They are quite irritating to the healthy flow of a human being's life force, and in my opinion the complexity of their by-products renders them a forbidding conundrum for use in creating kindly internal and external herbal

preparations. Sufficient to say for this manual, further discussion of these toxic substances draws to a close here. The original liquid seven, however, will receive a predominance of our focus, for they in the hands of the herbalist are the prime shakers and movers of the act of herbal extraction. As an introduction, I will make a cursory overview of them, then give more specifics in the following pages.

WATER

Water is a universal element. One of the most important products of nature, its presence or absence plays a major role in the economy of our planet. Water is more or less involved in almost all the changes that take place in inorganic matter, and it is quintessential to the growth and existence of all living beings, whether animal or vegetable. Chemically, water is extraordinarily talented, ingenious in its field, very stable, and predictable, and therefore a most versatile and reliable tool. Water, being immensely abundant, is an inexpensive ingredient. The only controversy limiting the free use of water in the current adolescent stage of our civilization is that we have to clean most of our water before we can consume it. Water's indefatigable solvent action has dissolved and is holding in solution much of our culture's discarded debris, slowly decomposing this litter (for water is fortunately not a preservative—except for soft contacts and pet fish) and depositing its elements back into the earth for the use of ongoing generative cycles. When we learn to stop making such large messes (and we are learning) and figure out how to clean up our neighborhoods, our ground water will become suitable again for extemporaneous use. Meanwhile, we often need to purify water by using assorted filtering and distillation techniques. This increases the cost of a gallon of water for consumption from when it was once abundantly free to currently around the average U.S. price of a gallon of gasoline. But aside from this pollution confusion, water is the best solvent we have. Its basic nature is absolutely consistent and reliable. We have used it from the very dawn of simple Homo sapiens' pharmacy, and its use as a primary menstruum has remained unchallenged on into the current alchemical shenanigans practiced within the labyrinths of today's high-tech pharmacy and commercial herbal product manufacturing.

ALCOHOL

Alcohol is the second most relied upon menstruum for most medicine-makers. It too is stable (at plus or minus room temperature) and is also reliably consistent in its actions as a solvent and preservative. As a solvent, it is so predictable that it is relied upon in pharmacy both for what it will eagerly dissolve as well as for what it definitely won't dissolve. And whereas we can depend on the fact that water acts the opposite of a preservative, medicine-makers know that alcohol is probably the best preservative. Aside from human party animals, not many life forms or enzymes can thrive for long when immersed in a volume of alcohol or even in diluted alcohol, and therefore changes due to disintegration and decomposition are greatly slowed down; shelf life is significantly increased.

WINE AND VINEGAR

The next two common menstrua that we will discuss, which have in other eras been eagerly employed by medicine-makers, are wine and vinegar. Both of these liquids do what water does, for H_2O is primarily what they are, but their total chemistry includes a couple of embellishments to their water body. Wine boasts of a mild touch of stimulating alcohol, and vinegar a little touch of sour-tasting acid. The amount of these "touches" from batch to batch is variable and therefore to a small degree inconsistent in different lots of these products. These variations are mostly determined by the nature of the vegetation used for production and the specific manufacturing process. The presence of the alcohol in wine and the acetic acid in vinegar supply a degree of preservation action to the waters of these liquids and also add a little different "bite" to their water-like solvent action. The inherent natures of wine and vinegar, however, also carry with them some other "uncontrollable" vegetable matter which during shelf time can begin to change their nature, affecting the chemistry and the preservation of the herbal components that have been dissolved in the extracts. The results are that the overall blend of these "variables," "uncontrollables," and "inconsistencies" renders these two menstrua less reliable in relation to sustaining long-range permanence. This is a feature which has greatly disturbed some medicine-makers in the past,

Set the tone for the new millenium, be a lay herbalist. Water, spirits, wine, vinegar and oil, culinary and medicinal herbs, common kitchen equipment, and one's unleashed passion are the shakers and movers of herbal medicine-making…that's all one needs to cook as a community herbalist.

especially those whose commercial preparations, and the marketability of such, demanded control, permanence, and a great deal of solvency predictability. This preoccupation with predictability, control, and permanence is orchestrated principally by the intensity and toxicity of the particular medicines they are manufacturing, whereas smaller quantities of gentler more benign medicinal and culinary preparations (which is what we will be making) don't demand such rigidity.

There is the story of two nineteenth century pharmacists, Lea and Perrins, who concocted an herbal digestive blend using a vinegar base menstruum. When completed, this infusion of Tamarind bean and other highly flavorful herbs turned out quite disgusting to the senses. Frustrated by the venture, the two men decided to trash the whole thing, but instead for whatever reasons some of it sat forgotten in their lab cellar. During this unpremeditated aging period the vinegar's inherent variables and inconsistencies, to the formulators' eventual surprise and delight, evolved the juice to a succulent compound solution that is well known today as Worcestershire sauce (the men obviously kept good notes during preparation for possible future reference). Wine and vinegar menstrua will receive considerable attention in later chapters of this manual.

MIXTURE OF WATER AND ALCOHOL

The next menstruum we will discuss is simply a mixture (in infinitely varying proportions) of the big two, water and alcohol. These proportions are determined by the nature of the components of the particular herb being extracted. This type of menstruum is also referred to as an aqueous-alcoholic menstruum, or other terms to that effect.

OIL AND GLYCERIN

The final two menstrua we explore are oil and glycerin. They are to me the chemical jesters of the show, sort of like Bozo and his pet bear. They are sweet, slow, and warm and seem to function in their own peculiar world. They are fun to play with, both commanding patience, heightened concentration (especially by those active members of Virgos Anonymous), and a light-hearted tolerance from the medicine-maker while she or he is working with these performers. The nature of the ensuing products derived from the actions of these two solvents are also pleasant, playful, soft, and comfort-enhancing companions to one's life, such as lip balms, body lotions, soothing therapeutic oils, pain-relieving, wax-removing ear oils, and balmy unguents.

Oil is a sensually unctuous solvent for the components of many herbs as well as itself, being a mild, protective component that carries herbal virtues to the skin quite comfortably. Oil carries these nutritional and therapeutic virtues to the outer skin of one's body as medicinal oils, ear drops, salves, and lotions, and to the inner skins as nourishing foods when swallowed by the upper end of the digestive tube, and as mildly coaxing boluses and suppositories when deposited in the lower end. As we all know by common experience, oil refuses to mix with water, and in like fashion it won't mix with alcohol. Fortunately, however, it does mix well with paper towels during and after spills, runovers, and other extemporaneously lubricious emergencies.

Glycerin is the sweet-tasting component of fats and oils. Most commercial vegetable glycerin is made available to us as a coconut oil by-product of the soap industry. After being initially derived from oil, glycerin will no longer mix with it; it's one of those odd generation gap things. At the same time, glycerin is a chemical cousin to alcohol, and an eager playmate with water. In direct contrast to oil, glycerin will mix quite willingly with both water and alcohol. Glycerin is the major component in any menstruum used to form glycerites. Glycerites are alcohol-free, sugar-free, sweet-tasting extracts popular with children, parents, and those who refuse to taste anything herbal unless it is sweetened.

Glycerin is often included as a small portion of an aqueous alcohol menstruum to modify the magnetic relationship that exists in nature between alkaloids and tannins whenever these two meet up in a liquid solution. The presence of glycerin generates a sort of love triangle, the inevitable results of which the tannins and the alkaloids practice ignoring each other, while the glycerin and tannins go off by themselves to be alone. This liberates the alkaloids to do what they pharmacologically do best without being distracted and ultimately precipitated by the amorous action of unfettered tannins. Further details of this soap will be disclosed later.

So, throw any, all, or an appropriate combination of the above seven liquids into a cauldron along with a harvest of wild and vibrant herbs and we have the initial makings of a fascinating, sensual, and colorful show — an Herbal Medicine Show.

SOLVENT ACTIONS OF MENSTUA

WATER

Water, the global menstruum that is forever dissolving the surface of our planet, has likewise, from time immemorial, been used by human beings as a solvent to enhance their lives. Water is called the universal solvent, for it has a more extensive range as a solvent than any other known liquid. It is also the cheapest and most abundant solvent available, and is therefore used in the extraction of plant essences whenever the advantage of using it outweighs any disadvantages.

Cold water is a good solvent for plant constituents, such as sugars, proteins, albuminous bodies, gums, mucilaginous substances, pectin, tannins or plant astringents, plant acids, coloring matter, many mineral salts, many glycosides, some alkaloids, most all alkaloidal salts, and, to a slight degree, a hint of essential oils.

Hot or boiling water causes plant tissues to swell and in so doing bursts the cells. This hot water then dissolves starches and disintegrates and extracts other vegetable tissues hardly affected by cold water. Heating a water menstruum permits the more rapid solution of a plant's soluble matter, but a frequently encountered disadvantage inherent with this phenomenon is that the heating process extracts substances which later separate out from the solution upon cooling. These precipitated substances can manifest as sinister-looking scum or foreboding foams and other frightening apparitions that float on the top of a solution or settle in strange ways at the bottom of the container. Although aesthetically disturbing to some, these precipitates are harmless unless you plan to store the liquid for a while, in which case they provide food for microorganisms. If you intend to use this tea to make a syrup, or are keeping it to use later for whatever reason, strain it as soon as it cools.

Plant tissues are made up of associations of complex bodies. As the extraction of these plant constituents with water is initiated, the sugars, gums, plant acids, mineral salts, and coloring matter, which are the most readily soluble constituents, dissolve first. The solution of these different substances in water produces a different menstruum which is now capable of dissolving constituents that were previously insoluble in pure water. As this phenomenon progresses, the ongoing compositions act as new extracting mediums one after another, with water no longer being the sole menstruum.

All this action instigated by bringing pure water to a boil evolves liquids of differing solvent capabilities than that of simple cold water, and in this way it is found that water solutions of plant constituents may produce important menstrua that are uniquely different from water alone. This is quite important to understand, because it gives the ultimate solvency power of simple water and the classic preparations that employ only water as a menstruum (teas) the regard they merit. As a result of these idiosyncrasies of a water menstruum, water may ultimately be made to dissolve water-insoluble substances that from their characters, at first assumption, would appear not to be soluble at all in a simple water menstruum. One finds that water may become a solvent for particles of such constituents as resins, oils, glucosides, and other plant constituents that, in a purified condition (isolated from the fully intact organic chemistry of the plant), are insoluble or nearly so in pure water. With this insight, water infusions and decoctions can be recognized (reinstated in home pharmacy) and relied upon as equally powerful or in many instances more powerful extraction processes as those processes that include alcohol and other solvents in the menstruum.

I've always felt that the humble cup of herb tea is a more overall potent and effective delivery system of herbal medicine than the most superlative power-products released by all our commercial herb industry. Chinese herbalists decocting their often severe-tasting herbal stews have been relying quite successfully on the potent alchemy of this simple aqueous delivery system for centuries.

There is a universal disadvantage, however, in using water by itself as a solvent. As one can affirm from experiencing the forces of nature, the conservation of status quo is not the work of water on the surface of this dynamic planet. Water is not one to preserve a static condition of any substance or being; and this salient characteristic is reflected by an herbal preparation when using water as a sole menstruum. Except in its own frozen state or glacial form, water is not at all a preservative. On the contrary, its presence stimulates change and is a prime mover in the perpetual transmutation of forms (and aqueous solutions). Therein, true to its fine nature, the greatest disadvantage in the use of water as a menstruum is that it is not a preservative. In fact, water in its passionate promotion of change is a near antithesis to a preservative. Its remarkable solvency extracts large amounts of diverse substances, while its tissue penetration excites plant enzymes (although these organic catalysts are usually destroyed by high temperature), and the resulting solution of plant constituents makes up a fertile soup that can be an excellent media for enzymatic action and the growth of molds, yeast, and bacteria. These opportunistic organisms, in their spontaneous feeding frenzies, radically alter the state of the extract, and this alteration is usually not on the side of sensory aesthetics or palatability. So one is required to either consume a water extract within a day or two, freeze it, or add another substance that can interfere with destructive enzymatic fervor and insidious multiplication of microorganisms; and that is what some of the following liquids do.

ETHYL ALCOHOL

Alcohol is more selective in its extraction action, and therefore does not have as wide a solubility range as water. Ethyl alcohol is a good general solvent for extracting resins, balsams, camphors (most of these three are thrown out of solution by diluting them with water), essential oils, alkaloids and natural alkaloidal salts, glycosides, organic acids, chlorophyll, most coloring matter, nearly all the acrid and bitter constituents of a plant, uncrystallized, amorphous vegetable sugars, and one fixed oil: castor oil. Some sugars, proteins, gums, mucilaginous substances, and albuminous bodies are, however, capable of being mixed with dilute alcohol (a mixture of 50 percent water, 50 percent ethyl alcohol).

Alcohol refuses, however, to abstract gums, mucilaginous substances, starch, albuminous materials, or many mineral compounds, and it does not dissolve any appreciable amount of crystallized cane sugar.

In addition to its selective solvent properties, alcohol paralyzes enzymes, and at the same time prevents the growth of yeast, molds, other fungi, and most bacteria; so alcohol solutions seldom if ever ferment or putrefy. As a consequence of these reliable preservative properties, alcohol more or less diluted has long been employed as a solvent in the making of tinctures, fluid extracts (which are merely concentrated tinctures), and solid extracts. Though not preferred by some people, alcohol as a preservative is efficient and often necessary for the following reasons:

1. To eliminate microbial activity and preserve preparations almost indefinitely

2. To inactivate enzymes which are destructive to alkaloids and glycosides

3. To control destructive chemical decomposition of glycosides and saponins due to the presence of water

Alcohol mixes well with water (and glycerin) in all proportions. As you will find in your medicine-making experiences, alcohol equals water in importance as a solvent for many active plant substances, many that water, especially cold water, does not readily dissolve. It is also a uniquely important agent for the very fact that (for manipulative pharmacy) it adamantly excludes many other plant substances which water does dissolve, such as albuminous matter (plant protein), plant starches, gums, and mucilaginous materials. This is sometimes referred to as alcohol's "negative strength." These plant components (which often refuse to be filtered out in certain solutions) when present in a solution will sometimes act as unsightly (opalescent, cloudy, gummy, jelly-like, ropy, or syrupy) solution disturbers as well as provide food for microbes.

Mix an appropriate amount of alcohol into an existing extract being "disturbed" by these components, and they will be thrown back out of the solution. They can then be

For those individuals who are concerned about the presence of alcohol in an herbal preparation, the following calculations based on a tincture containing 60 percent alcohol (most tinctures contain less) are given for your guidance:

• **A daily nutritional dosage:** For adults, 20 drops 3 times a day equals about 1/30th of an ounce of alcohol spread over 24 hours.

• **An acute dosage:** For adults, 20 drops per hour for approximately 12 hours equals about 1/7th of an ounce of alcohol spread over the day. Children are usually given 1/2 to 1/4 of this adult dosage.

removed, leaving the extract looking far more attractive. To illustrate this banishment of an offending component (in this instance slimy mucilage by alcohol) from an herbal solution, make a strong water infusion of Comfrey root, and when it is cool, pour some into a small container, add to it a substantial quantity of pure 190-proof ethyl alcohol, and therein you will behold the outcast. Add more water to this, thereby diluting the alcohol, and the mucilage will dissolve back into solution.

Often, however, the mucilaginous component of an herb is exactly what one wants to draw into solution. This is true in preparations of some of our most nourishing and therapeutic plants such as Comfrey, Marshmallow, Slippery Elm, and Cinnamon. But if one wishes to preserve an extract of these mucilaginous plants for any length of time, be well advised to use some alcohol as either a part of the extracting menstruum or as a later addition. Eighteen to 20 percent ethyl alcohol will be adequate, and usually this is not a sufficient amount to cause an eviction of the above-mentioned components.

Safe Storage of Ethyl Alcohol
• Keep alcohol packaged in bottles out of the sun and away from heat. I prefer to use high-density polyethylene (HDPE) plastic bottles; glass bottles full of liquid heat up faster and break too easily, and in this instance, are a most costly break.

• Keep container tightly closed to prevent leakage and evaporation.

• The boiling point of pure ethyl alcohol is 173° F.

• Be aware that alcohol containers can be hazardous when empty, for they retain residual vapor that is extremely flammable. Allow recently emptied containers to sit outdoors with the lid removed, so the contents will evaporate and dissipate completely.

• Alcohol is a flammable liquid.

• Spills: If a spill has not ignited use water spray to disperse the vapors and to dilute the spill to a nonflammable mixture.

• Fire-fighting procedure: Use dry chemical or carbon dioxide. Water may be ineffective, but should be used to keep the fire-exposed containers cool.

• Avoid prolonged inhalation of vapor.

ALCOHOL–WATER
Alcohol-water mixtures possess few, if any, of the disadvantages exhibited by water alone in the extraction and preservation of plant components. The blending of alcohol with water seems to be a consummate marriage for both extraction maneuvers in the lab and social merriment in the recreational arena. Some plant constituents are nearly as soluble in an alcohol-water menstruum as they are in strong alcohol, and in some cases the alcohol content of the menstruum can be as low as 25 percent. I recommend you strive for maximum extraction using a minimum percent of alcohol, keeping in mind that 15 to 20 percent alcohol by volume—of the end product—is probably the lowest alcohol content you can contrive that will preserve the extract for any length of time.

In pharmacy a mixture of 50 percent ethyl alcohol and 50 percent water is commonly referred to as dilute alcohol.

Vinegar

I am referring here to the use of apple cider vinegar or any other plant vinegar such as plum vinegar, rice vinegar, wine vinegar, balsamic vinegar, etc.

Vinegar is a sour liquid on account of its acetic acid content. It has valuable properties as a solvent as well as a preservative. As a solvent it provides a service that aids in the fixing and extraction of certain alkaloids and other water-soluble plant components, and it can be substituted for alcohol in the preparation of extracts, although this is not a common practice today. Medicinal vinegars await their renaissance in practical lay Herbalism, and it is intended that this particular manual will hasten that coming.

Vinegar's action as a preservative is considered to be excellent, though inferior to dilute alcohol, and for this reason pure vinegar preparations are said to be more liable to change than tinctures. In certain custom-prepared menstrua, vinegar is commonly added as 5 percent to 10 percent of an alcohol-based menstruum to adjust the pH when that is advantageous (i.e., for making extracts of Lobelia, Black Walnut, Goldenseal, Ephedra, etc.)

In the late 1800s medicine-makers felt that the state of solution of some plant components was at its best when vinegar was employed as the menstruum, at least as far as the medicinal action of these extracted components was concerned. This was particularly the case when the activity of the medicine depended on the presence of one or more alkaloids. A raw free-base alkaloid is often difficult to bring into solution, but by uniting it with the acetic acid of vinegar a free base alkaloid forms an alkaloidal salt. Alkaloid salts are readily soluble in water;

therefore, they may be more perfectly extracted in vinegar than by other menstrua.

However, the fact that vinegar contains inherent vegetable matter renders it liable to decomposition, and therefore these preparations are best made in small quantities and renewed at shorter intervals (annually) than alcohol-containing preparations. One can always, if desired, add a little alcohol to vinegar solutions to extend their preservation even further; this generates a medicine that is well preserved, and still greatly reduces the use of alcohol.

In chemistry, vinegar is generally classed among the derivatives of alcohol, as it is produced by the oxidation of alcoholic liquids, especially hard apple cider and wine. Vinegar is a very dilute solution of acetic acid containing what the pharmaceutical texts refer to as foreign matters. Why these matters are considered foreign I'm not quite sure, since they are inherent to and an actual part of what makes up whole vinegar itself. In the late 1800s the U.S. Pharmacopoeia's official description of vinegar is the same as mine. The Pharmacopoeia defined vinegar as "impure diluted acetic acid prepared by fermentation." A clue emerges as to the "foreign" mystery as it becomes clear that pharmaceutical activists focus solely on the action of the acetic acid in vinegar and not on the wholeness of vinegar itself; obviously, they are not at all impressed with or care about the fact that this wholeness gives vinegar its own inherent nutritional and medicinal virtues. Over time, vinegar fell into disfavor by pharmacists because not only was its acetic acid content found to be too variable, it was also relatively expensive and was said to be possessed by organic impurities (foreigners). Pharmacy eventually replaced vinegar with a much cheaper, more controllable product called acetic acid, nearly pure acetic acid prepared from wood by destructive fermentation and purification. Pure acetic acid is cheap, free from impurities, and unvarying in its intensity. In high pharmacy it is diluted to present a 6 percent acetic acid content (actually, 5.7 to 6.3 are allowable parameters—I guess even perfection has its slack side).

In light of all this, however, I think that the obsession with an acetic acid content that is exactly 6 percent (+ or − .3 percent) is a bit anal, and I, in addition to being comfortable with a little acidic variance, am rather fond of the synergy of many botanical impurities (even though they might lead to a faster change in a solution). I still prefer to use "crude" vinegar; I feel more comfortable with its vulgar character and variable acidity.

However, it is wholly understandable why vinegar fell into disfavor with the medical pharmacy establishment, for it is in the business of dissolving very heavy duty plant alkaloids and other intense and often highly toxic components into preparations, making the therapeutic use of the resulting drugs (as well as the survival of their patients) extremely dose specific. Responsible allopathic medical practitioners needed to be entirely sure of the strength of the extract, which in this case depended on the action of the acidic acid in the menstruum. So allopathic doctors did not discard vinegar because it was a poor solvent, but because it was (expensive and) relatively uncontrollable as almost all natural plant-derived things are. This is one reason why mainstream Western allopathic medicine does not use botanical medicines any longer. It has replaced these with chemical medicines and synthetically derived plant components. These are highly controllable and unvary-

ing. Moreover, there are no longer any foreign, impure matters to contend with that might shorten the stability of the products.

For those of us, however, who are not dealing in toxic materials and don't need an indeterminately long shelf life for our medicinals, vinegar remains an excellent solvent. We can revive its use because we are preparing tonics and therapeutic agents derived from gentler plants that are not dose critical. These plants may be extracted very well and are adequately preserved by vinegar and wine solvents.

It is important to realize that during the same era in our medical history, when the medical establishment made its decision to deal primarily with toxic botanical and non-botanical substances as their materia medica, the lay population concurrently surrendered its health and disease care to these same medical professionals and proceeded to lose their knowledge of self-medication using medicinal plants and stopped preparing herbal remedies as their grandparents and ancestors had done. We all lost touch with this (folk) technology of independence. As time passed, high-proof ethyl alcohol became the mainstream pharmacy's solvent of choice rather than wines, vinegar, and glycerin to a large extent. In the 1960s, when we saw the revival of homemade herbal preparations and self-medication, herbalists began to make their plant concoctions available in stores. They used ethyl alcohol (and water) as their primary menstruum probably because of the powerful influence of mainstream pharmacy and a desire for long shelf life. I don't think herbalists disregarded wines and vinegar as viable menstrua because they weren't good solvents and preservatives, but because they weren't as "strong" as alcohol, and therefore not the best menstrua to use for competitive commercial adventures. Glycerin, considered a "stronger" solvent and preservative than either wine or vinegar, has enjoyed a quicker revival in the modern herbal medicine-making world (maybe not as a star performer, but certainly as a popular supporting actor). So, although many herbalists today have experimented with and enjoyed making medicinal herbal wines and vinegars, not many have taken them very seriously. I think a greatly elevated regard for these (potentially homegrown) menstrua will transpire once we change our attitude to one that is based on experience rather than on the mainstream U.S. pharmaceutical history and literature. There is much to learn and appreciate about these excellent natural menstrua.

Lay herbalists (you and I) are in the process of reviving the foundations of Herbalism in our homeland. We have only just begun; we are relearning the language of Herbalism. Like aboriginal youths who return to their native homelands from the cities, it will take time to revive our traditional living skills. The language of Herbalism is unique among other medical languages. Its grammar and syntax are derived from the understanding and uses of Nature's organic phenomena. We can embrace this common language in our homes and communities as we focus on the wholeness and individual life cycles of local medicinal plants, redevelop our herbcraft, and recall how wonderful it is to dance barefooted in the green world.

Vinegar and wines are made from plants that can grow in most any garden, and their organic nature in turn can render remarkably efficient menstrua for us to use for making healthful foods, herbal tonics, and reliable medicines—at home. When you grow medicinal plants in your garden and also learn to use the wild plants that grow near your home, you don't need to preserve herbal extracts for years on end. These plants come to you anew every year, so you can make fresh extracts seasonally. You only need to preserve these for a relatively short time. This is a different rhythm of perception we can move to, a cyclic, seasonal rhythm that is unending. Herbalism encourages us to relax into a healthful sense of well-being with a deep awareness of Nature's nourishing, perpetual abundance.

GLYCERIN

Glycerin (a.k.a. glycerine) is the sweet fraction of a fixed oil. It is found in all true fats (except cholesterol, which is a fat containing no glycerin) and oils, of both vegetable and animal origin. Glycerin was discovered in the late 1700s and came into use in medicine and pharmacy in the mid-1800s. It is produced through a remarkably complex process that decomposes fats in a large digester. After several hours of a bizarre relationship between the fat, the water, and 150 pounds of steam pressure involving constant agitation, the fat's glycerin fraction is ultimately separated from its fatty acids. The glycerin is distilled out, purified, condensed, and collected for use. Much of the vegetable glycerin available to us is derived from coconut oil. There are also glycerin products derived from animal fat and synthetically contrived from trichlorpropane, which is a petroleum product. Investigate your sources.

Chemically, glycerin belongs to the class of alcohol, and is termed glycerol or glyceric alcohol. However it is a tri-atomic alcohol and contains no ethyl alcohol or methyl alcohol which are di-atomic

Glycerin is not a carbohydrate and contains no sugar. Taken internally it is slowly absorbed into the bloodstream, then slowly metabolized by the liver. Due to this slow process, glycerin does not cause any appreciable blood sugar imbalances.

alcohols having dramatically different characteristics. Glycerin is not a carbohydrate and contains no sugar. Taken internally it is slowly absorbed into the bloodstream, then slowly metabolized by the liver. Due to this slow process, glycerin does not cause any appreciable blood sugar imbalances. Glycerin is a valuable solvent and preservative agent in medicine-making. Some authorities say it is second only to alcohol in these respects, having a solvent power about half the strength of pure ethyl alcohol. This would make it an excellent choice as a solvent for herbs and roots that respond well to a menstruum having a lower solvent power. In my experience, I find its range of solvency less extensive than either water or alcohol. The beauty of glycerin is that it is capable of mixing with both water and/or alcohol, so its qualities can be easily combined with both. Glycerin is clear, odorless, has an agreeable sweet flavor, a thick, syrupy, stable consistency, produces a sensation of warmth to the skin and tongue, remains stable when heated, is antibacterial, and will extract a variety of constituents that make it useful in cases where neither water nor alcohol are appropriate. It is a notable substitute for alcohol in the menstrua of extracts given to alcohol-intolerant individuals. It can be used to prepare children's tonics or to use with plants that have relatively large amounts of ligneous (woody) fiber; water expands these gummy and/or glutinous materials far more than glycerin does — which is often an objectionable occurrence. Glycerin abstracts and holds tannates (it is said to have the capacity to absorb nearly its own weight of tannic acid), and therefore is exceptionally effective when incorporated as a portion of a menstruum for herbs containing tannins, as it reduces, if not elimi-

nates, the precipitating action in a solution where tannins contact alkaloids, a condition which can greatly interfere with the activity of the alkaloids. In many respects, glycerin resembles water as a menstruum more than it does alcohol. Glycerin will not dissolve or mix with resins or fixed oils, so it is not suitable for resinous or oily herb extracts. And although it is a good solvent for a few alkaloids, it is generally inferior to water, vinegar, and alcohol for extracting most alkaloidal structures. Glycerin does not extract volatile oils very efficiently, but it readily mixes with them and preserves them for a short time. When diluted with water or aromatic hydrosols (see Chapter Ten), glycerin is demulcent and emollient, lubricating, soothing, and protecting to the skin and mucous membranes. When used undiluted, it acts as an irritant that arouses activity. Glycerin readily absorbs water from the air and is useful for keeping substances moist. It does not ferment or evaporate at ordinary temperatures, but it does vaporize readily from a water solution at 212° F. Glycerin, when undiluted, boils at 329° F.

WINE

Wine as a menstruum can produce some delightful herbal infusions, as its solvent action is akin to an alcohol-water menstruum. Macerating herbs in wine is a highly creative arena in which to experiment. However, due to wine's naturally low alcohol content, a saturated wine extract might not hold up against the process of deterioration over an extended period of time unless more alcohol is added to ensure its stability, especially during warm weather.

At one time, there were several medicated wines and two natural wines considered official medicines in this country (meaning they were recognized in the official U.S. Pharmacopoeia and later in the National Formulary). Some of these medicated wines, such as Antimony wine and Colchicinum wine, were in fact very potent allopathic medicines, an improper dose of the later being fatal. But in time wines lost favor, due to the fact that it was found impossible to formulate tests whereby spurious wines could be positively recognized and distinguished from the pure ones. However, this is no longer an issue for us today with the vast array of legitimate local wineries currently in action.

Traditionally, white wines were preferred as menstrua for making medicinal wines because of their small proportion of tannins (sherry was the strongest white wine and therefore the most frequently used, and port was the most frequently used red wine). In the case of red wines, the skin of the grape is allowed to remain with the expressed juice during fermentation, and the astringent dark coloring-matter in the skin contains large amounts of tannin. This can be a problem when infusing herbs that are high in sought-after alkaloids because, as previously noted, tannins precipitate and therein pull out of solution these alkaloidal components. Official wine menstrua were required to contain 16 percent to 24 percent alcohol (which wine does not contain naturally), so these wines were fortified with pure grape brandy, which sounds to me like the makings of good medicine.

Oil

There are two kinds of oil, fixed oil and volatile. However, volatile oils (a.k.a. essential oils, aromatic oils) are not really oils at all. They are only referred to as oils because they blend with oil quite readily and they react with water much like fixed oils do. Chemically volatile oils have next to nothing in common with fixed oils, lacking both fatty acids and glycerin. They are referred to as "volatile" because, unlike fixed oils, they evaporate readily when exposed to air. We'll focus on volatile oils and their complementary aromatic hydrosols in Chapter Ten and continue this section with a discussion of the unctuous (smooth, slippery, and greasy) oils.

Fixed oils are obtained from both the vegetable and the animal kingdom and are often called fatty oils, as chemically they are fats. They are more or less smooth and greasy to the touch, and leave a permanent grease spot when in liquid condition and dropped on paper. They vary greatly in their point of congelation, olive oil becoming solid at a little above 32° F., whereas flaxseed oil can remain fluid at 4° below zero. Pure fixed oils have little taste or smell. They are lighter than water, and they do not evaporate easily; however, they do boil at about 600° F. and at this temperature are converted into vapor. Heated in open air, especially with the aid of a wick, fixed oils do take fire and burn with a bright and sooty flame. These oils are insoluble in water, but are capable of being mixed with water by the assistance of a mucilage, forming mixtures which are called emulsions (see Chapter Nineteen, "Lotions & Creams"). Fixed oils comprise most of the oils in common use such as Olive, Almond, Sesame, cod liver, and Castor oil (and mineral oils).

It is not commonly realized that fixed oils, especially when used as warm/hot infusions and decoctions, are good solvents for abstracting resins, oleo-resins, essential oils, and flavonoids.

Broadly categorizing, there are actually three kinds of oil. In addition to the aromatic essential oils and the vegetable- and animal-derived fixed oils there are the *mineral oils* (and paraffin wax). Mineral oils are a mixture of liquid hydrocarbons obtained from petroleum, and they may be highly volatile or non-volatile.

If you are so inclined, do not let these lists of plant constituents overwhelm you or put you off. They are important only when you care about them, and they are equally unimportant if you don't care. So, I include them in our discussions for the benefit of those individuals who are interested. Feel free to ignore them, for they are specialized information, not crucial information. Later, if you decide to focus on them for any purpose, they are here for you as a reference.

Chemically, in most cases, fixed oils consist primarily of three substances which are considered the three elementary parts of fat: olein, stearin, and palmitin. Olein is the liquid portion of fat, and stearin and palmitin are both solid portions; hence, the consistency of fixed oils and fats is due to the relative proportion of these substances. Thus, Almond oil, being composed principally of olein, is always liquid at ordinary temperatures, while butter, tallow, and lard, being largely stearin, are solid. Fixed oils are decomposed in the intestine by the digestive juices into fatty acids and glycerin and sometimes monoglycerides.

Decomposition and the resulting rancidity of fats and oils are due to exposure to heat, air, moisture, and/or light. This change is believed due to the presence of animal and vegetable tissue, protein, and other albuminous or mucilaginous compound substances which cause fermentation, induce decomposition, liberate the fatty acids, and produce volatile, odorous acids. Rancidity is noticeable by the oil giving a sharp, unpleasant taste and odor. The presence of water in a fatty oil favors the production of rancidity.

While you select and prepare your menstrua, keep in mind, regardless of which solvent or combination of solvents you choose, the "emptier" a solvent is, the more effective it will be as an extractant. In other words, a solvent that is not already floating a bunch of dissolved minerals within its liquid volume obviously has more room within itself to dissolve and hold the components of an herb that has been mixed with it. Likewise, once a solvent has dissolved components of the herb and brought them into solution, it is no longer as active because in this state it is more saturated and less hungry (although it might now dissolve components it

couldn't when it was pure). Therefore, for example, soft water (which by definition is empty of dissolved mineral content—that's why it's still soft) is overall more active in dissolving an herb than hard water (which is relatively full of dissolved mineral). Theoretically, distilled water is completely empty of dissolved minerals and is therefore a hungry, most powerful solvent, ready and eager to dissolve any water-soluble thing it can get its lusty molecules up against. Rainwater is the soft water I most like to use. It's more wild and whimsical than distilled water, but it's not always there for you when you need it. I'll talk more about the dynamics of active and saturated menstrua when I discuss "circulatory displacement" in the chapter on infusions (which will clearly illustrate why it's prudent to "shake your tinctures").

PRINCIPLE CONSTITUENTS OF PLANTS AND THEIR SOLVENTS

When speaking the language of the pharmacologist, these principal constituents are often called the "active ingredients" of the plant, or the isolated plant chemicals that have a salient, definable physiological activity on the body. If an individual has developed the insight to focus on the activity of the whole plant as a remedy within a wholistic framework for assisting a person to heal, specific knowledge of these ingredients is not of great importance. However, to formulate an efficient menstruum for making a plant extract, there is value in gaining a general knowledge of these constituents and an understanding of the specific menstrua in which they are probably soluble and insoluble. More whole, intact, and aesthetic herbal medicines can be prepared with this awareness.

When considering the solubility of individual constituents found in a particular herb, please remain aware that the solubility and insolubility of the various components I am about to outline for you come from data created in the reductionist science lab. This information was derived from each constituent in its isolated form, totally separated from the organic organization of the whole living plant. Due to this, Western science is often unable to explain why and how plant remedies work. Scientific method routinely inhibits a true understanding of the action of whole herbs or their individual constituents because the unique organization of the entire plant is rarely, if ever, tested. So when a plant constituent is said, for example, to be insoluble in water, this might not be and very likely isn't entirely true when that constituent is functioning in the dynamic context of the whole plant. Science is profoundly humbled by what actually goes on within the brilliant flesh of a whole herb. Therefore, in your study of plant constituents, beware of attempting to understand any medicinal plant by reducing it to its so-called "active ingredients." Again, the whole of the plant is the true reference, the one which one's whole body is most biologically familiar with.

Now, to assist you in formulating a suitable menstruum for your plant extracts, the following discussion of plant constituents and their solubility is given as a guide to help you make an educated guess as to what solvent or combination of solvents you will ultimately find to be your best menstruum for a particular plant. This discussion is not the final word, for to my knowledge no one, regardless of his or her credentials, knows the final word in any area of Herbalism.

Alkaloids

Alkaloids are organic bodies, derived chiefly from plants in which they are believed to exist in combination with organic acids, forming salts (a safer, more soluble form of the alkaloid). These alkaloidal salts are usually well-defined, colorless, odorless, crystalline, and soluble. Some are not colorless; for example, the bitter-tasting berberine in Goldenseal and Oregon Grape is yellow. Alkaloids may be unstable when heated. Most pure alkaloids are bitter, slightly alkaline, soluble in ether and chloroform, and often less readily in alcohol. In water they are comparatively insoluble. On the other hand, the solubility of the alkaloidal salts usually follow an opposite pattern: they are freely soluble in water and somewhat soluble in alcohol. The ready solubility of the salts of alkaloids have caused them to be preferred to the alkaloids themselves for therapeutic uses. For preparation of extracts with the highest levels of alkaloids, water/vinegar/alcohol menstrua having a 35 percent water, to 10 percent vinegar, to 55 percent alcohol content are recommended.

All the important alkaloids have profound physiological and pharmacological effects on the body, and some on the mind; many of them are the most poisonous plant substances known.

The chemical composition of alkaloids is not fully understood. All of them, however, contain nitrogen, which is a sort of "so what" bit of information to me, but all the other books mention this fact, so I thought I probably should too.

Please keep in mind, that while alkaloids and their salts have distinctive therapeutic properties of their own, they do not fully nor exactly represent the action of the whole plant from which they are derived.

Please keep in mind, that while alkaloids and their salts have distinctive therapeutic properties of their own, they do not fully nor exactly represent the action of the whole plant from which they are derived.

The names of alkaloids end in *ine*, such as morphine, caffeine, cocaine, and quinine. Nicotine, which is found in tobacco, is a true alkaloid. It is very similar to the alkaloids cicutine and coniine that are found in the seeds and root of Hemlock, a plant which can cause progressive paralysis of the nervous system and death. Nicotine is also quite similar to lobeline, an alkaloid found in Lobelia, which can help people stop smoking.

Balsams (Balsama)

Balsams are resins or oleoresins containing large proportions of benzoic acid, cinnamic acid, or esters of these acids. Balsams are soluble in alcohol and insoluble in water. In plants, balsams are a combination of resins and essential oils (see *"Oleoresins"*). Examples: Tolu balsam, Peru balsam, and Benzoin.

Bitter compounds

Physiologically, all bitters have a bitter flavor. This flavor stimulates the body into reflex action and sets the glands (especially of the digestive system) to work producing their various effects. In certain plants, the bitter principle prepares the way for the other active ingredients. In Hops, for example, a sedative is combined with the bitter substance. Most bitter compounds are soluble in water and, on the whole, soluble in alcohol. Optimal amounts of bitters are derived with menstrua having 30 percent to 60 percent alcohol. Other examples of bitter herbs: Wormwood, Dandelion, Mugwort, Feverfew, Gentian, and Globe Artichoke.

Camphors (Camphorae)

Physically and chemically, camphors are closely related to volatile oils. They constitute one of the elements of many of the volatile oils, and may be separated from them by subjecting the oils to a cooling process (for example, menthol from Peppermint oil). Camphors at ordinary temperatures are (mostly) solid bodies, but may be easily melted. They are soluble in alcohol, insoluble in water. Examples: menthol and camphor—from Camphor Tree wood (*Cinnamomum camphora*).

Essential oils, volatile oils

These components are volatile and aromatic at low temperatures. Essential oils are very soluble in alcohol, soluble in fixed oils and glycerin, very slightly soluble in cold water, and they are vaporized by boiling water. They form the basis of the various medicinal waters and hydrosols (see *"Oils and fats"*).

Enzymes

Enzymes are organic catalysts produced by animal and vegetable cells. An enzyme usually acts to break down or build up the molecules of one substance or group, since it is specific for a particular linkage. They are soluble in water, and insoluble in alcohol. Enzymes are rendered inactive in alcoholic solutions and are destroyed by high temperature. The addition of alcohol to a fresh plant extract containing glycosides prevents the destruction of the glycosides by enzymes.

Flavonoids

Flavonoids are a widely distributed group of plant constituents based on two phenolic rings. Because of their structure they are all anti-oxidants and are fundamental to all colors other than green in plants. Flavonoids are soluble in water, in alcohol, and in fixed oils.

Glycosides

Glycosides are organic plant principles which play an important role in the plant's protective, regulatory, and sanitary functions. They are a compound that contains a sugar part attached to a non-sugar part called the aglycone [sugar + aglycone = glycoside]. When the sugar part is glucose, the substance may be called a glucoside. Glycosides vary greatly in solubility, but nearly all are soluble in alcohol. Optimal amounts of glycosides are derived with menstrua having 30 percent to 60 percent alcohol. Glycosides are usually of a neutral character until hydrolyzed (reacting with water) in metabolism, at which point they become active. In plants, glycosides are frequently associated with alkaloids, and in many instances they are said to constitute the "active ingredient" of a plant medicine. Glycoside compounds can be broken apart by enzymatic action which can continue after a plant is harvested unless the plant is dehydrated or preserved in alcohol while fresh. Glycosides are distinguished from alkaloids by the ending *in*. Examples: hypericin — which is also soluble in fixed oil (St. John's Wort), arbutin (Uva Ursi), glycyrrhizin (Licorice root), aloin (Aloes) and salicin (Willow).

Gums (Gummata)

Gums are contained in great abundance in vegetation. They are exudates that are soluble in water, forming a mucilaginous liquid, or softening to form a jelly-like adhesive mass or paste. All softened forms are emollient or demulcent, and have a soothing, lubricating, and often nutritional quality. The dry concrete (unsoftened) state of this substance is more specifically referred to as a gum. Gums are insoluble in alcohol. When gums are undesirable in a preparation, a solvent such as alcohol is selected so it will inhibit solution of the gummy constituents. (This is an example of employing alcohol's "negative strength.") Examples: Acacia, Tragacanth.

Gum-resins (Gummi-resinae)

Gum-resins are milky exudates composed of (1) a gum or gums partly or wholly soluble in water and (2) a resin or resins soluble in alcohol. When triturated and admixed with water, gum-resins yield emulsions, the gum constituent more or less dissolving while the resin is mechanically suspended in the solution. Examples: Myrrh, Asafoetida.

Mucilages

Mucilages (like gums) are expressly soluble in water (they are best extracted in cold water) and insoluble in alcohol. Extraction of mucilaginous constituents must be done with as low an alcohol content as possible. Prove this principle to yourself sometime (intentionally rather than accidentally) by attempting to make a fresh plant Comfrey extract using 190-proof ethyl alcohol. Or, even more entertaining, blend a liquid Comfrey extract with a high alcohol content tincture — herbal escargot! You can salvage the results by adding sufficient water.

Oils (Olea) and fats

Oils are fluid substances, and fats are solid or semisolid bodies, both having a greasy or unctuous feel. Oils are of two types: non-volatile and volatile.

Non-volatile or fixed oils (Olea pinguia) are organic substances of a semisolid or solid consistency, readily soluble in chloroform and ether, in volatile oils, or other fats. Fixed oils are insoluble in water or glycerin. More than a small amount of fixed oil in a plant tissue will greatly reduce the solvent action of an alcohol or water menstruum. Heated in the presence of alkalis, fixed oils form soaps; an important by-product is glycerin, a tri-atomic alcohol. Glycerin is an excellent extractant and preservative component of a fixed oil. Examples of fixed vegetable oils: Peanut oil, Olive oil, and Castor oil.

Volatile or essential oils (Olea volatilia) are aromatic, flammable liquids obtained predominantly by steam distillation and to a lesser extent by expression (pressing). They are soluble in alcohol and in fixed oils; some essential oils are very slightly soluble in water. Essential oils are volatile, oxidizing, and evaporating upon exposure to air. Not all plants produce essential oils. Pure essential oils are the materia medica of aromatherapy (see "*Essential oils*"). Examples: Lavender, Jasmine, Orange blossom, Rose, Thyme, and Patchouli oils.

Oleoresins (Oleoresinae)

Resins often occur in more or less homogeneous mixtures with volatile oils; these mixtures are known as oleoresins. They are soluble in alcohol and fixed oils, and insoluble in water (see "*Balsams*"). Example: Turpentine from conifers.

Proteins

Albumin is a class of protein found in many vegetable tissues and fluids as well as in animal tissues. Albumin is soluble in water, insoluble in alcohol, and is coagulated by heat. Those individuals who believe that a plant's medicinal action is due solely to its so-called "active" principles regard these proteins along with other "inactive" substances (gums, etc.) to be inert, mostly useless, and, all in all, a bother, merely causing unsightly cloudy solutions and ultimate putrefaction of the preparation. Other experts disagree and revere the synergism of the natural organization of the whole plant as the active component. To avoid extraction or to remove proteins from a preparation, one can:

• Use 190-proof absolute alcohol as a menstruum;

• Precipitate the dissolved proteins from a water extraction by adding alcohol afterwards; or

• Coagulate and precipitate the albumin with heat by either boiling the plant as part of the extraction process, or by boiling the completed water extract and filtering the solution.

Resins (Resinae)

Resins are non-volatile excretions or secretions of very indefinite composition, and are chiefly oxidation products of essential oils. Resins are soluble in alcohol, fixed oils, and essential oils, and insoluble in water. Resins will melt at a temperature near to that of boiling water. Examples: Myrrh, Frankincense.

Saponins

Saponins are plant components that possess the unique characteristic of foaming when shaken with water, even when very dilute. They have the ability to hold finely divided fatty and resinous substances in perfect suspension in aqueous mixtures, producing emulsions of great stability. This is what a soap does that helps remove oil from hands and cleans greasy dishware. Internally, many saponins have direct medicinal effects such as those found in Ginseng, Horse Chestnut, Licorice, and Wild Yam. Other saponins are quite toxic (sapotoxins). With few exceptions, saponins are readily soluble in water and also soluble in dilute alcohol.

Starches

Starches are one of the most important derivatives of plant cells. They are insoluble in ordinary solvents, but swell in boiling water to form a peculiar jelly-like or mucilaginous paste (starch paste). Examples: Cornstarch, Arrowroot, Tapioca.

Sugars (Sacchara)

In their most basic form, simple sugars present themselves as single sugar units and are commonly referred to in science-lingo (not so simply) as monosaccharides. Saccharide comes from the Greek word *sakcharon*, which means sugar (around and around goes the scientific name game). These sugars have a sweet taste, are soluble in water, and soluble in dilute alcohol. Two to ten (or so) sugar units linked together are called oligosaccharides. A huge number of sugars linked together are referred to as polysaccharides. Polysaccharides don't taste sweet and are not very soluble. They are high molecular weight compounds found in almost all living tissue. They make up the skeletal substances in the cell walls of higher plants (i.e., cellulose), the food reservoirs (i.e., starches), or the protective substances (i.e., exudate gums or sap).

GAIA'S SWEET SUGAR-FILLED FORMULA FOR OUR LIVES

$CO_2 + H_2O$ (in the presence of chlorophyll and light) $= CH_2O + O_2$

I've been told this should actually be, $6\ CO_2 + 6\ H_2O = C_6H_{12}O_6$ (glucose) $+ 6\ O_2$ but I'm sorry, to me that's just not as poetic. So, in other words: Animal *out-breath* combined with pure water within the precious chlorophyll-full bodies of our herbs, in the presence of sunlight, yields food-full carbohydrates and free oxygen for animal *in-breaths*. Amen.

"Absolute alcohol" (100 percent ethyl alcohol) is hard to produce and maintain because when subjected to the atmosphere it quickly absorbs 5 percent water (absolute glycerin does the same thing). Therefore, when I use the term "absolute alcohol," I am really referring to the 95 percent ethyl alcohol/5 percent water mix that is commonly used by herbal manufacturers.

When in doubt, use "dilute alcohol" as a menstruum.

Tannins

Tannins are non-nitrogenous bodies that have an astringent taste and action on body proteins, rendering a protective layer on the mucous membranes and skin. They strike a blue-black or a green-black color with ferric (iron) salts. Widely distributed, especially in barks and leaves, most tannins form precipitates with alkaloids, albumin (protein), and many metallic salts, particularly iron salts. For this reason, they are of special interest to medicine-makers who would avoid the preparation of unsightly mixtures (for example, combinations of Goldenseal with Oak or Anemopsis) or of dangerous alkaloidal precipitates. Powerful alkaloids, thus precipitated, would be apt to be taken in the last doses of a bottle of medicine in which there had been a failure to "shake the bottle before using." The inclusion of glycerin in an extracting menstruum for a tannin-containing plant will bind the tannins, so they will not readily precipitate any accompanying alkaloids. Tannins are very soluble in water, soluble in glycerin, and somewhat soluble in alcohol. One can achieve an excellent "tannin tincture" using a menstruum of merely 20 percent alcohol, 80 percent water.

Waxes (Cerae)

Waxes are compounds of fatty acids with certain alcohols. They differ from fats in that they contain no glycerin. They melt when heated and are brittle at low temperatures. They come in varying degrees of solidity. Examples: beeswax, Carnuba wax.

SUMMARY

Since most medicinal plants are made up of representatives from several of the above-mentioned constituents, categorized as either active or ballast substances, the extraction agents should not be geared solely to any individual substance. Alcohol concentrations of 40 percent (sometimes less) to 60 percent (sometimes more) are customarily utilized, according to the official instructions given in most pharmacopoeia. Therefore, venturing resolutely into the risky arena of publicly stating a personal opinion in current herbal literature, I offer the following, experience-based summation of that which has gone before...to beginning students of herbal medicine-making who are faced with the task and awesome responsibility of formulating a suitable water-alcohol base menstruum for making an extract, I boldly suggest: when in doubt, use "dilute alcohol" as a menstruum. This is a very practical solution. There is sufficient amount of both water and alcohol to adequately dissolve the components of any plant and there is enough alcohol to preserve most any solution. One hundred-proof vodka is a dilute alcohol (approximately 50 percent absolute ethyl alcohol, 50 percent water) which is available at any liquor store for your use, whereas 190-proof grain ethyl alcohol is not so readily available.

For our purposes, merely divide the proof number (found on all commercial alcoholic beverage labels) by 2 to determine the percentage of absolute ethyl alcohol by volume contained in the product. An 80-proof vodka or gin, for example, is (approximately) 40 percent absolute ethyl alcohol, 60 percent other liquid; a 150-proof rum is (approximately) 75 percent absolute ethyl alcohol, 25 percent other liquid.

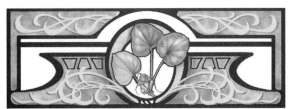

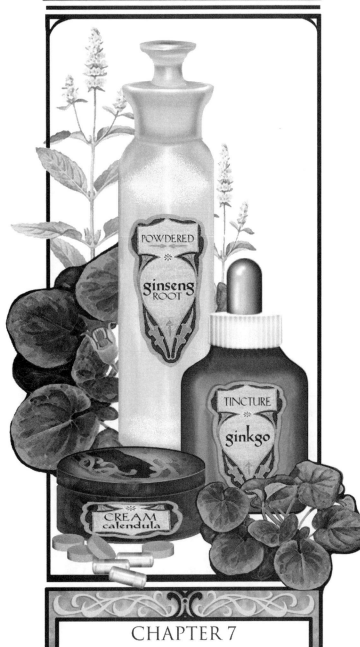

CHAPTER 7

FORMS OF
HERBAL MEDICINE

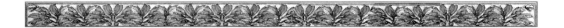

Herbal medicines can be prepared in different forms or "vehicles." These preparations are designed for efficient delivery of herbal actions and nutrients to the body and mind, and, if they are to be stored any length of time, for efficiency of preservation. It is not convenient to administer Saw Palmetto or Uva Ursi, for instance, in the form of berries and leaves, respectively. It would be a disagreeable task for an individual, an ailing person in particular, to chew these crude forms of the plant remedies. And likewise, it would be difficult for this person to obtain in this way the full nutritional and medicinal activity of these herbs. However, a water-alcohol tincture of Saw Palmetto berries or a cold water infusion of Uva Ursi leaves represents pretty much the true pharmacological activity of the herbs because the therapeutic and nutritional principles are held in solution, are easily administered (although in this case it doesn't do much to improve the flavor of the Palmetto berries), and ultimately assimilated, while the indigestible parts have been separated out and removed.

Some forms of herbal medicine are designed to be taken orally; others are prepared in forms suitable for topical application either directly onto the skin, in the ear, as an eye wash, or inserted vaginally or rectally. Some of these vehicles require a menstruum for the development of their unique design, others don't. Following is a working outline of these various vehicles that will give you an overall view of the major players in the theater of herbal pharmacy. Detailed instruction and supplementary information about the preparation and use of these herbal delivery vehicles is the subject of the following chapters.

HERBAL PREPARATIONS TAKEN ORALLY

PREPARATIONS USING A MENSTRUUM

Water-based menstruum
- Infusions, teas (one can also use fruit juice as a water-base menstruum)
   - Hot infusions
   - Cold infusions
- Decoctions
- Concentrates
- Jellos
- Hydrosols
- Flower essences

Alcohol-based menstruum

- Tinctures (maceration)
   - Folk method
   - Weight/volume method
- Tinctures (percolation)
- Fluid extracts (1:1 w/v extracts)

Wine-based menstruum
- Wine infusions

Vinegar-based menstruum
- Vinegar infusions

Glycerin-based menstruum
- Glycerites

Oil-based menstruum
- Oil infusions

Sugar or honey-based menstruum
- Syrups
- Oxymels
- Electuaries (honeys, confections)

PREPARATIONS NOT USING A MENSTRUUM
- Succus (expressed plant juice)
- Capsules
- Pills (tablets)
- Powders
- Lozenges (troches)

HERBAL PREPARATIONS FOR TOPICAL APPLICATION

i.e., Skin, vaginal mucosa, or rectal mucosa

- Liniments
- Lotions and creams
- Hydrosols
- Flower essences
- Medicinal oils and salves
- Ointments and balms
- Suppositories, boluses
- Fomentations (a.k.a. compresses or hot packs)
- Poultices
- Baths
   - Full body bath
   - Sitz bath
   - Foot and hand baths
   - Eye washes
- Douches

Parts of Plants Employed As Herbal Medicines

PLANT PART	EXAMPLE
Barks (Cortices)	Willow, Crampbark
Bulbs (Bulbi)	Garlic, Onion
Cellular	
Hairs	Cotton
Piths (Loose spongy tissue)	Sassafras pith
Spores (Primitive reproductive bodies)	*Lycopodium*
Glands	Lupulin (from the strobiles of the Hop)
Excrescences (An abnormal outgrowth)	Nutgall (highest source of tannic acid)
Corms (Cormi; a short, bulblike, underground, upright stem having a few scale-like leaves)	Trillium
Flowers (Flores)	Calendula, Chamomile, Hawthorn, Elder, Clove buds, Gumweed
Fruits (Fructi)	Cayenne, Vitex, Elder berry, Hawthorn berry, Saw Palmetto, Fennel
Fruiting bodies of fungi	Reishi, Maitake, Turkey Tail
Herbs (Herba)	St. John's Wort, Yarrow, Scullcap, Nettle, Peppermint, Mugwort
Juices (Succus; the fluid portion of a plant)	Cleavers, Plantain, Wheatgrass
Leaf and **leaflets** (Folia et Foliola)	Comfrey, Mullein, Ginkgo, Uva Ursi, Plantain
Lichen (Thallus; a composite organism consisting of a fungus living symbiotically with an algae)	Usnea
Rhizomes (Rhizomata; an underground root-like stem)	Ginger, Wild Yam, Goldenseal, Black Cohosh, Valerian
Roots (Radices)	Echinacea, Burdock, Yellow Dock, Comfrey, Dandelion, Marshmallow, Siberian Ginseng
Seeds (Semina)	Burdock, Echinacea, Psyllium, Chia, Flax (Linseed), Nettle
Thallus (A plant body showing no differentiation into distinct members, as stem, leaves, roots, etc.)	Kelp, Dulse
Tubers (Tubera; a short, fleshy, usually underground stem or shoot)	Aconite, Devil's Claw, Western Peony
Woods (Ligna)	Quassia, Sandalwood

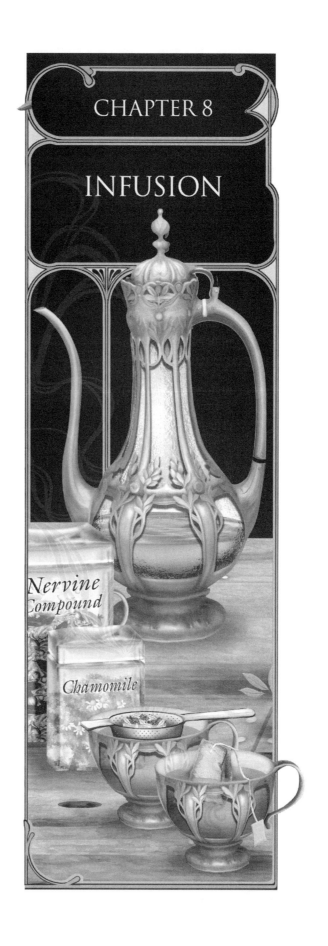

CHAPTER 8

INFUSION

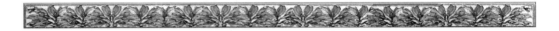

From the inception of herbal pharmacy, herbal traditions throughout the world have favored the simple infusion and decoction of medicinal plants as their predominant form of extraction. Only within this last 100 years has there been an emphasis on making concentrated alcohol and/or glycerin solvent tinctures and other highly concentrated fractional extracts. This compulsion has followed in the footsteps of those Western scientific interests who sought to isolate and concentrate pharmaceutically "active" constituents. Mainstream pharmacy secured its livelihood by catering to these flourishing medical practitioners who chose to rely on the drug qualities of botanicals. In current mainstream medical pharmacy (mimicked by today's predominant herbal mass marketing), these concentrated alcohol extracts continue to be considered more sophisticated; therefore, they are aggressively marketed as more potent.

After experiencing the energy of a wide variety of differently prepared extracts, it is my sense that our culture's current obsession with so-called "pharmaceutically active ingredients" has erroneously (and I suspect naively) disregarded as superfluous the remaining so-called "inactive" or "passive" components. The urgency and consistency with which twentieth (and now twenty-first) century medical pharmacists and herbal product marketers have acted to isolate and concentrate the "active" components as a method to establish increased "potency" in their products has heedlessly eliminated vast amounts of each medicinal plant's complementary "ballast," or so-called "inert" components.

In my opinion, these "inert" constituents—common residents in infusions and decoctions—are carriers of a plant's "tonic" mineral stash which a human body requires for successful digestion, assimilation, elimination, repair, toning, and overall health maintenance. And equally important (in fact, profoundly essential to physical health), many of these "passive" components, especially the non-digestible ones that slide into our colon untouched by our erosive stomach secretions, supply food for multi-millions of beneficial microorganisms that dwell in our gut. These microorganisms have been recently termed "pro-biotics," for they are the good-guy germs that live (and ideally are thriving) in our digestive tract.

Microbiologists have observed many nutrients taken into the human body as food are not used by the body, but instead appear to be eaten by friendly bacteria that live in colonies lining the human intestine. The formidable presence in our gastrointestinal tract of these beneficial organisms is essential for our physical well-being, because they participate in the chemistry of digestion and prevent non-beneficial pathogenic organisms from capitalizing on any opportunities to establish colonies in our digestive tube. The pathogens are so overwhelmingly outnumbered that they can't secure any intestinal real estate to colonize as home. In other words, the "inactive" constituents of a plant make up the fodder that feeds the pro-biotic organisms which render healthy digestion possible and constitute the substrata of the geography of our entire physical immune system. With this information, it requires little imagination to speculate that the "inactive," "inert" ingredients in whole herbs are also used as food for these bacteria in the GI tract, and this allows these microorganisms to assist the body to assimilate the nutritional components along with the "active" components of the herb.

Stemming from this insight, I contend that the Chinese style of low heat, slow decoction, and to a lesser extent our own culture's historic use of infusion-pots (see illustrations, page 107), yield medicinal-tonic extracts that are overall superior to other methods of extraction. These simple techniques supply us with extracts that deliver not only the pharmacologically active components of an herb, but their nutritive components as well, along with the fodder that is used by beneficial intestinal flora to help us digest and assimilate all of this. And subsequently, these same flora, well-fed, go about their life cycle, thrive, and therein lay the primal groundwork for our physical immune system. In other words, except for those folks who prefer to use herbs simplistically as drugs rather than as herbal tonic foods and medicines, I fail to see how

we (in spite of the revered evolution of technologically sophisticated alternative forms of extraction) have improved much on (unfiltered) herbal tea (or capsules of powdered truly whole herb) as a potent tonic beverage and plant medicine—I rest my rant.

A properly prepared herbal infusion or decoction is not merely a cup of tea. These extraction processes are quick, efficient methods for preparing and administering an easily assimilated herbal tonic/medicine/food, and they help supply water for keeping the body properly hydrated, as well as provide appropriate materials for abundant pro-biotic proliferation.

The term infusion is derived from the Latin *infundere*, meaning to pour in. An infusion is a liquid preparation made by treating fresh or dehydrated vegetable substances with either hot or cold water to extract the medicinal and nutritional principles. Herbalists also use other fluid menstruums for preparing infusions, such as vinegar, dilute glycerin, wine, juice, etc.

Infusions can be made in three ways:

• *Maceration* (soaking a properly ground or chopped herb in a menstruum until it is thoroughly penetrated and the soluble portions softened and dissolved)

• *Digestion* (maceration subjected to moderate continual heat below boiling temperature, the heat quickening the solvent powers of the menstruum)

• *Percolation*

Because infusions are generally extemporaneous preparations, and are frequently needed immediately, the process of maceration is the most simple, practical, and usually preferred method. In this chapter I will discuss primarily the maceration method of preparing herbal infusions.

By definition, herbal infusions represent the solvent action of boiled water (or in some instances, cold water) on herbs for a given time period. This period of time varies according to the degree of extractability of the principles to be dissolved. During the infusion process, the herb is not subjected to boiling, although it is common to pour boiling water over the plant material. The infusion process is particularly suitable for substances with a light structure and comparatively soft tissue easily exhausted of their principles, such as flowers, most leaves, soft stems, and some roots. This process of extraction is also most suitable for those plant tissues containing volatile or other principles which would be dissipated or injured by boiling, such as Chamomile and Red Clover blossoms, Peppermint leaves, or Valerian root. Because the constituents of many of the plants that are normally infused are volatile, infusions should always be conducted in closed vessels.

HERB PREPARATION

Herbs are best prepared for extraction with water as a menstruum by cutting them into thin slices or grinding to a coarse powder, especially harder parts you want to infuse (like volatile roots such as Valerian which, unlike most roots, should not be boiled as a decoction). In this form, they can be easily permeated by the liquid. If you are wanting to separate all undissolved particles (pro-biotic fodder) from the final infusion (which I do not recommend, but some folks insist on relating only to clear liquids), the use of fine powders should be avoided for they are difficult to remove. Fresh, undried herbs should be cut into small pieces and/or bruised. Flowers can be infused whole.

WATER

Clear soft water, rainwater, or distilled water are best for making infusions. Hard or limestone water from springs or wells are often unfit, for they are apt to foster precipitation. While the common practice of using hot water has time-saving advantages, in some cases, depending on the herbalist's preference and intent, it can be inefficient. This is because (for those insisting on clear liquid) many inert components in an herb are dissolved by the hot water, and as the infusion cools, these components separate out in a finely divided condition. When one wants to, it is often difficult to remove them even by filtration. This mainly affects the appearance and preservation of the infusion. However, infusions are usually used directly, and one doesn't normally intend to preserve them for very long. Of the inert components found in plants, starch is extracted by hot water and albumin (plant protein) by cold water, while gum, sugar, and other extractives are dissolved by both. When infusions are made with boiling water, starch and other principles are often taken up, and their presence over time disposes to acidity or moldiness. Hot water also coagulates plant albumin, which can materially impair the extraction process. In these instances, cold water infusions would be preferable. In light of this phenomenon, plant materials that are high in albumin, such as most roots and barks, are ordinarily decocted rather than infused. Decoctions are initiated using cold water, which is then slowly heated as a means to circumvent problems stemming from the coagulation of albumin; but we'll discuss all this in Chapter Nine, "Decoction."

Consider selecting cold water for the menstruum when:

• The herb contains a valuable volatile constituent (i.e., essential oil, frequently found in blossoms and leaves). As beverage teas, however, we all use hot water for making Peppermint, Chamomile, Lemon Balm, and the like.

• The desirable principles are readily soluble in water of ordinary temperature (such as Slippery Elm bark, Marshmallow root) or would be deteriorated by high temperatures (such as Wild Cherry bark).

• The herb contains a constituent that is not desired and not readily dissolved by cold water (such as the safrol in Sassafras root bark or the tannins in Uva Ursi).

CONTAINERS

The most suitable vessels for infusions are made of glazed earthenware, porcelain, or glass. Tinned iron, aluminum, or metallic vessels are unsuited for infusions, and are particularly objectionable when the herb contains tannin, gallic acid, or an astringent constituent.

The vessel to be used should be warmed before the infusion process, so it does not chill the hot liquid menstruum.

An infusion-pot with a design that retains the herb within the top section of the solvent, similar to one of the accompanying illustrations, is best suited for preparing an herbal infusion.

The advantage of these designs is that the material is efficiently exhausted by circulatory displacement. Circulatory displacement occurs as the molecules of the liquid menstruum in direct contact with the herb become charged with the soluble ingredients of the herb and acquire an increased specific gravity. As each charged molecule sinks to the bottom of the pot, its place is taken by an unattached molecule (the unsaturated "empty" portion of the menstruum), which has risen to the top to further extract the remaining soluble ingredients in the herb. The herb is therefore constantly subjected to the solvent power of the least impregnated portion of the menstruum, and this circulation goes on until all of the soluble matter is extracted or the menstruum becomes fully saturated.

You can demonstrate the process of circulatory displacement for yourself if you take a clear glass jar (a pint to a quart size) and fill it with hot water; then lay a tea bag (preferably a dark-colored tea, so the process will be most visible) on the very top of the water and keep it there by tightening down the lid of the jar onto the string close to the bag. Now leave the jar untouched and observe the extracted constituents as they descend to the bottom of the jar, displacing the less dense unattached water molecules. Eventually the entire menstruum will be equally impregnated with the extracted herbal constituents. Provided there is sufficient water in the jar, the herb in the bag will become depleted of its soluble constituents which have gone into solution.

Whenever using a tea bag or a tea ball, suspend the herb-filled apparatus in the upper part of the menstruum in order to take full advantage of the principles of circulatory displacement (stirring is never required). This is particularly important when using cold water menstrua, as there are no heat currents to help promote the infusion.

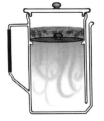

Alsop's Infusion Jar

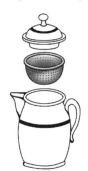

Infusion Pitcher

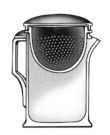

Squire's Infusion Mug

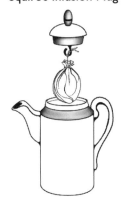

Homemade Infusion Mug

It will help to keep in mind that a pint is approximately equivalent to 500 ml, a quart is approximately equivalent to a liter (1000 ml), a fluid ounce is approximately equivalent to 30 ml, and an ounce is approximately equivalent to 30 Gm.

PRESERVATION AND STORAGE

Infusions should not be made in large quantities unless it is for immediate use. They are generally difficult to preserve because the herbal principles extracted by the water begin to decompose fairly quickly. Infusions soon spoil if special precautions are not taken to preserve them. Ideally, they should be used within a 12-hour period with about a 24-hour maximum limit, if stored in a very cool place.

DOSAGE

Dosage varies according to type of herb(s) and the size, age, and condition of the person drinking the infusion. Normally, the recommended adult dosage is one cupful three times a day. When an individual appears to have a kidney condition that does not readily allow adequate urine production, or when there is evidence of extreme weakness, a reduced dosage is usually recommended.

METHODS OF PREPARATION

The U.S. has distinguished itself as the only major country on planet Earth that has not officially adopted the metric system as its conventional system of weights and measures. (By god, no one is going to tell us what to do!) Outside of our scientific community, we (and also the people of Burma) still embrace an archaic measuring system that originally disgorged out of the egocentrism of a long line of ancient French monarchs, and our esteemed leaders apparently lack the presence of mind or more likely the political courage to seriously suggest that we modernize ourselves. Hear me out now; I'm not suggesting we throw away our current system, that would be too much like throwing away one's treasured old toy (or newest electronic device). No way! I'm simply suggesting that we make ourselves bi-scale (teach metric in schools) and learn to measure reasonably well in both systems. Therefore, in the spirit of this suggestion, I will try to make the measurements referred to in this manual as user-friendly as possible for us avoirdupois devotees, and us metric geeks. (It's tough, though; I grew up avoirdupois.) Please see Chapter Twelve, "Tincturing by Maceration," and Chapter Twenty-Five, the section *"Weights and Measures,"* for further discussion of this voluminous controversy.

The method of preparation that follows is based on standard measurements and procedures directed by official pharmacy manuals for preparing herbal infusions. It is a clear illustration for explaining how to make an infusion. This method produces 500 ml (1 pint) of tea which if consumed in its entirety delivers the activity of 25 Gm (1 ounce) of dried herb. However, one would normally not be directed to drink 500 ml of this tea in one day but perhaps 90 ml (3 fluid ounces) of tea 3x a day which would deliver the activity of 13 to 14 Gm (approximately 1/2 ounce) of dried herb for the daily dose. Most herbalists today tend to make their infusions and decoctions more dilute, recommending for example 3–5 Gm of dried herb in 250 ml (approximately 1 cup) of water 3x a day. This delivers the activity of 9 to 15 Gm of dried herb (and more liquid than the official method does) for the daily dose. Bear in mind that the amount of liquid used to prepare a medicinal tea is not so important, *the weight of herb used is.* (It is this latter method I will be referring to when giving recommended dosages in the final section of this chapter.)

HOT INFUSION

Unless otherwise appropriate, hot infusions are made of 1 part coarsely ground herb (2 parts if using fresh undried herb) to 20 parts of boiling water (or other hot menstruum), or, for example, 25 Gm (1 oz.) of herb [50 Gm (2 oz.) of chopped fresh herb] to 500 ml (1 pint) of boiling water.

1. Put the herb into a suitable vessel (with a lid). (It is not essential but preferable to pre-warm the vessel or enclose the herb in a suitable container to employ the circulatory displacement technique discussed above.)

2. Pour boiling water upon the herb.

3. Stir well (do not stir if using the circulatory displacement technique).

4. Cover the vessel tightly, and let it stand for 20 to 30 minutes in a warm place.

5. Strain and, if possible, press out the marc (pulp). It is obvious that bulky herbs and flowers (i.e., Chamomile, Red Clover blossoms, Mullein leaves) will retain a considerable proportion of the extract, and this will be lost if the marc is not pressed.

6. Add enough hot water (pour it through the pressed marc) to make the infusion measure 500 ml (1 pint).

Bitter herbs do not require quite as large a quantity of crude herb as other herbs do, and only a pinch of a very intense herb like Cayenne is needed for an effective infusion (use more if you like the heat wave).

COLD INFUSION

Cold infusions are made using 1 part of herb to 20 parts of water, or 25 Gm (1 ounce) of coarsely ground herb to 500 ml (1 pint) of cold water. (Depending on the quality of the herb, a small amount of Slippery Elm bark or Marshmallow root can provide an abundance of mucilaginous slime—experiment with this.)

1. Put the herb into the water and let it remain overnight at room temperature. With cold infusion it is recommended that the herb be contained in a small cotton pouch, suspended in the water overnight, and squeezed out when the infusion process is completed.

2. Strain, and press the marc.

3. If necessary, add enough cold water to make the infusion measure 500 ml (1 pint).

HERBS ON THE "35 HERBS AND A FUNGUS" LIST THAT ARE WELL PREPARED AS AN INFUSION

Including a recommended dosage—ex. 3–5 Gm (grams) dry herb. This amount would be infused in approximately 1 cup water.

As recommended in Chapter Four, "Kitchen Pharmacy Equipment," it's best to obtain a scale that measures gram weight. Using this scale, you can easily prepare the following recommended dosages; it is impractical and maddening to attempt to measure these as fractions of ounces or portions of a spoonful.

HOT INFUSION

Cayenne	A pinch to a tolerable amount
Chamomile	3–5 Gm: 3x a day
Cleavers	3–5 Gm: 3x a day or as needed
Comfrey leaf	2–4 Gm: 2x a day (See discussion of Comfrey in Chapter Two.)
Dandelion leaf	3–5 Gm: 3x a day
Elder flower & berry	2–5 Gm: 3x a day
Fennel, crushed seed	2–4 Gm: 3x a day
Ginger, dry	2–3 Gm: fresh a few slices
Ginkgo	2–4 Gm: 3x a day
Goldenseal leaf, dry	1–3 Gm: 3x a day
Hawthorn leaf, flower, & berry	2–5 Gm: 3x a day
Mugwort	2–3 Gm: 3x a day
Mullein leaf	3–5 Gm: to 4x a day
Nettle herb	3–5 Gm: 3x a day
Oat spikelets and straw	3–5 Gm: 3x a day
Peppermint	3–5 Gm: 3x a day
Plantain	2–5 Gm: 3x a day
St. John's Wort	3–5 Gm: 3x a day
Saw Palmetto berries	2–5 Gm: 3x a day
Scullcap recently dried	2–5 Gm: 3x a day
Valerian	2–5 Gm: 3x a day
Yarrow	2–5 Gm: 3x a day

COLD INFUSION

Burdock root	3–5 Gm: 3x a day
Chamomile	3–5 Gm: 3x a day
Cleavers	3–5 Gm: 3x a day or as needed
Comfrey root	2–4 Gm: 3x a day (See discussion of Comfrey in Chapter Two.)
Crampbark	3–5 Gm: up to 4x a day
Marshmallow root	3–5 Gm: 3x a day
Mugwort	2–3 Gm: 3x a day
Nettle root or whole herb	2–5 Gm: 3x a day
Peppermint	3–5 Gm: 3x a day
Uva Ursi	2–4 Gm: 3x a day
Slippery Elm★	2–5 Gm: 3x a day

★Slippery Elm has to be included in this section for it is such an important and commonly prepared cold infusion.

The properties of Goldenseal *root* are not soluble enough in water to be efficiently prepared as a tea.

CHAPTER 9

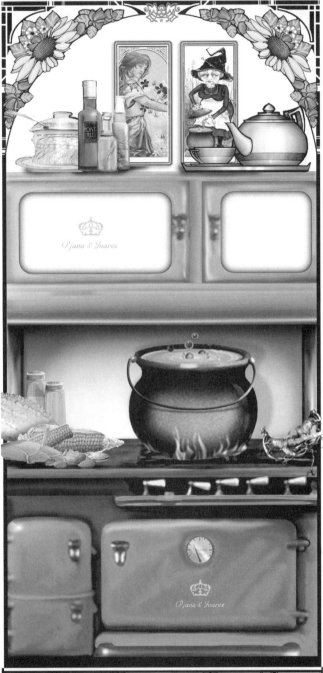

DECOCTION

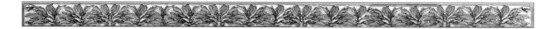

Decoctions are liquid preparations made by boiling either fresh or dehydrated herbal substances with water or other fluids. Along with infusions, decoctions are a standard method for preparing medicinal teas. Decoction is also the chief method used to extract herbal constituents for use as fomentations, syrups, and enemas.

Decoction, from the Latin *decoquere*, meaning to boil down or away, is normally reserved for herbs that will not yield their active virtues at a lower temperature and for situations in which no loss of volatile principles need be feared (for example, with Fenugreek seed, Astragalus, Sarsaparilla, or Licorice). The object of preparing decoctions is to secure, in aqueous solution, the soluble active principles of herbs that are hard and woody and have a close, dense texture. Their tissues are softened more readily by boiling than by merely steeping in hot water, and are not injured by heat. This would be especially hard, ligneous, wood-like herbs such as most roots, barks, and some seeds.

Herbs whose activity depends on resinous constituents (like Gumweed and Yerba Santa), or herbs that contain substances liable to be changed into insoluble and inert materials under boiling heat (like Marshmallow and Slippery Elm), should never be subjected to decoction. Likewise, herbs containing volatile principles should never be subjected to decoction (i.e., Valerian root, Peppermint, Fennel).

In *compound decoctions* where several herbs are employed together, it is probably best to add different types of herbs at different points in the process. The hard, ligneous herbal ingredients that need to be boiled for extended periods should be added first, while the herbs which more readily yield all their virtues should be added toward the end of the process. The aromatic herbs, or those containing volatile oils, should be added after the decoction has been removed from the heat, so that the volatile oils will not evaporate. A decoction that includes aromatic herbs should be kept closely covered until it has cooled down.

HERB PREPARATION

The herbs to be decocted should be cut or ground, the degree of fineness depending upon the nature of the tissue. Woody, ligneous herbs may be reduced to a moderately fine powder and/or soaked in cold water for 12 hours before bringing the water to a boil. Leaves, however, and other parts of the herb that consist mainly of loose parenchyma (pulpy or pithy portions) are better used in the form of a moderately coarse or very coarse powder. When fresh undried herbs are used in a decoction, the roots should be cut into very thin slices, barks and woods should be shaved down to small pieces, seeds lightly crushed, and leaves and whole herbs only moderately cut.

WATER

Clear, naturally soft water, rainwater, or distilled water should be used in making decoctions, since hard or limestone water from springs or wells is often apt to cause precipitation.

CONTAINER

Glazed earthenware, porcelain, or glass vessels are the best choices for preparing decoctions, as they will bear the heat of boiling water if heated gradually. Iron vessels are not well suited because the tannin of astringent herbs will react with the iron, causing discoloration.

PRESERVATION AND STORAGE

Decoctions are intended for immediate use—ideally within a 24-hour period, with about a 72-hour maximum limit if stored in a very cool place. As with infusions, the difficulty in preserving decoctions arises from the decomposition of the starches and the mucilaginous and albuminous principles that have been extracted by the water and retained in the preparation. Except when demanded for immediate use, decoctions should not be made in large quantities.

DOSAGE

As always, the proper dosage depends on the age, body weight, and temperament of the individual. In general, give a wineglass to a cupful of liquid three times a day.

METHODS OF PREPARATION

[Restated (minus the accompanying preliminary rant) from Chapter Eight, "Infusions"]

The method of preparation that follows is based on standard measurements and procedures directed by official pharmacy manuals for preparing herbal infusions. It is a clear illustration for explaining how to make a decoction. This method produces 500 ml (1 pint) of tea which, if consumed in its entirety, delivers the activity of 25 Gm (1 ounce) of dried herb. However, one would normally not be directed to drink 500 ml of this tea in one day, but perhaps 90 ml (3 fluid ounces) of tea 3x a day which would deliver the activity of 13 to 14 Gm (approximately 1/2 ounce) of dried herb for the daily dose. Most herbalists today tend to make their infusions and decoctions more dilute, recommending, for example, 3–5 Gm of dried herb in 250 ml (approximately 1 cup) of water 3x a day. This delivers the activity of 9 to 15 Gm of dried herb (and more liquid than the official method does) for the daily dose. Bear in mind that the amount of liquid used to prepare a medicinal tea is not so important, *the weight of herb used is.* (It is this latter method I will be referring to when giving recommended dosages in the final section of this chapter.)

The amount of liquid used to prepare a medicinal tea is not so important, the weight of herb used is.

Decoctum Taraxaci—
DECOCTION OF
DANDELION

Slice and bruise 1 oz. of
dried dandelion root, and
boil it in 1 pint of distilled
water for 10 minutes.
Strain, and pour upon the
residue in the strainer
enough distilled water to
make the finished product
measure 1 pint. A little orange peel added at the end
of the boiling period is
said to increase its useful-
ness. This preparation does
not keep well and must be
freshly prepared.

DECOCTION

If the strength of the decoction is not otherwise directed:

1. Place 25 Gm of herb (approximately 1 ounce) into a suitable vessel with a cover. (Use half to three quarters this amount of herb if you want a weaker decoction.)

2. Pour upon it 500 ml (approximately 1 pint) of *cold* water. It is important to begin the process with cold water in order to ensure the complete extraction of all soluble principles from the herb by the gradually heated water. The albuminous matter is subsequently extracted out of the cells and slowly coagulated outside the herb as the heat is increased to near the boiling point. If the herb is immersed in boiling water, the albumen contained in cells will possibly coagulate at once and can interfere significantly with the extraction of the other constituents.

3. If time allows, let the herb macerate—soak—a few hours prior to heating.

4. Cover the container well and bring the ingredients slowly to a boil.

5. Decrease the heat and simmer it for approximately 10 to 15 minutes. The harder the material, the longer the simmering time of extraction needed. If not specified, this extraction time must be determined by observation, common sense, and experience.

6. After decoction, press the herb hard to make sure all the solution is removed from the marc (the remaining undissolved pulp).

7. Allow the pressed decoction to cool to a temperature below 104° F. (40° C.), and strain the liquid. If you wish, after it cools, this decoction can be further strained using a filter paper. By then, principles which are soluble only in hot water are mostly precipitated and, if desired, generally can be removed without weakening the medicinal value of the preparation. However, even with this precaution, the strained liquid may become unsightly due to further deposition of matter that is soluble only in hot water or by the development of apotheme (the dark deposit which sometimes appears in vegetable infusions and decoctions once exposed to air). None of this matter is harmful to drink (some would even contend that it is highly beneficial—see previous chapter). It just looks disagreeable to some folks, however, and it is kind to cater to the consumer's aesthetic preference.

8. Pour enough water through the marc to return the volume of water to 500 ml.

HERBS ON THE 35 "HERBS AND A FUNGUS" LIST
THAT ARE WELL PREPARED BY DECOCTION

Including a recommended dosage—ex. 3–5 Gm (grams) dry herb. This amount would be decocted in approximately 1 cup (250 ml) water.

As recommended in Chapter Four, "Kitchen Pharmacy Equipment," it's best to obtain a scale that measures gram weight. Using this scale, you can easily prepare the following recommended dosages.

Blackberry root bark	2–5 Gm: 2-4x a day
Black Cohosh root	1–3 Gm: 3x a day
Burdock seeds	2–5 Gm: 3x a day
Comfrey root	2–3 Gm: 3x a day (See discussion of Comfrey in Chapter Two.)
Crampbark	2–5 Gm: up to 4x a day
Dandelion root	2–6 Gm: 3x a day (King's decocts for 10 min.; I decoct it 30 min.)
Echinacea root	2–5 Gm: 3x a day
Ginger fresh slices, dry	2–3 Gm in warm water
Mullein root	3–5 Gm: up to 4x a day
Reishi	3–6 Gm: 3x a day (Decoct 45 minutes.)
Siberian Ginseng	2–4 Gm: 3x a day
Willow bark	2–10 Gm: 3x a day
Yellow Dock root	1–3 Gm: 3x a day

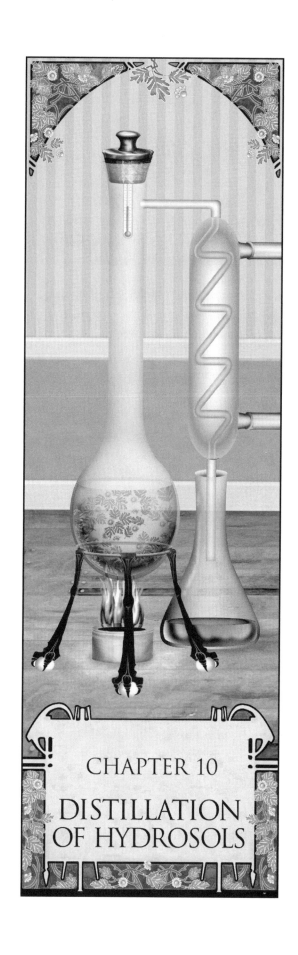

CHAPTER 10

DISTILLATION
OF HYDROSOLS

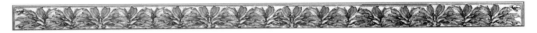

Oil and water aren't miscible, this fact being the inspiration for one of our culture's most popular clichés. And while the accuracy of this statement is experienced time after time by most of us in our daily lives, there is a particular situation in which an aromatic volatile oil and water reach out to one another and create a dramatic bond. I know! I know volatile oils aren't really oils—give me some slack; I'm taking a little license here. The story of this chemical cohesion is a phyto-aqueous enactment of Shakespeare's *Romeo and Juliet*, wherein the youthful opposites of two ego-immiscible families fall deeply in love and give themselves wholeheartedly to one another within the heat of a steaming social environment. But unlike Shakespeare's grand finale, wherein Romeo and Juliet choose to leave their uncompromising world and continue their romance in the nonphysical realms, oil and water sustain their affair in an ethereal oneness on this physical plane as a delightfully aesthetic anomaly, and this aromatic coupling is what aromatherapists refer to as a hydrosol or a hydrolate.

A true hydrosol is a particularly pleasant offspring of the steam distillation of aromatic plants. The initial introduction and coupling of water and oil occurs in a heated vessel wherein water as steam ascends, carrying with it volatile oil molecules dissolved from the plant material. The two components of this vaporous blend sustain an ardent embrace until they enter a cooling process, whereupon the oil soluble components separate out once again from the water. However an abiding remembrance of the torrid union forever lingers as the departing aromatic molecules pass on an intimate part of their qualities to the water, and this amiable water maintains a subtly delicious memory of the passionate intimacy of the distillation process being indelibly transformed into an aromatic hydrosol. Therein, simple steam distillation of certain organic material results in the production of two complementary liquid assets: an aromatic volatile oil and a true aromatic hydrosol.

Most volatile oils are derived from plants in which they exist ready formed. Upon completion of the distillation process the distillate is usually milky, and on standing separates, with most of the oil rising to the top, while the water (hydrosol) continues charged to saturation with the oil. Except for Rose water and Orange blossom water, throughout the history of volatile oil production, most hydrosols were disposed of as waste. Only in very recent times have these fascinating waters been valued as carriers of a rarefied form of the volatile oils, coexisting in combination with many mild and soothing water-soluble components of the plant that are not present in volatile oils. And whereas most volatile oils contain bitter substances and some harsh components which if not adequately diluted before application can cause irritation to the inner and outer skin of the body, the complementary hydrosol simply does not. Instead, these lotions present soothing, anti-inflammatory acids and other compounds that gratify the skin, and these agents are exclusive to the singular nature of aromatic hydrosols.

Hydrosols are applied directly to the skin or taken internally, as their flavor is far milder than that of volatile oils; and hydrosols are much safer to drink, provided they have not been derived from a toxic plant. Hydrosols make excellent base waters for preparing syrups, lotions, fomentations, culinary exotica, etc. When applied to the skin, hydrosols are mildly astringent and highly effective tonics to be used daily. Not only are they not drying to the skin, but they pleasantly counteract the drying effects of natural atmospheric conditions, as well as the adverse conditions contrived by rampant household, office, and in-flight air-conditioning technology. Hydrosols are used as skin toners or added to other ingredients to form compound lotions and hydrating masks. Hydrosols comfort and nourish ultra-sensitive and/or inflamed skin where other agents might be too strong. Many hydrosols are good for use on normal and oily complexions, and on acne skin, and most are suitable for moisturizing dry skin.

It is important to understand the contrast between true aromatic hydrosols and commercial products labeled as "flower waters," "floral waters," etc. Whereas hydrosols are a direct product of the distillation process (a process which gives birth to complementary sisters, a gentle aromatic water and a more acute volatile oil), flower waters are generally fragrant liquids made by adding aromatic volatile oil(s) to distilled water. These waters will not contain the same hydrophilic (water fond) compounds as hydrosols, and though often erotically aromatic (if that kind of behavior is allowed on retail shelves), they are less effective as anti-inflammatory, moisturizing agents.

In order to accumulate any appreciable quantity of volatile oil, one must gather and manipulate an enormous amount of plant material. This is one reason most volatile oils (essential oils) are so costly. Volatile oils are a particularly precious component of the plant: the plant manufactures only a diminutive amount of this substance, granting only a small yield to the anticipative distiller. However, with a relatively small amount of plant material, one can readily produce a sufficient quantity of aromatic hydrosol for home use. Once you contrive and assemble a still and get it functioning, you will be able to feed it adequately from humble garden harvests and make an abundance of a variety of hydrosols for yourself and others. I used to grow a few plants of Catnip (*Nepeta cataria*) in my yard, and by distilling their leaves, make enough Catnip hydrosol to put just about every cat in the neighborhood into deep kitty stupor; they loved it, couldn't get enough. Alice's Cheshire Cat is no longer the only feline that can grin and fade away. And likewise, a Lemon Verbena (*Aloysia triphylla*) hydrosol originating from the same garden was (is) a human olfactory dream come true.

Another joy inherent in distilling hydrosols is that it requires only a small amount of aromatic plant material to produce a sufficient amount of this holy water to annoint one's home and body throughout the year.

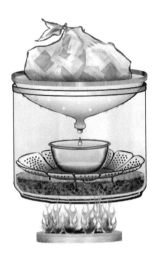

Homemade Still

STORAGE AND PRESERVATION

Refrigerate your hydrosols. Store them in sterilized, tightly capped bottles.

METHOD OF PREPARATION

As pointed out previously, hydrosols are a product of steam distillation. Distillation is a process involving the conversion of a liquid into a vapor subsequently condensed back to liquid form (the distillate). This is exemplified at its simplest when steam from a kettle becomes deposited as drops of distilled water on a surface. Distillation is used to separate liquids (for our purposes, water and volatile oils) from non-soluble solids (plant material). It's apparently an age-old process utilized by the early experimentalist Aristotle (this man must have never slept), who mentioned that pure water is made by evaporation of sea water.

The apparatus needed to perform this operation is a *still* or retort in which a liquid is heated, a *condenser* to cool the vapor, and a *receiver* to collect the distillate. This simple apparatus is sufficient to separate volatile liquids from non-volatile materials, which is what we will be doing here. The pieces of equipment used for distillation in a lab are commonly made of glass and connected with corks, rubber bungs, or ground glass joints. This equipment can be purchased from a laboratory supply house (for megabucks). However, one can contrive a variety of ingenious homemade contraptions. I am going to share an example of this down-home technology with you forthwith. It may not qualify as "ingenious," but it is assuredly illustrative and unquestionably loveable.

This is a severely simple still that you can put together using kitchen paraphernalia. Subsequently, if you get hooked on distillation, you will undoubtedly want to contrive, acquire, and assemble a more sophisticated apparatus. The rustic design illustrated in this chapter works reasonably well, belonging to the same league as the funky skateboards I used to build as a kid by separating the two halves of the old metal-wheeled roller skates and nailing them to the front and back of the bottom of a 2 x 6 piece of wood; they got me down the road...eventually. And damn it, this still will get you some aromatic hydrosol!

The Still

The still is a common enameled 20.4 L (21.5 quart) canning pot that is designed to can fruit and vegetables. It's normally dark blue or black with white flecks all over it. It can be purchased in most department stores.

The Condenser

The condenser is the lid of the canning pot placed upside down on the pot. At the appropriate time, a mass of ice is placed on top of this.

The Receiver

The receiver is a bowl that is placed inside the pot. It, in turn, is sitting on a metal veggie steamer basket which has had its center post removed and is standing in the center of the pot. This elevates the receiver bowl, so that it is not jostled around by the rumbling action of the boiling water and herbs during distillation.

To Make an Aromatic Hydrosol

1. Clean all the equipment.

2. Place approximately 3 liters (3 quarts) of water in the pot.

3. With the water, mix approximately 200 Gm (10 oz. or so) of the selected plant or the parts of the plant containing volatile oil. When appropriate, it is certainly okay to use more plant material than suggested here; follow your judgment; weigh it out and make notes.

4. Let this macerate for a couple hours.

5. Remove the center post from the metal veggie steamer basket and stand the steamer, spread fully opened, in the center of the pot.

6. Place the receiver bowl on the center of the steamer.

7. Put the lid right side up on the pot.

8. Put all this on the heat and bring it to a boil; keep watching!

9. As soon as the water begins to simmer, turn the lid upside down on the pot.

10. Lay a thick plastic bag full of ice on the lid. (This way, when the ice melts, the ensuing bag of water can be easily removed and dealt with.) This step is semi-optional; the steam will condense on the condenser lid without using the ice, but the hydrosol seems to have a little more "something" when you cool the lid with ice.

11. Adjust the heat to a moderate level. Keep the heat just high enough to maintain the vaporization of the liquids.

12. Inside the pot, the water/aromatic oil vapor will rise to the cooler lid, condense back to liquid, flow down to the low point of the lid, and drip into the receiver which will collect the hydrosol and volatile oil. **Beware of steam whenever lifting the lid of the pot. Escaping steam enjoys hot-licking unsuspecting finger skin.**

13. Place a wetted filter paper in a funnel.

14. Place the funnel into a jar or bottle that has a lid.

15. When the hydrosol is cool, pour it through the filter paper. The hydrosol will pass through; if any appreciable volatile oil is present, it will collect in the bottom of the filter paper cone. You can collect this volatile oil with a dropper bottle pipette.

16. Cap the jar and refrigerate.

For best results, harvest the plant to be used at the time of year and the time of the day when it is highest in volatile oils.

Using this system, as the steam makes it to the lid, much of it escapes out of the pot. Most of the volatile oil probably escapes with this portion of the vapor. When you use a more sophisticated still that is sealed, you avoid this loss of vapor and the volatile oil ends up floating on top of the hydrosol which has been deposited in the receiver vessel. In other words, don't expect to collect much volatile oil using this method. Aromatic hydrosol, however, you will get, and I suspect you will be delighted with it. You will probably want to make more, and soon you will probably want to upgrade your still…journeying ever nearer and nearer to the megabuck equipment zone…and no telling where this might lead you. Follow your fascination and enjoyment, all will be well and available to you.

Herbs on the "35 Herbs and a Fungus" List That Are Well Prepared As Hydrosols

Chamomile

Elder blossoms

Fennel

Peppermint

Yarrow

Other common garden plants that present excellent hydrosols are:

Catnip (for the meowmaster)

Lavender

Lemon balm

Lemon verbena

Orange blossoms

Rosemary

Rose petals

And, of course, experiment with other aromatic plants.

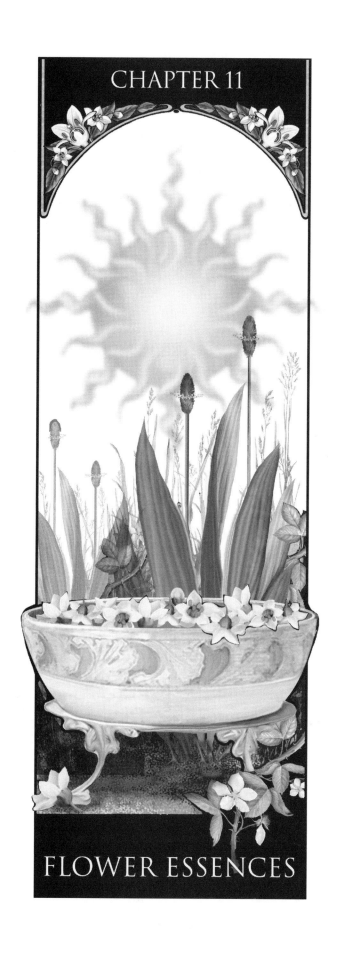

CHAPTER 11

FLOWER ESSENCES

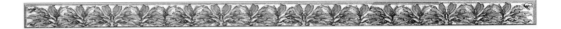

In Chapter Three, in the section on harvesting, I suggested that the Earth's plants are a perpetual source of unconditional love. That probably came over a little schmaltzy to some readers, and, at risk of losing any fragments of cool-'n-macho status that might remain in my account, I must avow that conclusion once again in this chapter, with a further assertion that this love is most luminously expressed by a plant's flowers—sensual, uplifting communication with members of the animal kingdom is a flower's essence. And as herbal medicine-makers, we can bring this pure positive energy into solution—a most subtle aqueous solution.

It has been my recurrent experience and observation that floral vibrations that have been infused in water that is sitting on the Earth in a clear glass bowl, floating blossoms in the warm sunlight of a clear blue sky, can profoundly affect the subtle disposition of an ailing (or even more promising, a pre-ailing) being. Like a music master's hand tuning the eager strings of a perfect Stradivarius, the pristine clarity of a flower's uplifting vibrations adjusts the tone of one's thoughts and respondent feelings, bringing them back in harmony with the richness of one's true nature. When our thoughts and feelings are in line with our spirit's unique

path, we resume our journey as a vital creator of a prosperous, healthful, joyous life—the intrinsic dynamics of a human being's essence.

The life work of Dr. Edward Bach (1886–1936) pioneered understanding of the subtle energy and actions of flower essence medicine. Dr. Bach created a bouquet of subtle, water-infused floral essences, each of which embraced and treated a being's subtle nonphysical nature, ultimately relieving manifested physical symptoms. More importantly, the essences helped individuals establish ease in their life, thereby preventing unpleasant physical manifestations entirely. Edward Bach's vision was to develop a system of herbal medicine that anyone, when feeling out of sorts, could use to diagnose and prepare his or her own medicines, and treat himself or herself, thereby allaying illness before its physical symptoms are made manifest. In a short period of seven years, Dr. Bach succeeded brilliantly, and developed a system of herbal therapeutics the core of which is pure simplicity. I'm convinced that the principles underlying this and other forms of subtle energetic medicine will guide the practical course of mainstream medicine and the art of self-medicating in the very near future.

One can illustrate Dr. Bach's insight and

technique for treating an individual whose illness has progressed to the manifestation of physical symptoms by reprinting a short quotation taken from his book, *The Twelve Healers and Other Remedies*: "Take no notice of the disease. Think only of the outlook on life of the one in distress. The same disease may have different effects [varying states of mind or moods] on different people; it is these effects that need treatment, because they guide to the real cause…as one becomes well by gaining increased happiness and interest in life, the disease goes, having been cast off by the increase in health. Health and disease are caused by how we think, how we feel within ourselves. Health and disease are the consolidation of mental attitude."

This chapter explains how to prepare a flower essence infusion for one's personal use. At the end of the chapter, I will list the 38 essences, the flowers of herbs, trees, and bushes, and the one non-flower essence (Rock Water) that Dr. Bach included in his original materia medica. I have arranged them in the diagnostic fashion I use them. Therefore, at the conclusion of this list, you will find a bibliography of books that can be used to study others' insights and their systems for using flower essences to alleviate and prevent human as well as plant and animal illness.

METHODS OF PREPARATION

There are three stages in the preparation of flower essence infusions before a dose is administered to an individual: the first preparation is what I will refer to as the Mother Essence; the second is the Stock Water; and the third is the Medicine Water.

There are two basic methods for preparing the Mother Essence: the sun method, used for flowers that bloom during the late spring, summer, and early autumn when the sun is often overhead, full and hot, and the boiling method, used for the flowers and twigs of plants that bloom at times other than when the sun is at the most intense phases of its solar cycle.

Wildflowers growing in their natural habitat rather than cultivated flowers are preferable (with the exception of Cerato, Olive, and Vine found in Dr. Bach's materia medica).

Each individual essence should be made with blossoms gathered from as many different plants of the same kind as possible.

ABOUT THE EQUIPMENT

When preparing flower essences by either the sun method or the boiling method, all equipment to be used must be first sterilized by placing it in a container of cold water, slowly heating it, and gently boiling it for 20 minutes, then carefully drying it and wrapping it in a clean cloth. Dr. Bach felt it was important to tend to these details.

Simply, one first prepares a Mother Essence from wildflowers by using either the sun method or the boiling method; from this essence one prepares the Stock Water; from this one prepares a Medicine Water; from which one takes daily doses.

PREPARING THE MOTHER ESSENCE BY THE SUN METHOD

Equipment

- One thin-gauge, plain glass bowl, approximately 8 fl. oz. (Do not use an etched, cut glass, or otherwise ornate bowl or a Pyrex type oven glass bowl.)

- A quart jar with a lid to carry water to the flower site

- A 30 ml (1 oz.), amber dropper bottle with a glass pipette

Method

1. When the dropper bottle and pipette have cooled from the sterilizing process, fill half the bottle with brandy (or half fill many bottles with brandy; you will be creating a relatively large amount of Mother Essence), cap it tightly, and label it with the name of the flower to be prepared. Note on the label that this is the Mother Essence. Dr. Bach preferred to use brandy as a preservative, considering it a purer and more natural agent than rectified spirit.

2. Decide beforehand which plant community you are going to harvest, and choose a perfectly sunny morning when there are no clouds in the sky that might obscure the sun's light, therein immersing the bowl and its contents in the most animated energy of Earth's crystal clear air element.

3. Take your bowl, jar, and dropper bottle and arrive at the site a little before 9 A.M. (Pick the flowers at about 9 A.M., so they are floating in place as the sun is gaining intensity during the hours between 9 and noon. By 9 A.M. the flowers will be freshly opened in full bloom, and most airborne, pollen-spreading creatures will have not yet arrived.)

4. Sit with the flowers for a few minutes and focus on your intent; honor and extend gratitude to the plant community. You'll probably be feeling pretty good right now; you couldn't be in a better place than you are at this moment.

5. Place the bowl on the ground near the flowering plants, thereby connecting the subtle essence to the stabilizing energy of the Earth element. Choose a location for the bowl that is well away from trees, bushes, tall grasses, fences—anything that might cast a shadow over the bowl of basking flowers as the sunlight brushes across the Earth's surface.

6. Fill the bowl to the brim with the water you transported in the jar, or water from a clear stream, if one is nearby. Empty any unused water from the jar. Do not drink from this jar; it needs to remain sterile, as it will be used again later.

7. Pick some leaves, preferably from the plant you are preparing, or from some broadleaf plant, and place them on the palm of your hand. A Mullein leaf or one of similar dimensions is ideal.

8. Select the most perfect blossoms and carefully pick the flower heads just below the calyx (the external, usually green part of the flower that attaches to the stem) from as many plants or bushes of the same kind as possible. Let the flowers fall onto the leaf in your hand.

9. Quickly, carry the flowers to the bowl and float them on the surface of the water, thereon uniting everything with the fertile, receptive energy of the water element. Continue this process until the surface of the water is thickly covered. Overlap the flowers, but make sure each flower touches the water. (Throughout this process avoid casting your shadow over the bowl and avoid touching the water with your fingers. Eliminate the human vibrations as much as possible from the flower vibrations in the subtle infusion.)

10. Leave the bowl in full sunshine for 3 to 4 hours to absorb the resplendent energy of the fire element.

11. After about 4 hours, there will be slight signs of the petals fading, giving evidence that their subtle properties (vibrations) have been transmitted to the water. With a stalk from the plant you are preparing, or with a rigid portion of grass, lift the flower heads from the water. *Do not touch the water with your fingers.* The water will be crystal clear and full with minute, vibrant bubbles. Many herbalists confess to feelings of elation at this point.

12. Pour this Mother Essence into the jar that has been previously emptied, and from this fill the remaining half of the labeled dropper bottle (or as many bottles as you wish to prepare with this mother load). Cap it tightly.

Equipment

- One 4-quart enamel pot and lid
- 2 quart jars
- A 1-ounce, amber dropper bottle with a glass pipette
- A funnel
- 2 or 3 pieces of filter paper

Method

1. Sterilize the jars, funnel, and dropper bottle in the enamel pot. When this equipment has cooled from the sterilizing process, half fill the dropper bottle with brandy, cap it tightly, and label it with the name of the flower to be prepared. Note that this is the Mother Essence.

2. A sunny morning is chosen whenever possible. For the same reasons you chose 9 a.m. for the sun method, gather the flowers and twigs at that time.

3. Decide beforehand which plant community you are going to harvest and take the enamel pot, covered with its lid to keep out any dust and debris, to the location. Sit with the flowers and focus on your intent; communicate with the plant community.

4. Fill the pot about 3/4 full with flowering sprays, including the leaves, buds, and twigs. Also gather two extra twigs of the same species of plant. These will be used later.

5. Place the lid on the pot, grab the extra two twigs and the pot filled with flowering sprays, and quickly return home.

6. Upon returning home, cover the plant parts with approximately a quart of cold water. Use rainwater, stream water, pure well water, bottled spring water, or, if nothing else is available, tap water that has been allowed to sit in an open container overnight. (Dr. Bach didn't like the energy of distilled water; he referred to it as "dead water." If you want to use distilled water, let it first sit in a clear glass bottle in the sunlight for a day. This should resurrect it.)

7. Place the pot uncovered over heat, and bring the water to a gentle boil. If necessary, press the flowers beneath the water with one of the twigs you brought home with you to prevent touching the water with your fingers.

8. Boil the plants over low heat for 1/2 hour.

9. At the end of a half hour, remove the pot from the heat and set it outdoors to cool.

10. When it is cold, remove all the twigs, leaves, and flowers, using one or both of the extra twigs as tools to help you. *Do not touch the water with your fingers.*

11. Cover the pot with its lid and allow the water to stand long enough for any sediment to settle to the bottom of the pot.

12. Line the funnel with a filter paper and place this in one of the two empty jars.

13. Fill the other jar carefully with the flower water from the pot. Pour slowly not to disturb the sediment.

14. Pour the liquid from this jar into the filtered funnel that is sitting in the first jar. This will take a while. Often, there is much sediment and you may need to filter the liquid twice.

15. From this filtered water, fill the remaining half of the labeled dropper bottle containing the brandy.

16. Cap tightly.

PREPARING THE STOCK WATER

This is the second stage in the preparation of a flower essence infusion. Later, from this Stock Water, a person's Medicine Water is prepared.

To prepare a Stock Water from a Mother Essence which has been prepared by either the sun method or the boiling method:

1. Sterilize and dry a 1-oz. amber dropper bottle.

2. Label it with the name of the flower essence. Note that this is the Stock Water.

3. Fill the bottle with brandy.

4. Add merely 2 drops from the Mother Essence bottle.

5. Cap it tightly and succuss it (shake it vigorously) for a few moments.

PREPARING THE MEDICINE WATER

This is the third stage in the preparation of the flower essence, and it is from this one the individual takes the doses suitable for a human, an animal, or a plant.

1. Determine which essence or combination of essences an individual requires. (Using 2 or 3 in combination is ideal, and from my experience, I recommend using no more than 5 at a time.)

2. Into a sterilized dropper bottle, put 2 drops from the Stock Water of a selected essence, or 2 drops from each of the essences selected for use in combination (making a compound essence).

3. Add a teaspoonful of brandy as a preservative to inhibit the water from going cloudy.

4. Fill the bottle with water.

5. Cap it tightly and succuss it.

6. Label with the flower(s) name and note it as a Medicine Water. Include the recommended dosage.

DOSAGE

Focus on the positive aspects for taking the flower essence(s); clarify and focus on your intent; visualize the experiences of joy and health you are reviving.

A dose is 4 drops. Taking more than 4 drops per dose does not increase the benefit.

Hold the dose in the mouth for a few moments before swallowing to gain the full effect of the flower essence(s).

Normally, an individual takes four doses a day: one first thing in the morning, one last thing before retiring at night, and two more times during the day, ideally before meals.

When necessary, doses can be given more frequently, every 15 or 30 minutes, and then hourly until the individual feels uplifted and more at ease within.

If it is difficult to take the doses each time, place 16 drops of the Medicine Water into a glass or thermos of water or juice each morning and take frequent small sips throughout the day.

ANIMAL DOSAGE

Flower essences can be used for pets large or small displaying emotional perplexities, farm animals, wild fauna, or plants who have experienced a trauma or shock of any nature.

• Horses and other large animals: Put 8 drops of an essence (from the Medicine Water) into a bucket of water or 4 drops onto fruit or a piece of bread that they will eat.

• Dog- and cat-size animals: Put 4 drops of any essence (from the Medicine Water) into the food or drinking water. The essences can be put onto paws or directly into the mouth if the animal agrees.

• Or apply essences to beaks, snouts, noses, muzzles, on plumage, on scales, on tails, on Prancer, on Dancer…, behind ears, or into the fish bowl.

• Administer doses 4 times daily.

PLANT DOSAGES

• Place 16 to 20 drops of an essence or combination of essences in a gallon watering can full of water and water the plant's soil.

• Put 8 to 10 drops of the same essences in a spray bottle and spray the plant's foliage.

PRESERVATION AND STORAGE

The Mother Essences and the Stock Waters, when prepared as directed above, will retain their strength indefinitely. If they are kept for several years, a slight sediment may form at the bottom of the bottle; this is not harmful. Sometimes, over a lengthy period of time, the rubber bulb on the dropper top will soften and lose its tone; it should be replaced with a new sterilized one.

When using the boiling method a large quantity of sediment may form. This should be filtered twice. Then, even though you have filtered the liquid a couple of times, after some months more sediment may form again at the bottom of the Mother Essence bottle; this should be re-filtered and rebottled.

The Medicine Water will be preserved quite adequately during the relatively short time it is used by the individual.

It is best to sterilize the bottle each time it is refilled.

SELECTING AND USING FLOWER ESSENCES

My approach to manifesting anything, whether it is health, friendship, stuff, travel, whatever, is to focus my attention on what it is I want, rather than on the absence of it, and I give very little thought to what I don't want or to anything that doesn't feel good to me. Therefore, when I use flower essences to assist other people to enhance their life processes, I ask him or her to get in touch with how they want to feel within themselves. I ask them to identify what feels most like their true nature, to envision their most desired self-concept, to ascertain who they truly are and what they want to express.

To assist this process, I have arranged the following list of Dr. Bach's particular flower essences by homogeneous positive aspects of personality. I have assembled word pictures individuals can use to help form a clear vision of what they feel defines their nature most closely and how they want to function. I note the corresponding flower essence whose vibration resonates most closely to this inspiration. I also include the related "shadows" of that nature, those traits no longer wanted, and those contrary states of mind and moods one can slip into that cast a shadow over inner light and joy. But clouds can merely hide the sun for a while. The light is the enduring reality that is soon revealed with the gently effective assistance of flower vibrations. I trust this will be of assistance to those who are attracted to using this subtle and remarkably effective vehicle of herbal medicine.

ONE'S TRUE NATURE	FLOWER ESSENCE	SHADOW
• I am a genuine optimist, cheerful, and carefree • I am a peacemaker at heart • I make light of discomforts • I have a fine sense of humor that I express freely and joyfully without pretense	**Agrimony** *(Agrimonia eupatoria or odorata)*	• Tortured mental state • Carefree veneer • Hides symptoms and woes, never discussing problems with others • Distressed by quarrels • Worries • Restlessness caused by churning thoughts
• I participate in life with true joy, beyond worry or fear • I am adventurous and enjoy the journey of my creative path without regard of difficulty or danger • I am fearlessly in touch with well-being	**Aspen** *(Poluus tremula)*	• Apprehension, inexplicable • Fears by day or night for no known reason • Fear accompanied by sweating & trembling
• I am a tolerant, lenient, and understanding of others • I have strong convictions with high ideals • I see the good in all, and with unconditional love I appreciate the paths others choose for themselves	**Beech** *(Fagus sylvatica)*	• Intolerant • Critical of others • Lonely • Lacks humility and sympathy • Annoyed • Taskmaster • Must have precious and order
• I am a strong individual • I mix well with others wherein I know my true self and set my own tone • I serve wisely and quietly	**Centaury** *(Centaurium umbellatum)*	• Timid • Weak-willed • Servile doormat • Too persuaded by others and by convention • Vitality is sapped by overdoing favors for admired others
• I am intuitive and in touch with the wise guidance of my own inner-being • I am a visionary and hold definite opinions • Confidently, I stick to my own desires and decisions once I've made them	**Cerato** *(Ceratostigma willmottiana, Plumbago)*	• Doubts own ability • Tends to imitate • Lacks confidence in own judgment • Seeks advice from one and all • Talkative
• I am calm, quiet, and courageous • I hold a strong mental focus on the positive aspects of life	**Cherry Plum** *(Prunus cerasifera)*	• Fear of losing control of mind and reason • Desperation • Violent impulses • Suicidal • Fear of insanity or doing fearful things

ONE'S TRUE NATURE	FLOWER ESSENCE	SHADOW
• I am keenly observant and most appreciative of contrast • I focus my attention in the present where my creative power lies • I reap knowledge of self from every observation and experience • I change my creative mental focus quickly and easily	**Chestnut Bud** *(Aesculus hippocastanum, White or Horse Chestnut Bud)*	• Repeats mistakes due to lack of observation • Impatient • Habitual negative thought • Tries to forget the past • Slow to learn how one's own thoughts and beliefs are that which creates all unwanted experiences
• I appreciate others, and I enjoy their diversity • I allow and encourage others to be who and as they are • My unconditional love is generous and caring • I inspire others with warmth and gentleness • I am selfless in my care for others	**Chicory** *(Chicorium intybus, Wild Succory)*	• Bossy • Overpossessive of others • Directs affairs of others • Fussy • Argumentative • Greedy • Interferes by nagging and criticizing • Martyr • Self-pity • Domineering • Intolerant • Discontent • Fretful
• My mind is sensitive to inspiration • I have a lively, passionate interest in all things • I am master of my own thoughts and set my tone in life • I am full of appreciation for life • I have zestful desires and a wonderfully creative imagination • I travel my inner dimensions well	**Clematis** *(Clematis vitalba, Traveler's Joy)*	• Dreamy hope of a better future • Uses impractical thoughts to escape from world • Diminished vision and desire • Lack of passion and vitality • Apathetic • Exhaustion • Homesickness • Lack of interest in present circumstances • Indifference • Led and influenced because thoughts are elsewhere
• I maintain complete control of thought • I see things in correct perspective and proportion • I'm broad-minded • I realize that any physical disorder is due to internal disharmony	**Crab Apple** *(Malus pumila)*	• Feelings of uncleanliness • Despair • Disgust • Despondency • Congestion • Self-hatred • Mental obsession and concern with trivia • Finicky fussiness • *The cleanser essence*

ONE'S TRUE NATURE	FLOWER ESSENCE	SHADOW
• I have unshakable conviction • I'm confident, responsible, and reliable • I have powerful creative focus • I'm self-assured, and my abilities are generally directed toward the well-being of others	**Elm** *(Ulmus procera, English or Common Elm)*	• Overstriving for perfection • Temporary feelings of inadequacy • Feelings of failure • Exhausted by overwhelming feelings of responsibility
• I have faith in my ability to attract what I want • No obstacle is too great or any task too big to be undertaken with conviction that it can be accomplished • I integrate contrast to give me clarity of desire • I have strong ability to hold a vision and to appreciate and enjoy the journey to its fulfillment • I am a bearer of the light in darkness	**Gentian** *(Gentiana amarella, Felwort or Autumn Gentian)*	• Reduced desire • Discouraged by setbacks • Skeptic • Doubt • Discouragement • Deflated by delay • Negative outlook • Deep depression due to a known cause • Dark melancholia • Attracts negativity due to negative state of mind
• I have positive faith that my visions will be realized • I am uninfluenced by statistics, judgments, opinions, or advice of others • I am certain I can overcome all obstacles to realize my desires	**Gorse** *(Ulex europaeus, Whin or Common Furze)*	• Loss of heart • Diminished vision and desire • Hopelessness • Despair • Given up • Negative attitude • Dark melancholy • Resigned • Lack of ambition or interest due to hopelessness
• I am an uplifter who is genuinely interested in others • I am caring, understanding, and helpful • With tolerant good humor I radiate well-being	**Heather** *(Calluna vulgaris, Ling or Scotch Heather)*	• Rapid incessant talk • Always bringing any conversation to themselves • Saps vitality of others by excessive self-centeredness • Shunned and avoided
• I am deeply connected to my inner joy • I love others and myself • I recognize and appreciate the achievement of others • I can give without need of return • I am loving, tolerant, and happy, and I rejoice in others' well-being and joy	**Holly** *(Ilex aquifolium)*	• Hatred, envy, jealousy, or suspicion of another's abilities and success • Intolerant • For the active, intense, extrovert type who wants to open his or her heart—for whom very man essences are indicated—this will help identify the exact essences that are best

ONE'S TRUE NATURE	FLOWER ESSENCE	SHADOW
• I am fully alive in the present, the place of my creative power • I use my past and present experiences to assist in forming clear visions to prepare my future experiences • I retain the lessons taught in the past, letting the experiences pass from mind	**Honeysuckle** *(Lonicera caprifolium)*	• Dwells upon thoughts of the past and holds a pessimistic outlook both for the present and the future • Loss of interest in the present due to homesickness or chronic nostalgia • Regretful • Stagnation that diminishes vital, creative life force
• I am certain of my abilities and strengths even in the fact of overwhelming tasks • My mind is alert • I am able to call up reserves of strength for mental and physical fortification in moments of self-doubt • Fatigue passes as I become interested in normal activities	**Hornbeam** *(Carpinus betulus)*	• Weariness of the mind • Doubt of strength • Suffers fatigue through dislike of work that one is doing • Monday morning or morning-after feeling • Disinclined to face future or even daily routine • Mental and physical exhaustion which often passes when mental focus is taken off of self
• I am patient and efficient • I am spontaneous and quick in mind and action • I am gentle and sympathetic toward others, understanding and tolerant with those slower than me • I feel very capable, decisive, and intuitive • I work well alone and with others and I enjoy doing both	**Impatiens** *(Impatiens glandulifera, Policeman's Helmet)*	• Impatient and irritable with those who are slower • Active and nervous • Quick flaring and subsiding anger • Mental tension, manifesting as muscular tension and pain • Injury through bad temper or own impetuousness • Exhaustion from frustrating nervous effort when things are moving too slowly
• I plunge into life, taking risks, and I'm never discouraged by results • I never think that, "I can't" • I am a powerful intentional creator of my own experiences • I am determined and confident • I use any experience of failure as a tool for a clearer, more focused vision and stronger determination	**Larch** *(Latrix decidua)*	• Lack of confidence in self and abilities • Anticipation of failure • Despondency due to failure to even try • Seldom attempts anything due to self-assurance of inevitable failure • Convinced can't do as well as others • Wistful feeling of inferiority, though lacking jealousy or envy of others' success

ONE'S TRUE NATURE	FLOWER ESSENCE	SHADOW
• I face all contrast, trials, and difficulties with equanimity, courage, and humor • I deal with life with wise anticipation, spontaneity, and enthusiasm • With understanding, intuition, and knowledge I work fluidly with the universal law of attraction	**Mimulus** *(Mimulus guttatus, Monkey Flower)*	• Fear and anxiety of a known origin • Mental emotional focus on that which one does not want • Shy and retiring, prone to hide anxieties • Deterred by chronic fears such as fear of dark, injury, poverty, etc., which retards the joy of freely creating
• I have an inner serenity and knowing which nothing can shake or destroy • I set my own tone in all situations coming from an inner stability and connectedness to my joy, freedom, and overall well-being • In every moment I am keenly aware of the harmony that abounds throughout all	**Mustard** *(Sinapis arvensis, Wild Mustard or Charlock)*	• Experience of a black depression, almost a hopeless, despairing melancholia which suddenly closes down upon one without apparent cause or reason; it can lift just as suddenly of its own accord • A gloominess which from out of the blue temporarily shuts down all one's joy and pleasure
• I persevere in face of all contrast and difficulties without loss of faith or slackening of confidence • I'm keenly aware that the visions and mental focus of one's creative energy are far more effective for accomplishment than action alone • Joyfully I inspire others • I am helpful to others while always remaining in harmony with myself	**Oak** *(Quercus robur)*	• Ceaseless in efforts even when depleted • Disappointed, despairing, and discontent with self when unceasing effort fails • Can suffer breakdown due to enduring too much strain of responsibility • Reliable, dependable, and loves to help others; characteristically taking on too much responsibility
• I maintain interest in life and peace of mind even when required to be inactive • I depend fully on my inner-self • I understand that mental visualization is a far superior channel of creative power and healing than action • I attract happiness and pleasure in spite of temporary weariness	**Olive** *(Olea europaea)*	• Depleted • Complete exhaustion of mind and body due to long-endured stress or illness • Suffered a long time under adverse conditions • Lack of effort due to lack of vitality • Feels no pleasure in life • Fear of losing friends and support • *The convalescence essence*

ONE'S TRUE NATURE	FLOWER ESSENCE	SHADOW
• I acknowledge my mistakes, but do not dwell on them • I see what I want by observing the contrasting experiences of what I do not want; and then I focus on a fresh, positive vision • I am compassionate • I appreciate myself and others • I inspire and uplift others, helping them to thrive • I have great perseverance • I use "failures" to increase my passion and desire to manifest my visions	**Pine** *(Pinus sylvestris, Scots Pine)*	• Self-condemning • Never content with achievements • Blames self for own and others' mistakes and for everything that goes wrong • Overworks and stresses self to "improve" and become "better" • Feels guilt and despondency • Has high ideals and does one's best, but is too humble and apologetic, which disallows creative life force to flower easily through self
• I broadcast thoughts of well-being to all • I am keenly aware of the well-being that abounds, and I see others in their natural state of health and wellness • I am a true uplifter and healer • I am able to remain calm, mentally and physically in any emergency, peaceful and assuring to others	**Red Chestnut** *(Aesculus carnea)*	• Excessive fear and anxiety for others • Worries and anticipates troubles for others • Over-protective of another • Negative mental visions with regards to others • Foresees trouble and broadcasts fear and anxiety
• I am a calming and soothing individual even in the most terrifying conditions • With courage, I can rise to emergencies in an instant • I can assume a selfless state of mind in moments to focus on another's well-being • I have no fear of death, and I am willing to risk my life to aid others	**Rock Rose** *(Helianthemum nummularium)*	• When panic and extreme fright are experienced, placing the vibrations of terror in the atmosphere • Extreme fear caused by facing an unexpected or unfamiliar experience or by any fear induced by a terrifying sight or nightmare • Whenever great fear or panic is experienced

ONE'S TRUE NATURE	FLOWER ESSENCE	SHADOW
• I have high ideals and a flexible, creative mind • I am readily open to changing my beliefs when convinced of a higher truth • I'm not easily influenced by the beliefs of others, because I know I will find greater, deeper truths from the inspiration of my own internal connection to life • My experience of joy, freedom, and growth uplifts and encourages others to trust and respond to their inner guidance and to follow their own unique path	**Rock Water** *(H₂O, Healing well or stream water)*	• Inflexible mind • Inflexible, prideful opinions about religion, politics, or reform • Mind and life is ruled by cherished theories • Hard master on self (yet not on others) • Enjoys suppressing one's own faults • Strict in way of living, cannot deflect from ideals, forcing self to live up to them • Self-denial, a martyr to ideals • Self-domination • Does not understand that such practices as diets are the result, not the cause, of spiritual growth
• I am open-minded, quick to make a decision and prompt to act on it • I am calm and determined • I am attentive and responsive to my inner guidance, and therefore, I set my own tone • I keep my poise and balance under all conditions • I observe contrast, and from this I make clear decisions of what I want • My clear visions come forth from these decisions and give me great ability to manifest my desires	**Scleranthus** *(Scleranthus annuus, The annual Knawel)*	• Indecision, lacking ability to make up mind • Swayed between two things • Experience swings between joy and sadness, energy or apathy, pessimism or optimism, clarity and confusion • Unable to concentrate due to constant changing of mind • Conversation jumps from subject to subject • Erratic body functions (symptoms come and go, pulse, pain, temperature are here and there) • Magpie mind, full of bits and pieces
• All shock has been neutralized, and my mental and physical recuperation has been accelerated • All is well • I am comforted and soothed of all my mental and physical pains and sorrows • I have strength and quick recovery in spite of shock	**Star of Bethlehem** *(Ornithogalum umbellatum)*	• Emotional or physical illness due to residual shock from a current or past experience or accident • All shock has an effect; this effect can manifest at some point even after the incident has been forgotten • *Useful for nonresponsive folks*

ONE'S TRUE NATURE	FLOWER ESSENCE	SHADOW
• I have full control of my emotions • I know all is well in the midst of the intensity of any experience • In light of intense contrast, I learn clearly what I desire, and I can focus on the uplifting thoughts of what I want to change in my experiences	**Sweet Chestnut** *(Castanea sativa, the edible Spanish chestnut)*	• Acute hopeless despair • Feelings that one has reached the limit of one's endurance • Focus on feelings of great anguish • Suicidal state of mind • Intense feelings of abandonment and the void of inner darkness • "Lonely dark night of the soul"
• I am a calm, wise person • I keep my mind fluid • I know that all persons have a right to their opinions, and I will listen to them open-mindedly • I have strong ideals, but I do not impose them on others • I am inspired, enthusiastic, and knowledgeable • My mind is alert and full of interest • I know that by feeling good and flowing creative thought, rather than by strong action, great things are accomplished effortlessly and harmoniously	**Vervain** *(Verbena officinalis)*	• Over-effort, stress, and tension • Lives on nerves, resulting in breakdown • Fanatic reformer, convert, and/or martyr • Imposing will on others • Over-enthusiastic, high-strung, fretful and fussy • Impatient, tense, and anxious • Takes on too much, leaving no time to relax and enjoy life • Depleted mental and physical vitality through overuse of effort and strong will • Strict, violent temperament • Over-aggressive and persistent • Argumentative
• I am a natural teacher and leader • I am wise, loving, and understanding • I am able to organize and delegate power and service with no need to dominate • I enjoy helping others to know themselves and to find their path in life • I can inspire others with my unshakeable confidence and certainty • I am efficient, certain, and ambitious, a quick thinker who can be depended upon in an emergency to direct others with confidence	**Vine** *(Vitis vinifera, Grape vine)*	• Tendency to crave power and dominate others • Rides roughshod over the opinions of others • Makes no attempt to convert others, but instead is demanding and dominating, often hard and cruel without compassion • Loses interest in those that cannot be dominated • Rigid, inflexible attitude which manifests in extreme tension with stiff, rigid physical pain, and disability

ONE'S TRUE NATURE	FLOWER ESSENCE	SHADOW
• In direct response to my inner guidance, I employ constancy and determination as I pursue my beliefs and carry out my life work • Conventions that might impede my self-fulfillment are easily ignored • I am unaffected by adverse circumstances • I'm neither hindered nor discouraged by the opinions or ridicule of others • I am a creative pioneer • I change my beliefs and habits fluidly as I feel appropriate • I am a free individual, and I offer no resistance to my inspiration	**Walnut** *(Juglans regia)*	• Swayed by a stronger or more dominating personality or forceful circumstance • Inspired course is altered by some link with the past, family tie, habit, or other outside influence • A "link breaker" from any influence from the past or circumstances of the present • An ally for advancing stages of maturity (teething, puberty, menopause) or for big life-change decisions for taking any step forward and breaking conventions, leaving all old limits and habits
• I have great gentleness and poise • I am a tranquil, objective, sympathetic, and practical counselor • I am self-reliant and dignified • I am an example of integration and confidence to others • I do not interfere with the affairs of others nor do I tolerate interference in my affairs • I create a serene environment for myself and others	**Water Violet** *(Hottonia palustris)*	• Feeling of superiority to others • Proud and aloof • Disdainful and condescending, which can manifest as mental rigidity and physical stiffness and tension • Disapproving of others, though tolerant and never interfering • Bears grief and sorrows in silence • Prefers to be alone when ill
• I have a quiet and calm mind, undisturbed by outside influences • I am at peace with myself and with the world • From the serenity of my mind comes the solutions to my problems • I have a strong ability to direct my thoughts where I want them • I have learned to control thought and imagination and put them to my conscious creative use	**White Chestnut** *(Aesculus hippocastanum, Horse Chestnut)*	• Persistent mental arguments and conversations with self, reoccurring like a stuck record • Worries racing around and around in the mind • Tortured mind • Insomnia • Seeks to escape thoughts and get back into the world • Overactive mentality results in depression and fatigue • Headaches due to chronic over-anxious thoughts

ONE'S TRUE NATURE	FLOWER ESSENCE	SHADOW
• I am energetic, talented, and able to do things well • I have definite ambitions and focus • I know just what I want to do with my life • I do what I want to do, and I let nothing interfere with my purpose • My life is filled with feelings of usefulness and happiness • My heart is open to joy and freedom and growth • I have the ability to do many things well, and I am successful and satisfied in my undertakings	**Wild Oat** *(Bromus ramosus, Hairy or Wood Brome-grass)*	• Undecided as to what to do with life • General but unclear ideas of what is wanted • Despondent and dissatisfied due to feelings that life is passing by • Frustrated and unhappy due to a tendency to drift into uncongenial environments and occupations • Indefinite due to so many ideas and ambitions • For those weak, introverted, despondent type of persons from whom very many essences are indicated—this will help identify the exact essences that are best
• I have a lively interest in all happenings, both in my life and in the lives of others • My very interest and vitality attract excellent conditions into my life, so I enjoy happiness, good health, prosperity, growth, and friendship • I accept and appreciate life with good humor, and I respond to my inner-being's constant guidance and wisdom • I realize and fully exercise my power to create all my life experiences	**Wild Rose** *(Rosa canina, Dog Rose)*	• Resignation to illness, uncongenial work, debilitating relationships, and/or to a monotonous life • Diminished desire • Makes little effort to heal, improve life, or to envision and enjoy the abundant pleasures of life • Feels one "might as well get used to it" and "learn to live with it all" • Observes conditions and surrenders to them without realizing that they have created them • Weary, lack vitality, and are dull companions • Not depressed, but resigned to their apathy and colorless life
• I enjoy my sense of humor and well-being • I know that all my experiences proceed from my thoughts • What is outer is a clear reflection of the sum of my thoughts and beliefs • I am optimistic about life, because I am the master of my own fate • I am fully self-empowered, for I blame no one else for my experiences • With my offerings I attract unto me • I appreciate my life and the lives of others	**Willow** *(Salix vitellina, Yellow Willow or Golden Osier)*	• Resentment and bitterness • Self-disempowerment by blaming all one's self for whatever misfortune or adversity is being experienced • Lack of appreciation • Feels life is unjust • Begrudging and resentful of all good fortunes and success of others • Sulking and gloomy • Pessimistic • Takes without giving • Stuck in feeling of discontent; loath to admit any improvement

Sources of Other Perspectives

1. *The Collected Writings of Edward Bach*, ed. Julian Barnard, Flower Remedy Programme, 1987, P.O. Box 65, Hereford, HR2 oUW, Great Britain.

2. *Handbook of the Bach Flower Remedies*, Dr. Philip M. Chancellor, Keats Publishing, Inc., 1980.

3. *The Medical Discoveries of Edward Bach, Physician*, Nora Weeks, C.W. Daniel Company, Ltd., London, 1973.

4. *The Bach Flower Remedies Illustration & Preparation*, Nora Weeks and Victor Bullen, C.W. Daniel Company, Ltd., London, 1976.

5. *Heal Thyself*, Edward Bach, C.W. Daniel Company, Ltd., London, 1973.

6. *The Twelve Healers*, Edward Bach, C.W. Daniel Company, Ltd., London 1973.

7. *The Bach Remedies Repertory*, F.J. Wheeler, C.W. Daniel Company, Ltd., London, 1970.

8. *The Original Writings of Edward Bach*, J. Howard and J. Ramsell, The Dr. Edward Bach Healing Trust and Centre, Mount Vernon, Sotwell, Wallingford, Oxon., OX10 OPZ, England, 1990.

9. *Questions & Answers Clarifying the Basic Principles and Standards of the Bach Flower Remedies*, J. Ramsell and N. Murray, The Dr. Edward Bach Healing Trust and Centre, Mount Vernon, Sotwell, Wallingford, Oxon., OX10 OPZ, England, 1986.

10. *Bach Flower Therapy: Theory & Practice*, Mechthild Scheffer, Torsons Publishers, Inc., 1987.

11. *Flower Essences: Reordering Our Understanding and Approach to Illness and Health*, Machaelle Small-Wright, 1988.

12. *Flower Essence Repertory*, Patricia Kaminski & Richard Katz, The Flower Essence Society, P.O. Box 459, Nevada City, CA 95959, 1994.

13. *Choosing Flower Essences: An Assessment Guide*, Patricia Kaminski, The Flower Essence Society.

14. Alaskan Flower Essence Project, P.O. Box 1369, Homer, Alaska 99603-1369.

15. *Healing with Australian Flowers*, Va'sudeva Barnao, Living Essences, P.O. Box 355, Scarborough, Western Australia, 6019, 1988.

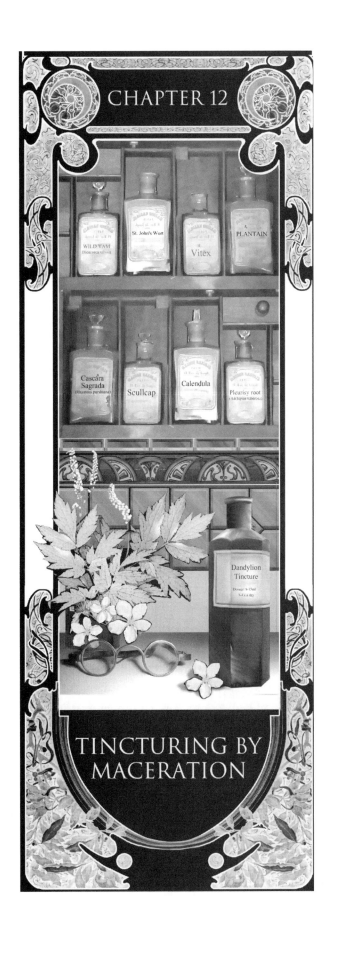

CHAPTER 12

TINCTURING BY
MACERATION

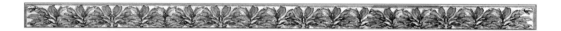

Herbal tinctures are alcoholic or water-alcohol solutions prepared from fresh or dried botanicals. It is believed by many that alcohol is a better solvent than water for extracting plant constituents and that a mixture of alcohol and water will dissolve nearly all the desired constituents of a plant, while at the same time acting as a highly efficient preservative. The term tincture commonly refers to these alcohol preparations, but it is also used to refer to preparations that are vinegar, wine, or glycerin based. The glycerin-based tinctures are more often referred to, however, as glycerites or glycerates.

All official tinctures (as determined by an official U.S. Pharmacopoeia) are made with an alcohol and water solution or pure alcohol, the majority of herbal tinctures containing around 60 percent alcohol. The official definition of a tincture is stated to be a solution that contains at least 45 percent alcohol and has an herb/menstruum ratio of at least 1:4. Of course these ratios can always vary and this definition is supplied more as a means to distinguish concentrated infusions and decoctions which are sometimes preserved using up to 25 percent alcohol, and "fluid extracts," which usually have an herb to menstruum ratio of 1:1.

Aside from those plants that require dehydration such as Pleurisy root (*Asclepias*

tuberosa) or Wild Yam (*Dioscorea villosa*), and those that require a year or more of aging to develop their full therapeutic potential such as Cascara Sagrada (*Rhamnus purshiana*) and its relatives, the therapeutic potency of tinctures made from fresh "green" herbs and roots are thought of by some individuals to be stronger than those of dry plant equivalents. Even though I tend to prefer fresh plant preparations, I can't hold to a generalization like that, but it is interesting that homeopathic mother tinctures of herbs are almost always made from the fresh plant, since the dry plant products provide less satisfactory potencies.

There are two fundamental processes for tincturing an herb: *maceration* and *percolation*. Maceration requires no expensive or unusual equipment or complex procedures, whereas percolation usually does. And of course each method has its pros and cons, but then all things being relative, what doesn't? We will discuss the maceration method in this chapter and deal with percolation (and the pros and cons of each) in Chapter Thirteen.

There are two basic methods for making a tincture by maceration; one requires measurements, the other doesn't. The first method we will discuss is simple and very effective. I will refer to it as the "folk method." It requires no measuring and is good for general use. The fact there is no measuring of substances, however, makes it somewhat vague as to the resultant "tincture strength." Tincture strength refers to the amount of herb that has been concentrated into a given measure of solution.

When one prepares a tincture that will be dispensed by others, it is important to state on the label the tincture strength of the preparation, so it can be dispensed in appropriate and accurate doses. In order to prepare these tinctures for professional use (or as required by the FDA for all tinctures sold in commerce), use the method I will refer to as the "weight to volume (w/v) method." In this method the weight of the herb and the volume of the menstruum are measured and noted in order to produce a specific tincture strength.

The metric system of measure is most convenient for this purpose because it offers us a working 1 to 1 relationship between a *weight* of a solid material with a *volume* of a liquid. The avoirdupois system of weight and measure that we normally use in the U.S. doesn't readily supply us this convenience.

Simply put, one cubic centimeter of water weighs one gram. For our practical purposes, we can allow that this holds true for all the liquids (water, alcohol, wine, vinegar, glycerin) we use to formulate our menstrua. This is a relationship we can access in our weight to volume (w/v) method of making tinctures. The relationship of plant material to menstruum is known as the weight (of herb) to volume (of menstruum) ratio of the tincture, or the tincture strength. The most commonly found tincture strengths used in commerce and in mainstream medicine are 1:5 and 1:10 for dry plant preparations and 1:2 for fresh plant preparations.

There is a historical precedent for this phenomenon.

In September of 1902 in Brussels, Belgium, a "Conference Internationale pour l'Unification de la Formule des Medicaments Heroiques" was held. This gathering brought together delegates from nearly every "civilized" country. The purpose of this body was to formulate standards for potent remedies which would be adopted by the various pharmacopoeias of the world, and therefore secure the principal object of an international pharmacopoeia. The protocol agreed upon at this conference was adopted and made official in the U.S. Pharmacopoeia VIII (1906) and has remained as a standard. Conforming in principle to the standards recommended by the International Protocol adopted at Brussels in 1902, these are the ratios of herbs to menstrua:

• Tinctures of dried non-toxic botanicals represent the activity of 20 Gm of dried herb in each 100 cc of tincture (a 20% or 1:5 w/v tincture).

• Tinctures of dried toxic or intense botanicals represent the activity of 10 Gm of dried herb in each 100 cc of tincture (often called a 10% or 1:10 w/v tincture).

• Tinctures of fresh undried plants are made to represent the activity of 50 Gm of fresh herb in each 100 cc (a 50% or 1:2 w/v tincture). Pure, undiluted (190-proof) ethyl alcohol is used for the fresh plant menstruum.

In other words, if you take 100 cc (which is equivalent to 100 ml) of a 1:5 tincture of dried Stinging Nettle into your body, theoretically, you receive the same activity as if you ate 20 Gm of the dried herb. Or if you take 100 ml of a 1:2 tincture of fresh Nettle, theoretically, you are receiving the same activity as

Ideally, a 1:5 tincture of dried herb delivers the action of 20 Gm of herb for each 100 ml of tincture taken; a 1:10 tincture delivers the action of 10 grams of dried herb; while a 1:2 tincture of fresh plants carries the action of 50 grams of fresh herb with each 100 ml of tincture taken.

if you ate 50 Gm of fresh Nettle (you might want to steam those fresh Nettles first).

Of course these international standards, though excellent, are not sacrosanct and a lay herbalist can make his or her tinctures in any strength desired. I usually make my dried Nettle extract at 1:4, my fresh St. John's Wort at l:1.5, and my fresh Mullein flowers at a 1:1. I often start out using the suggested standards, but frequently alter them as I prepare successive batches. My current preferences have evolved based on my experience with these plant extracts. View all these processes and standards as principles to use as initial guides, but ultimately do adjust them according to your own preferences.

It is important to note that, provided one is using good-quality herb, both methods, the folk and the w/v, make high-quality tinctures. Neither method is superior to the other (that statement will draw some debate); the choice is merely a matter of the medicine-maker's needs and preferences. Some folks like to measure ingredients when cooking, some don't. We will discuss both methods for preparing tinctures in this chapter.

Regardless of which method you choose for making tinctures, remember that maceration is floating time, when the alluring qualities of the liquids have their way with the herbal solids; the waters and alcohols of the menstruum gently coax the essence of the plants into solution. This is a time of quiescence as the earth, air, fire, and water elements of the herb surrender themselves to the receptive liquid of the menstruum. Inevitably, however, this relationship will fall into deep slumber as we are all prone to do within the delicious wetness of a tranquil bath. So, it is the task of an attentive medicine-maker to shake his or her tinctures routinely, thereby re-arousing the active part of the extraction process.

PRESERVATION AND STORAGE

Store all tinctures in airtight, light-resistant containers and avoid exposure to direct sunlight and excessive heat.

DOSAGE

Tinctures are normally more concentrated than either infusions or decoctions and therefore stronger. The dosage to be taken can be much smaller. The dosage again depends on the herb at hand. When I use a mild tonic herb such as Nettle, Dandelion, or Hawthorn, I will take up to five droppersful in a glass of water 2 to 3 times a day. When taking a more intense herb, such as Echinacea or Chaparral, I take anywhere from 10 to 25 drops, 3 to 4 times a day. With Cayenne, sometimes 1 drop is plenty.

SUMMARY

Since most medicinal plants are made up of representatives from various types of constituents, categorized as either active or ballast substances, the extraction agents should not be geared solely to any individual substance. When extracting dehydrated plant material, alcohol concentrations of 40 percent (sometimes less) to 60 percent (sometimes more) are customarily utilized, according to the official instructions given in most pharmacopoeia. This range of alcohol to water varies widely among experienced herbalists. Therefore, as I suggested in a previous chapter, when formulating a menstruum for conducting an herbal extraction process of dried plant material,

When in doubt as to a suitable menstruum, choose "dilute alcohol" as a solvent.

Tincturing by Using the Folk Method

Tincturing dry plant material

1. Grind dried herb to a moderately coarse powder (mcp).

2. Place the powder into a large jar that can be tightly closed.

3. Add prepared menstruum (see page 150.)

4. Stir the mixture well, so that all of the herb is wet.

5. Add sufficient menstruum to the wet herb so that about 1/4 inch of extra menstruum sits atop the herb; if the herb is floating, 1/4 inch below the herb.

6. Cap jar tightly.★

7. Check the jar after 12 hours. If the herb has absorbed the menstruum, add a sufficient amount of menstruum to re-establish the 1/4 inch of extra liquid.

8. Shake the tincture frequently for 14 days, then let it sit another day.

9. Pour off (decant) the clear tincture from the top, press the remaining wet pulp, and combine these two liquids (see methods for decanting and pressing in Chapter Twenty-Five).

10. Filter if desired.

11. Bottle, tightly cap, and label.

Tincturing fresh plant material when using 190-proof alcohol

1. Chop the fresh plant into small pieces and stuff them into a canning jar, filling it to the top. Pack the herb into the jar very tightly. Get as much into the jar as you can, especially when working with a light herb.

2. Add 190-proof ethyl alcohol, filling the jar to the top. Make sure all the herb is covered by the alcohol.

3. Cap jar tightly.★

4. Agitate the tincture frequently for 14 days.

5. Decant the liquid, press the remaining wet pulp, and combine these two liquids.

6. Filter if desired.

7. Bottle, tightly cap, and label.

★ It is important to clean and wipe off the rim of the jar thoroughly before placing the lid on the jar and tightening it down. It is even advisable after wiping the rim to place a piece of waxed paper between the rim and the lid of the jar as a gasket. This assures that a tight seal will be made preventing the loss of any menstruum that can occur due to constant shaking of the liquid contents. You will know if there has been any leakage by the discovery of narrow streams of extract appearing on the outside surface of the jar.

Tincturing fresh plant material when using diluted alcohol (less than 190-proof)

1. Chop the fresh plant into small pieces and stuff them very tightly into a canning jar, filling it to the top.

2. Add menstruum (see below), filling the jar to the top. (See *Preparing the Menstruum* below.)

3. Pour the entire ingredients (herb and menstruum) into a Vita-Mix or some other suitable blender and blend it like a smoothie. (You will have to make a large enough batch, so that the volume of menstruum required is sufficient to completely cover the blender blades.)

4. Pour the liquefied ingredients into a jar and cap tightly.★

5. Agitate tincture frequently for 14 days, then let it sit another day.

6. Decant, press, and filter.

7. Bottle, tightly cap, and label.

Preparing the menstruum

The nature of the folk method is simplicity. This means using what is commonly at hand and readily available. The easiest menstruum to obtain is probably a commercial 80-proof or 100-proof vodka. Eighty-proof vodka is (approximately) 40 percent alcohol by volume; 100 proof is (approximately) 50 percent alcohol by volume. Twenty to 30 percent alcohol is sufficient to preserve a tincture. Therefore, when making a dried plant preparation, 80-proof vodka is adequate. When making a fresh plant preparation, which always incorporates the juices of the plant (which dilute the menstruum), maybe 100-proof vodka is more judicious (as noted above, 190-proof would be the most efficient).

Of course, one can always prepare a custom-made menstruum (as discussed in the next section on weight to volume method) and use it as a menstruum for this folk method. Make notes on your decision and on the results that manifest.

Tincturing Using the Weight to Volume Method

Tincturing dry plant material

1. Powder and weigh dried plant and place the powder into a large jar that can be tightly closed.

2. Prepare custom menstruum (see page 152).

3. Be sure to mix together all the liquids of the menstruum thoroughly in a separate container before adding them to the powdered plant material.

4. Add the menstruum to the powdered herb.

5. Stir well, making sure all of the powdered herb is wet. (After stirring the herb and menstruum together, some plant parts—usually the seeds, barks, or roots—will be very wet, showing a considerable amount of liquid, while some other parts—certain leaves, flowers—will appear merely dampened by the menstruum. Do not be concerned about either extreme condition. Leave them as they are and continue with the following steps.)

6. Cap jar tightly.

7. Shake tincture frequently for 14 days, then let it sit another day.

8. Decant, press, and filter.

9. Bottle, cap tightly, and label.

Tincturing fresh plant material

VARIATION 1

1. Chop and weigh the plant and place it in a large jar.

2. Prepare custom menstruum (see page 152).

3. If you chose not to use an undiluted (absolute) 190-proof ethyl alcohol menstruum, be sure to mix together all the liquids of the menstruum thoroughly in a separate container before adding them to the plant material.

4. Add the menstruum to the herb.

5. Cap jar tightly.

6. Shake the tincture frequently for 14 days, then let it sit another day.

7. Decant the tincture, press the remaining wet pulp, and combine the two liquids.

8. Filter if desired.

9. Bottle, cap tightly, and label.

VARIATION 2

1. Chop the plant into small pieces and place them into a Vita-Mix or some other suitable blender.

2. Prepare custom menstruum (see below).

3. Cover the herb with menstruum and blend it like a smoothie. (You will have to use enough of the menstruum to cover the blender blades.) Use as much of the measured menstruum as you can to make the mixture churn actively in the blender. (In some instances, you may not be able to fit in all the menstruum during this blending stage.)

4. Pour the liquefied ingredients into a jar and cap tightly. Be sure you have added all the measured menstruum to the herb at some point during or after the blending process, in order to maintain the intended weight to volume proportion.

5. Shake the tincture frequently for 14 days, then let it sit another day.

6. Decant, press, and filter.

7. Bottle, cap tightly, and label.

Preparing the custom weight to volume menstruum

Two problems need to be addressed in preparing a custom weight to volume (w/v) menstruum: (1) determining the total volume of menstruum needed for the quantity of herb at hand; and (2) determining the "correct" (based on your judgment) combination and proportion of solvents within the menstruum.

To Determine the Total Volume of Menstruum

Example 1: To determine the total volume of menstruum required to make a 1:5 w/v tincture (also called a 20 percent tincture) of 400 Gm of powdered dried herb, simply multiply the weight of the herb by 5 (400 x 5 = 2000). This tells you that you need to prepare (a volume of) 2000 ml of menstruum to add to (the weight) 400 Gm of herb to give you a tincture strength of 1:5.

Example 2: To determine the total volume of menstruum required to make a 1:10 w/v (10 percent tincture) from 260 Gm of powdered dried herb, multiply 260 by 10 = 2600. You will need to prepare a volume of 2600 ml of menstruum for the weight of 260 Gm of herb.

Example 3: To determine the total volume of menstruum required to make a 1:2 w/v (50 percent tincture) from 215 Gm of fresh undried herb, multiply 215 by 2 = 430. You will need to prepare a volume of 430 ml of menstruum for the weight of 215 Gm of fresh herb.

When tincturing a fresh plant, one ordinarily makes a 1:2 w/v (50 percent tincture) and usually, but not necessarily always, uses a menstruum of pure 190-proof ethyl alcohol (according to the standards recommended by the International Protocol adopted at Brussels in 1902).

To Determine the Proportion of Solvents in the Menstruum

WHEN TINCTURING DRIED PLANT MATERIAL

This step requires some simple research. You need to look up the unique characteristics of the plant to become acquainted with its salient organic constituents (to later determine overall how much is water soluble and how much is alcohol soluble). As you involve yourself in the art and science of Herbalism, you will accrue a good working library of herbal references. Refer to these herbals to give you a list of the constituents found in commonly used herbs. (See Resources at the end of this book for references.) Also learn to trust your senses to give you a plant's constituent picture. Does it taste bitter (bitters) or sour (acids), is it astringent (tannins) or demulcent (mucilage), is it aromatic (volatile oils), etc.?

Using the list of constituents and their prime solvents given to you in Chapter Six, you can begin to get a sense of the proportions of water to alcohol that might be best used to bring most of the properties of this plant into solution. This will also prove helpful to determine if the plant contains tannins that would be well managed by the addition of some 10 percent glycerin in the menstruum. If the plant is high in alkaloids, you might want to add 5 to 10 percent vinegar to help convert these free alkaloids into alkaloidal salts which are far more soluble in water and alcohol.

The results of this research will give you a good foundation for a well-educated guess as to the best initial menstruum to formulate. There is no one right answer; there is, however, the "correct" answer for your requirements and preferences. Make your first batches small; make notes on your decisions and the results of these decisions; and continue to modify your menstruum until you have developed the one you like best (see "*The Sensual Approach to Successful Tincturing and Other Methods of Herbal Extraction*" in Chapter Five). The joy of good herbal medicine-making evolves with the willingness to experiment and the delight of discovery.

Ultimately, it's your decision as to what is the best menstruum for your herbal tincture. A good principle to follow when formulating a menstruum for dried plant material is to make the proportion of water as large as possible while still efficiently dissolving all soluble matter and not endangering the permanency of the preparation. One special advantage of this, beside the obvious economic one (alcohol is expensive), is that such tinctures may be added in small proportions to teas, baths, and other aqueous preparations without causing serious precipitation.

Whenever using more than one single solvent for your menstruum, be sure to mix together all the liquids of the menstruum thoroughly in a separate container before adding them to the plant material.

WHEN TINCTURING FRESH PLANT MATERIAL

Use the same method to determine total volume of menstruum for a quantity of the fresh herb as you would for a dry, powdered herb. The major difference here is that when tincturing a fresh plant one ordinarily makes a 1:2 w/v (50 percent tincture) and most often uses a menstruum of undiluted 190-proof ethyl alcohol (according to the standards recommended by the International Protocol adopted at Brussels in 1902).

Example: Find the volume of menstruum required to make a 1:2 w/v (50% tincture) from 454 Gm of fresh herb. Multiply 454 by 2 = 908. You will need to prepare a volume of 908 ml of menstruum for the weight of 454 Gm of fresh herb.

Note: Most pharmacopoeias, having adopted the standards of the 1902 International Protocol, hold to using a menstruum of pure 190-proof (95 percent ethyl) alcohol for tincturing fresh plants. This standard was established by pharmacists based on the theory that ethyl alcohol, when in contact with the fresh plant tissue for an adequate length of time, dehydrates the tissue and in so doing draws into solution all plant constituents that are dissolved in the plant juice. This leaves behind merely the cellulose and other insoluble tissues to be discarded. Some herbalists feel it is unnecessary to blend or shake these macerating mixtures because this dehydration process occurs automatically and completely without the need for any other action. Obviously if one chooses not to blend or shake a tincture of this nature, every part of the plant material must be immersed in the pure alcohol for the extraction process to act upon the entire mass.

Keep in mind if you use 100-proof vodka (or any diluted ethyl alcohol), you need to blend the fresh herb with the menstruum and shake the macerating tincture regularly.

Herbs on the "35 Herbs and a Fungus" List That Are Well Prepared As a Tincture

See the *"Dosage"* section in Chapter Twenty-Five for calculating dosages for children.

	PLANT PART	WEIGHT TO VOLUME	% OF ALCOHOL IN MENSTRUUM	ADULT DOSAGE
Black Cohosh	fresh rhizome/root	1:2	100%	.5–2 ml: 3x a day
	dry root	1:5	60–80%	.5–2 ml: 3x a day
Baneberry[1]	dry root	1:5	70–80%	10–20 drops: up to 3x a day[2]
Burdock	fresh root	1:2	100%	2–4 ml: 3x a day
	dry root	1:5	40–60%	2–4 ml: 3x a day
	seed	1:5	60–70%	1–2 ml: 3x a day
Calendula	fresh flowers	1:2	100%	1–2 ml: 3–4x a day
	dry flowers	1:5	60–80%	1–2 ml: 3–4x a day
Cayenne	dry fruit	1:5 or 1:10	80–95%	1–8 drops
Cleavers	fresh whole plant	1:1.5	100%	2 to 4 ml: 4x a day
Crampbark	dry bark	1:4	50–60%	2–3 ml: up to 4x a day
Dandelion	fresh root	1:2	100%	8 to 15 ml: 3–4x a day
	dry root	1:5	35%–65%	8 to 15 ml: 3–4x a day
Echinacea	fresh root	1:2	100%	1–3 ml: up to 5x a day
	dry plant root	1:5	50–75%	1–3 ml: up to 5x a day
Fennel	crushed seed	1:3	60%	2–4 ml in warm water as needed
Ginger	fresh root	1:2	100%	2–4 ml in warm water as needed
	dry root	1:4	80%	
Ginkgo	leaves	1:5	55–70%	2–3 ml: 3x a day
Goldenseal	fresh root	1:2	100% alc./5% vinegar	.5–2ml: up to 3x a day
	dry root and/or leaf	1:5	60–75% alc./5% vinegar	.5–2ml: up to 3x a day
Gumweed	fresh flowering tops	1:2	100%	1–2 ml: 4x a day
	dry tops	1:5	65–80%	1–2 ml: 4x a day
Hawthorn	fresh leaf, flower, berries	1:2	100%	1–3 ml: 3x a day
	dry	1:5	40–70%	1–3 ml: 3x a day
Mugwort	dry herb	1:5	40–60%	.5–2 ml: 3x a day
Mullein	fresh flowers	1:1	100%	2–3 ml: up to 4x a day
	dry	1:5	50–60%	2–3 ml: up to 4x a day
Nettle	fresh herb	1:2	100%	1–3 ml: 3x a day
	dry herb or root	1:4	40–50%	1–3 ml: 3x a day
Oat	fresh "unripe milky" seed	1:1.75 or 1:2	50–75%	2–5 ml: up to 4x a day
Peppermint	dry herb	1:4	40–60%	1–3 ml: 3x a day[3]
Plantain	fresh herb	1:2	100%	2–3 ml: 3x a day
St. John's Wort	fresh flowering tops	1:2	100%	1–3 ml: 3x a day

	PLANT PART	WEIGHT TO VOLUME	% OF ALCOHOL IN MENSTRUUM	ADULT DOSAGE
Saw Palmetto	fresh berries	1:2	80–100%	
	semi–dry	1:5	60–80%	2–5 ml: 3x a day
Scullcap	fresh herb	1:1.75 or 1:2	100%	1–3 ml: 3x a day
	recently dried	1:5	45–60%	1–3 ml: 3x a day
Siberian Ginseng[4]	powdered root	1:5	60%	2–4 ml: up to 4x a day
Uva Ursi	leaf	1:5	50–65%	1–3 ml: 3x a day
Vitex	berries	1:4/1:5	45–65%	1–2 ml: 3x a day
Valerian	fresh root	1:1.5 or 1:2	100%	1–3 ml: up to 3x a day
Yarrow	fresh flowering plant	1:2	100%	1–3 ml: 3x a day
	dry	1:5	40–60%	1–3 ml: 3x a day
Yellow Dock	fresh root	1:2	90% alc./10% glycerin	1–2 ml: 3x a day
	dry	1:5	40–50% /10% glycerin	1–2 ml: 3x a day

1. *(Actea Rubra)* used as a substitute for Black Cohosh

2. As per Michael Moore, *Medicinal Plants of the Pacific West*

3. Excellent flavoring agent

4. Very difficult to find authentic herb best to buy the authentic extract. Otherwise use powdered root.

TINCTURING
BY PERCOLATION
CHAPTER 13

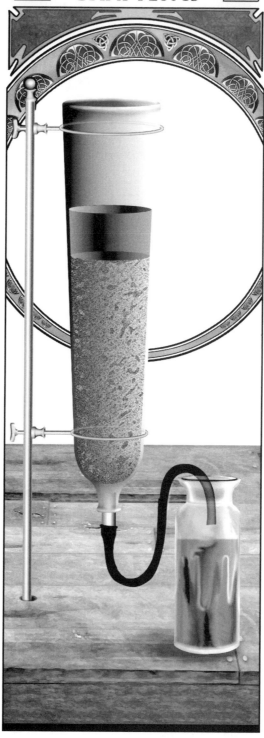

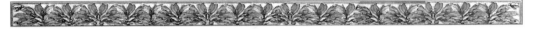

There is a perennial debate amongst herbal medicine-makers and herbal extract manufacturers as to the superiority and practicality of percolation versus that of maceration. We probably won't resolve the issue in this chapter, but as you will see, we'll definitely grapple with the question. Maceration (extracting soluble constituents by simply soaking them in a solvent) is one of the oldest methods of extraction known to human medicine-makers. Percolation is a process having a relatively late introduction into Western pharmacy, but which quickly caught the fancy and blazing fervor of professional pharmacists and erudite herbalists. It is a process of extracting the soluble constituents of an herb by the slow passage of a solvent (mainly, but not entirely, due to the pull of gravity) through a column of dried powdered plant which has been packed in a special form of apparatus known as a percolator. Percolation is sometimes called *displacement*, because the solvent after becoming charged with the soluble part of the herb is displaced by fresh portions of the solvent liquid.

The question of which of these methods of extraction is the better, I guess, is best answered by stating that each has advantages and disadvantages over the other.

The percolation process can be found advantageous because:

• It offers a means of making a tincture in 24 hours (when in a huge rush, as little as 3 or 4 hours), whereas maceration ordinarily takes 10 to 14 days, sometimes longer.

• It is easier and faster to prepare more highly concentrated dry plant tinctures (1:2, 1:3) and fluid extracts (1:1).

• The soluble constituents of an herb can be removed and collected more completely by percolation than by the soaking, pressing, and filtration processes used in maceration. (However, this assertion probably incites more heated debate than the creation vs. big bang and evolution contest.)

• The liquid left in the residue (marc) and discarded after completion of a successful percolation is pure menstruum, which is a bit bothersome, but at least all the plant's constituents dissolved in the proceeding percolate and have been collected in there entirety for use. In maceration, the liquid left in the residue is a finished full-strength tincture, which is never completely removed, and that is even more irksome.

• One does not have to press the marc. Maceration requires pressing in order to remove as much of the saturated solvent (tincture) as possible from the marc. With more highly concentrated tinctures (1:3. 1:4), 20 to 25 percent of the extract can remain in the mark if it is not pressed thoroughly, and, even when pressed thoroughly, some of the tincture (regardless of its w/v concentration) is always lost to the marc.

• Well-made, efficient presses, when available, can be expensive (percolation requires no pressing).

• Percolation offers a fascinating challenge and carries a discerning air of status for those who can do it consistently, like those few surfers who can ride the big ones—the mountain riders. Actually, percolation's not quite as demanding as riding a 40-foot wave.

Maceration is more advantageous in the following circumstances:

• For the extraction of plants containing large amounts of gum or mucilage which swell considerably when moistened. Percolation is only suited for the extraction of close-grained plant materials which swell only a small amount.

• For the extraction of fresh undried plant material.

• For the extraction of plant materials that contain a high proportion of resins and gum-resins. Neither highly resinous or gum-resinous plant materials nor fresh plant materials can be extracted by the percolation method. Due to the physical nature of these materials, they cannot normally be packed properly to allow an effective flow of menstruum essential for efficient percolation.

• For the making of glycerates or the use of menstrua containing glycerin.

Other practical advantages that are inherent in maceration:

• The process of maceration is decidedly more simple, requiring less aptitude, dexterity, and judgment in conducting it, and it requires little or no practice.

• It is uniform, always done in the same way.

• The results are quite predictable in that all of the derived tincture will be of uniform strength.

• It requires less constant attention during the process (just shake it once or twice a day). This is quite significant when dealing with large quantities.

• The apparatus required is less complicated and more easily acquired.

• It works every time, and it produces excellent tinctures.

With regard to our immediate situation, wherein we are communicating solely by illustrations and written word, percolation evokes a significant problem because to learn and develop a semblance of success in this process of extraction, physical demonstration and hands-on practice are usually needed. However, after some deliberation, I decided to pursue this introductory discussion and instruction in the performance of the percolation method for the benefit of those who have heard of it and wonder what the heck it's all about; for those who are fascinated by the fabrication and manipulation of apparatus; for those feral spirits who will take to the challenge of an untutored attempt; and for those who have previously experienced the making of a tincture by percolation, but can use a mental review. Ergo…

PERCOLATION

Equipment

You need a percolator cone. This can be a relatively costly Pyrex® glass cone purchased from a lab equipment supply house, or it can be a clear glass funnel, or a homemade device manufactured by removing the bottom of a glass (don't use a plastic bottle) 1-liter Crystal Geyser® or Calistoga®-like water bottle (which is what most of us do). This is done by using a glass cutter. The idea, design, and popularization of this homemade percolator is directly attributable to the practical brilliance of Mr. Michael Moore, herbalist and director of the Southwest School of Botanical Medicine in Arizona. The transmogrified water bottle will sit upside down in a wide-mouthed Mason® canning jar and the screw cap of the bottle is used to control the rate of drip from—what has now been converted to—the bottom of the bottle. For percolating smaller batches of tincture, a Perrier® bottle is better used, as its diameter is narrower, allowing a small amount of herb to create a longer column of powdered herb for the menstruum to percolate through. This can often make for better extraction. Use a narrow-mouth Mason jar with the Perrier bottle.

You also need a packing rod. This can be any device having a broad, flat end that can be used to tamp down the powdered herb while packing it into the cone. A 10" length of 3/4" to 1" diameter wooden doweling sawed off squarely at the end works well.

In addition to some of the kitchen pharmacy equipment I have recommended in Chapter Four, you will also need:

- unbleached filter paper
- a small container that can be closed airtight
- plastic bags and rubber bands
- a small weight like a quartz crystal or a rock that is fairly impervious to liquids
- a couple of 1-quart canning jars (when using the homemade type percolator)
- well-dried plant material
- alcohol and water

For a detailed description of the "technical" approach to percolation, you can read Remington's *Practice of Pharmacy* or *Remington's Pharmaceutical Sciences*. The following method is a variation of the "lay" method popularized by Michael Moore, who wheeled onto the campus of our herb school one afternoon and started cutting the bottoms off of a bunch of glass Perrier bottles. At the time, we weren't exactly sure why.

Herb Preparation

You will need to grind and sift your dried plant material to allow for smooth easy extraction. A coarse #20 powder will do (see "*Powdering,*" Chapter Twenty-Five). The

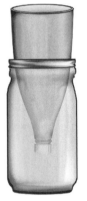

Standard Percolation Cones

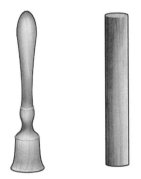

Homemade Percolator

Packing Rods

nature of the plant being percolated is the prime factor as to how finely it should be powdered in order to be efficiently extracted by percolation. National Formularies direct anywhere from #20 to #60 powders depending on the herb, with #30 and #40 seeming to be the most often directed. Vary the fineness of the powder you use as you experiment with each herb. This is why, over the long run, note-taking is so helpful. Run the powder through your sifter and remove all chunks and clumps, leaving a uniformly textured powder. When making a tincture by percolation, the evenness of the texture of the powder is probably as important as how finely it is powdered.

Preparation of the Menstruum

Suppose you have decided to prepare a tincture at 1:5 weight/volume in a 60 percent alcohol menstruum:

1. Weigh the freshly ground herb. Let's say you have 180 Gm.

2. I'll be referring back to this step at the latter part of the process. Pack the herb into a measuring cup to determine the compressed volume that the herb fills. Let's say it is 300 ml (10 oz). This is approximately the volume of menstruum that will be retained by the marc and discarded along with the marc at the completion of this percolation. This amount varies depending on the herb being used. At the end of this process it may be found some plant material retains more liquid than this estimate, some may be less; when finished with the percolation, one should make note of the actual amount retained by this herb for the next time it is percolated. Therefore, that amount of (estimated) menstruum (300 ml) must be added to the full volume of menstruum that is required to produce a 1:5 w/v tincture (which in this example will be 900 ml—5 x 180). So, you will need to prepare 1200 ml (300 ml + 900 ml) total volume of menstruum for this percolation (See details for calculating a w/v menstruum in Chapter Twelve).

3. Prepare 1200 ml of 60%:40% menstruum, 60% (720 ml) of 190-proof ethyl alcohol, 40% (480 ml) of distilled water.

4. Mix the alcohol and water together, and set it aside in a closed container.

Moistening the Herb

This is a preliminary moistening that is done before the herb is packed into the cone. It allows the dampened powder to swell upon absorbing the liquid. Some plant powders, if dampened and packed in the cone before swelling occurs, can expand to such a degree that the cone ends up being packed too tightly to allow the liquid that is added later to flow down through it.

1. Add approximately 200 ml of menstruum to the 180 Gm of powdered herb and mix it thoroughly. (This is about 2/3 to 3/4 of the 300 ml volume calculated—in

Step 2, on page 161 — to saturate the marc. Remember, we are only dampening the powder at this time, not yet saturating it). Make the consistency such that you can pinch some of the moist powder between your fingers, and it will hold together. Precaution: *Moisten the herb slowly*; if it is not moist enough you can always add more liquid. However, if it gets too moist, the ball game's over, maceration wins.

2. Place the moistened powder into a container that can be tightly sealed to prevent evaporation and let it sit for 1 hour to over night, depending on your time urgency.

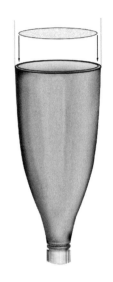

Diameter of Cut Paper

Packing the Cone

1. First cut two round pieces of coffee filter paper. Make their diameters roughly equivalent to the inside top opening of the cone.

2. Make a cone out of one of the papers by folding it into fours (in half twice) then opening it up to form the cone.

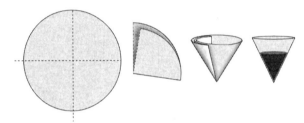

Making the Cone

3. Pack this paper coffee filter cone with some of the moist powder. (Pack it lightly at this point.)

4. Slide the filled paper cone down into the neck of the glass percolator cone. You may need to use a chopstick to get it in place. (If you experience some difficulty, relax and hang in there, you'll get it.) Once it is in place, make sure the paper cone is adhering to the glass and is sealed completely around the circumference.

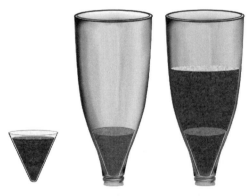

Packing the Filter Paper Cone and
Positioning It in Glass Cone

5. Now that the packed paper cone is in place, gradually add more of the moist powder (about 1/3 of what is left to pack) on top of this first batch, and tamp it down evenly with the packing rod.

6. Now put in the second 1/3 of the powder and tamp it down a little harder and evenly.

7. Follow this with the final 1/3 of the herb. Each successive portion being pressed a little more firmly than the proceeding portion. Compress and compact the column of powder very evenly. When this is done correctly, the packing will look uniform from the top to the bottom of the cone. It will not look like three separate layers.

8. Be sure the top surface of the final layer is flat and level. *This is the judgment portion of the operation that will take some practice.* If the column is packed too hard, the menstruum that is poured on later will not flow at all. If it is packed too loosely, the herb will redistribute itself as the menstruum flows through it, creating fissures that disturb the flow of the menstruum, causing an incomplete extraction. If the column is not packed evenly throughout the width and depth of the cone, the flow will descend unevenly, causing an incomplete extraction. Packing the percolator so that the best results will be realized is a skill that is acquired only by the experience of trial and error.

9. Lay the second round piece of filter paper on top of the packed herb, and on top of this put the quartz crystal or the rock to weigh the paper down. This is done to protect the top stratum of the packed powder when the rest of the menstruum is being poured in.

Adding Some More of the Menstruum

1. Remove the bottle cap from the bottom of the cone so air can escape as the body of solvent descends. If this is not done, when more menstruum is poured on, air will bubble up through the herb instead and mutilate the packing job.

2. Set the packed percolator down into the wide-mouth Mason jar, making sure the top surface of the powder is level, horizontal, parallel, perpendicular to vertical, straight across, etc.

3. Slowly pour the menstruum onto the column of herb. The menstruum should progress slowly and evenly down the herb column throughout each successive layer of the moistened herb. If it does this successfully, this is when the fat lady sings; this is when you get your wings — or not (till the next time).

4. When the menstruum reaches the bottom of the percolator, the herb is saturated and the menstruum will begin to drip out of the bottom. Gently pick up the bottle and replace and tighten the cap to completely stop the flow of liquid. Place the cone back into the Mason jar.

5. Be sure to leave a layer of an inch or more of menstruum sitting on top of the packed herb. *This layer must be maintained throughout the entire percolation until the last portion of the menstruum has been added.* If instead, the column of powder is exposed to air, the air at once enters the powder; then when more liquid is poured on, the air must escape and forces its way to the surface disarranging the well-packed powder (bummer).

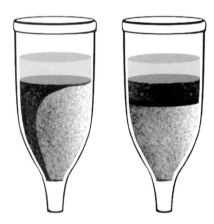

Properly Packed and Imperfect Packed Cones

Let me attempt to illustrate this more clearly for you with the following comparison. Visualize, if you will, a soiled and sweaty, battle-worn soldier who, after having just survived the most gruesome combat episode of a high-budget, Dolby sound, war film (or if you prefer, just moments after the hottest love scene in motion picture memory) lying back and taking a long, slow, deeply satisfying drag on a svelte, name-brand cigarette. Now, zoom in for a close-up shot of the cigarette's burning end. See it glowing brightly as the fire moves gracefully and evenly down the cigarette's chemical-laden, nicotine-enhanced, firm and uniformly packed cylindrical shaft? That's the move we want the menstruum to make on the powdered herb as the solvent flows deftly down a firm, uniformly packed, percolator column. Now, compare that picture to a scene wherein a small group of colorfully clad people are sitting in a circle drumming, talking, and laughing amongst themselves while one of them takes a lengthy toke on a rather hastily assembled home-rolled unit. See the fire sputter and crackle unruly as it speeds down one side of the unevenly packed cylinder leaving the rest of the paper and its herbal contents, for the time being untouched. That's the kind of movement you don't want to see the menstruum make. Get the picture? Maybe you have to be there. But I'm confident a significant number of readers can relate to the experiences and appreciate my analogies.

The Maceration Period

1. Having made sure that a one- or more-inch layer of menstruum covers the top of the moist powder, so no air gets into the column, cover the cone with a plastic bag and secure it with a rubber band.

2. At this point, the herb is left to macerate for at least 12, but preferably 24 to 48 hours.

Percolation, the Dripping Period

1. After the period of maceration is completed, remove the plastic bag and loosen the bottle cap. Allow the menstruum, carrying with it the extractive (this is called the *percolate*), to drip slowly into the Mason jar(s). In fact, the volume of 900 ml will require two Mason jars. While dripping, before the accumulating tincture reaches the cap of the percolator, slowly lift the cone and set it in a second jar to continue dripping. The drip rate should be approximately 1 drop each 3 seconds (20 drops per minute). The rate of flow can be adjusted by tightening or further loosening the cap.

2. Continue to add fresh menstruum until it all drips through. This can take up to two hours and sometimes longer. The actual drip rate will depend on the constituents of the herb, the firmness of the packing, the tightness of the cap, and the nature of the menstruum used. The higher the menstruum's alcohol content, the easier it passes through the herb.

3. When the percolation has finished, there will be approximately 900 ml of tincture in the Mason jar(s) and approximately 300 ml of menstruum remaining in the marc, to do with as you will. The first time you "do" the herb at hand, you may or may not end up with 900 ml of tincture because the "300 ml" of extra menstruum you added in Step 2, on page 161, at the very beginning of this procedure may not have been an accurate estimation due to the nature of the herb and the nature (alcohol water proportion) of the menstruum. If the percolate proves to be more or less than 900 ml, so be it. It won't be off by more than a few milliliters. Make a note and adjust the amounts the next time you do this herb. Each herb will be different.

SUMMARY

For a successful percolation, one that extracts all the constituents from the entire column of powdered herb, the dampened herb has to be packed uniformly firm (but not too firm) throughout the entire length and width of the glass column (this takes some practice and judgment) and the menstruum must be poured onto the packed powder ever so gingerly, so it will flow slowly, evenly, and regularly throughout each successive horizontal layer to the next. The menstruum must not scoot down one side of the column in a narrow trail leaving the remainder of the powder untouched, for this will result in an incomplete extraction. If this does happen (and it does!), or if you packed the column too firmly and nothing happens (in extreme circumstances, it can take up to an hour for the dripping to start, so don't throw it out too soon), just dump everything (all the herb and all the menstruum) into a jar and simply macerate it instead (a point for maceration). You'll end up with a fine tincture having a 1:5 (plus the extra menstruum, in this case, +300 ml) tincture strength. Or if while pouring the latter portions of menstruum into the cone, you see that the flow isn't going well, withhold 300 ml of the menstruum; now when you dump everything into the maceration mode, you will have a 1:5 strength tincture and 300 ml of high-proof cocktail to drown your tears in.

If any or all of my explanations, illustrations, and candid analogies remain unclear to you, I'm not too surprised. Percolation is difficult to put in words; but I tried. You might want to reread the final point I made in the beginning of this chapter on page 159. But certainly persevere; take the challenge—inevitably glorious success awaits you. It could be worse; you could be trying to toilet train a thirsty puppy. So practice packing, and pouring, and dripping by using inexpensive powdered Fennel seed or like material and relatively inexpensive 80-proof vodka. Powdered seeds pack easier than most leaf or flower material, which tend to be a little spongier when packed, and many roots, which tend to contain a relatively large amount of albumen and are, therefore, a little more difficult to begin with. Better yet, find a bulk Chai tea blend (like the one discussed in Chapter Twenty-Two for making a Chai syrup), and use plain water as the menstruum. Percolation is a method commonly used in pharmacy to make aqueous infusions. This will give you good practice having little financial risk and will render a delicious Chai tea beverage with which to celebrate your suc-

cesses, or toast the lessons of your mishaps. Pure water is more difficult to flow through a packed cone than pure alcohol or alcohol/water mixtures; so once you successfully percolate using pure water, you can flow and drip any menstruum thereafter. Obviously, hold off on percolating ultra-precious Black Cohosh, or Goldenseal, etc. (or using relatively expensive high-alcoholic menstruums) until you've got the process mastered.

A final indication as to how successfully you exhausted the plant material, thereby rendering a full-bodied extract, is reflected by the taste of the last drops of the percolate. If these final drops have merely a faint flavor, you can assume that you extracted nearly all the constituents from the plant material. If these drops are, however, highly flavorful, there is probably a major portion of the constituents still remaining in the marc. Do something different next time. Pack the cone a little more firmly to slow down the flow of solvent and extend the extraction time, or use a finer powder for this particular plant, or slow down the drip rate by keeping the cap tighter. Enjoy the challenge! Be fortified by your failures; celebrate your success.

DOSAGE

Dosage varies according to type of herb(s) used and the size, age, and condition of the individual. Refer to the suggested adult dosages found at the end of Chapter Twelve, "Tinkering by Maceration." Also see the "*Dosage*" section in Chapter Twenty-Five for calculating dosages for children.

Herbs on the "35 Herbs and a Fungus" List That Are Well Prepared by Percolation

To help determine a good menstruum formula, refer to the suggested range of percent of absolute alcohol for dried plant tinctures found at the end of Chapter Twelve, "Tincturing by Maceration."

Fennel, Nettle, and Peppermint	These are inexpensive and abundant—good practice plants for developing your percolation dexterity.
Blackberry	This is usually better used as an astringent infusion or decoction, however.
Black Cohosh	
Burdock	
Cayenne	
Crampbark	
Dandelion	
Echinacea	This is best used as a fresh plant tincture, but if you are using very recently dried root it can be well percolated.
Fennel	
Ginger	
Ginkgo	
Goldenseal	
Siberian Ginseng	It is difficult to find reliable, authentic dried herb; for this reason, it is probably better to buy a reputable imported extract.
Uva Ursi	This is usually better used as a cold in-fused tea.
Valerian	
Vitex	
Willow	This is usually better used as a tea.
Yarrow	It is a little tricky to render this plant into a uniform powder.
Yellow Dock	

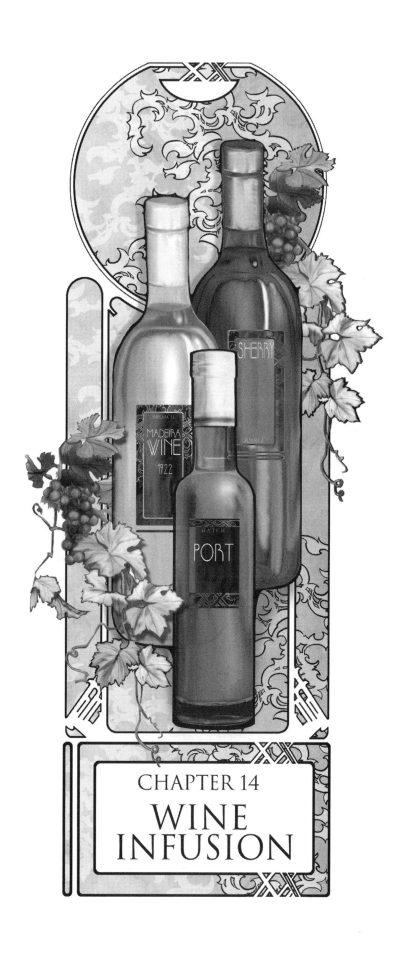

CHAPTER 14

WINE
INFUSION

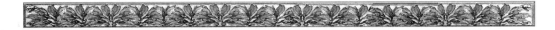

The history of the human race abounds in grapes and finds humanity romping merrily through the history of wine. Arabian physicians, as well as Hippocrates, Galen, and Pliny, heartily acclaimed the medicinal virtues of wine, and modern medical science is heard singing its praise as well, consistently finding it an active agent in disease prevention.

Throughout the history of herbal medicine-making, wine was commonly employed as a menstruum to coax into solution the virtues of several plants, and the preparations formed were called *vinous tinctures* or *medicated wines*. In the U.S. and Britain, the wines most often used for menstrua were the official wine sherry, together with port, madeira, teneriffe, and claret.

Our ancestors found certain advantages in the use of wine as a pharmaceutical menstruum: it dissolves substances normally considered insoluble in water, and, to a large extent, resists their tendency to spontaneous change. At the same time, wine is less a stimulant than rectified or proof spirit, both from its smaller proportion of alcohol and from the modified state in which the alcohol exists in wine's composition.

Medicated wines are one of the oldest class of Galenic preparations. They are hydro-alcoholic solutions made from various plants and employing white (sherry) or red (port) wine as the principal solvent or menstruum. In 1906, the official U.S. Pharmacopoeia VIII recognized red wine, white wine, and 8 medicated wines. In 1916, the National Formulary IV included formulas for 15 wines, all of which were made with sherry, but none have been official in later editions.

Herbal or medicinal wines are tinctures in which the menstruum is wine. The solvent power of wines on herb material depends primarily on the water and alcohol they contain. The acid that wine usually contains serves in some instances to increase its solvent power. The absence of uniformity in the proportion of alcohol to water in commercial wines renders the preparations made with them of unequal strength. The availability of other preparations such as tinctures and fluid extracts, which can render a more standardized strength (at a precision which can seldom be attained when wine is used), and the legal restrictions affecting the use of wines during the period of national prohibition, accounted for the decline in popularity of medicinal wines and their eventual deletion from official compendia. However, in spite of the heightened degree of pharmaceutical precision attainable from mixtures of grain alcohol and water, and the applauded preservative action of these high-alcohol content extracts, to me they are somehow less consonant with the human body than medicinal wines, and for my nature they often vibrate a bit too…medical. Herbal wines come across more as flavorsome foods and genial tonics. In contrast to the use of grain alcohol extracts, the employment of which often stems from a rather solemn, clinical, and renovating perspective, herbal wines seem to have a more festive relationship with the human mind and body. In my experience, the spirit of imbibing an herbal wine lends itself more to the mental and spiritual celebration of health and wellness.

As discussed later in the vinegar monologue (Chapter Fifteen), hyper-extractants and perpetual-preservatives served the medical/pharmaceutical establishments well in the manufacturing and marketing of their uniform strength, high potency, heroic products, but we lay herbalists need not rely so heavily on these qualities as we create a home pharmacy of herbal tonics. Because we have made ourselves more independent and can recreate our herbal preparations annually if we wish, they don't have to last "forever" on a shelf. And our handmade meds need not always present a precise strength or be pharmacologically mega-potent to touch our health. In addition to their abundant herbal actions, they provide other components in their overall tonifying therapeutic effect not found in the use of commercial products. Inherent in their handmade character are the seasonal joys we experience by nature of going outdoors into the wilds, along a pathway, and into the garden, seeking, visiting, and harvesting moderate amounts of our herbal allies and creating our own premium products. The handmade nature of our herbal preparations supplies us a considerably broader spectrum and more wholistic emplacement of health-enhancing therapeutic actions. So, for all herbal medicine-makers who agree with my meanderings, wine shines once again as a welcome solvent/preservative for common use.

THE UNIQUE RELATIONSHIP OF WINE WITH THE HUMAN BODY, MIND, AND SPIRIT

It would be a sober error to conclude that a given quantity of wine is equivalent to an equal quantity of water containing a like percentage of distilled grain alcohol. The peculiar effects of a true wine depend upon its ethereal and saline elements, such as its volatile oils, sugar, or acids, which modify materially those effects that would be produced by its alcohol alone. The grape-derived, naturally occurring accessory components of pure wine help the body metabolize and eliminate the wine's alcohol more gracefully, excreting it more benignly. Whereas purified alcohol is blunt in its nature, seeming to bump and bruise the organs and the brain as it transits through the body. Understand, of course, that any alcoholic liquid, be it grain alcohol or fine wine taken in excess on a regular basis, may bump, bruise, and break livers, careers, and families.

In various circles, discussion swings back and forth on the benefits and evils of imbibing alcohol of any nature. Traditionally it was believed that the physiological actions of wine on the human experience afforded many benefits. It was held that genuine unadulterated wine is essentially a stimulant of the nervous and circulatory systems, but its mode of stimulation is quite unlike that of other alcohol. In moderate proportions, wine increases activity and freedom of action, quickens and brightens the intellect and imagination, warms the feelings, invigorates the digestive powers, and it diffuses a cordial satisfaction throughout the whole being. No wonder Bacchus has always been humanity's most favored god.

In contrast, the action of distilled alcohol tends to benumb the faculties even while stimulating them, so that subjectively and objectively they seem to be struggling under a brute force; the exhilaration they produce is usually fierce and maudlin and they often leave in their wake a dull and torpid feeling. Quality wine, when taken in excess (which occasionally happens), affects the body less harshly (though harshly none the less) than distilled alcohol; the latter leads to complications with the liver, heart, and kidneys, while the former engenders gout, gravel, and nervous affections.

Wine, especially when used medicinally, needs to be of premium quality, and fortunately the California wine industry (and I assume other regions of the U.S.) is providing some excellent quality beverage and vinum menstrua for our humble domestic use.

During convalescence from fatigue or disease, wine taken in moderation with food is uplifting and can be an agreeable aid to recovery. It can also be of significant assistance in chronic conditions which waste the strength by profuse discharges, or by pain, or by inducing an anemic condition. In all of these cases, red wine seems to be more helpful than white. Sparkling wines have been used to help allay seasickness and other motion sickness.

The primary properties of pure wine are stimulant and antispasmodic. In convalescence from prolonged fever and the sinking of one's vitality, wine is potentially one of the finest remedies. In some convulsive and spasmodic conditions, wine, liberally imbibed, can be quite useful. There is evidence that one glass of red wine a day is beneficial.

THE NATURE AND VARIETY OF WINE

Wine is characterized as a spirituous liquid, the result of the fermentation of grape juice (the fruit of numerous varieties of *Vitis vinifera*), containing natural coloring matter and other substances, either combined or intimately blended with the spirit. All wine's other qualities vary with the nature of each particular wine.

The "spirit," the intoxicating ingredient in all wine, is alcohol; hence their relative strength depends upon the quantity of this substance entering into their composition. Wine's other ingredients, aside from water and alcohol, are sugar, gum, extractive, coloring matter, tannic, malic and carbonic acids, bitartrate of potassium (tartar), tartrate of lime, aenanthic ether, and volatile oils. The volatile oil is reportedly the cause of the delicate flavor and aroma of wine, which is called the "bouquet." The constituents on this list are not necessarily present in every wine. Thus sugar is present in sweet wines, tannic acid in rough wines, and carbonic acid in effervescent wines. The different kinds of wine derive their various qualities from their mode of fermentation, the nature of the grape, the soil, and climate in which it may have grown. Following is a brief review of those wines that were commonly used in pharmacy for making medicated wines.

SHERRY

Sherry (*Vinum Xericum*, from Xeres, Spain) is of a deep amber color, and when good, possesses a dry aromatic flavor and fragrance without any acidity. It ranks among the stronger white wines and contains between 15 and 20 percent by measure of alcohol. The U.S. and British pharmacopoeias at one time agreed on indicating it as the official wine. This was due to the fact that this wine, along with port wine, are the two varieties of wine most nearly resembling pure alcohol in their operation. When sherry was official, it was often made to order by dealers and could in these instances, by the addition of brandy, range from 20 to 35 percent of alcohol. This wine, when of good quality and being free from all acid, is the recommended one to use whenever the stomach is delicate or has a tendency to acid indigestion.

PORT

Port (*Vinum Portense*, from Portugal) is of a deep-purple color, and when young is a rough, strong, and slightly sweet wine. When kept a certain length of time in bottles, it deposits a considerable portion of its astringent matter, loses the greater part of its sweetness, acquires more flavor, and retains its strength. If kept too long, it deposits the whole of its astringent and coloring matter and becomes deteriorated. Port is not considered a natural wine due to the practice of adding to it considerable quantities of brandy, which causes its heating quality to the palate. This makes it the strongest of the wines in common use, and its alcoholic strength can be raised to 30 or 40 percent (keep in mind when choosing a menstruum that this is 60 to 80 proof). Port can be useful in cases of deep debility, especially when there is also a condition of loose bowels and

inflammation. This wine can act as a tonic stimulant increasing the strength of all functions, digestion in particular. A white port is available to us as well. I have not yet used it, but I assume it is free of the astringency compulsions found in red port. White port contains 18 to 20 percent alcohol.

MADEIRA

Madeira is the strongest of the white wines in use. It is a slightly acid wine and when of proper age and in good condition has a rich, nutty, aromatic flavor. As it occurs on the market, however, it is of variable quality because less care is taken in its manufacture now than formerly, and it is subject to adulteration after importation. It is 6 to 7 percent alcohol, unless fortified. Nutritionally, this is the most generous of the white wines and is particularly adapted to the purpose of reviving weakened constitutions and of abetting the declination of vitality in old age. The slight acidity of Madeira may disagree with some stomachs, and, as with all acidic wines, this makes it contraindicated for those who tend to gout.

CLARET

Claret is also a red wine and from its moderate strength is ranked as a light wine. It has a deep purple color and, when good, a delicate taste in which the vinous flavor is blended with slight acidity and astringency. It is 12 to 17 percent alcohol. This wine is much less heating than port, and is useful as an aperient and diuretic.

SPARKLING WINES

Sparkling wines, such as Champagne, are more or less sweet (but can be dry), charged with carbonic acid, bottled before fermentation is completed, and before the grape

A favored herb—say Damiana (*Turnera aphrodisiaca*), for example, infused in a fine wine with some mildly mischievous spices and a few plump raisins touches one's amorous spirit and feelings of well-being in a very special way.

sugar is all converted into alcohol. Alcohol content is 12 percent.

APPLE CIDER

Apple cider is 5 to 10 percent alcohol. This is a nutritious wine carrying with it the apple's unique spectrum of nutrients.

MEAD

Mead is a wine made from honey. This is a fascinating beverage having a rich history of enhancing merriment while festively benumbing medieval maidens and raucous warriors. Spawned by honey bees—our planet's most brilliant herbalists—mead is a particularly appropriate menstruum for making herbal extracts. This fermented flower nectar is 9 to 11 percent alcohol.

METHODS OF PREPARATION

Medicated wines are relatively low alcohol content tinctures prepared usually by maceration, in which the menstruum is wine. They have the advantage over water-based infusions and decoctions since they are much more permanent preparations.

Wine infusions lend very well to the folk method of extraction, but are also perfectly suited for the weight/volume method. (See Chapter Twelve for details on these two methods of tincturing.)

DOSAGE

In general, the dose when taking a medicated wine is a tablespoonful to a wineglassful, two or three times a day.

PRESERVATION AND STORAGE

In the choice of a wine to use as a men-

struum, the purest and most generous in alcohol should be selected. Sherry, port, madeira, and teneriffe were preferred by the official pharmacopoeias; sherry and port having the highest alcohol content.

Medicated wines are liable to undergo a change with time, and hence it is best that they be made:

• in small quantities

• without heat

• and kept in well-capped bottles, in a cool dark place like other fine wines

---

TO PREPARE A MEDICATED WINE

1. Reduce the dried herb to a moderately coarse powder.

2. Combine with pure undiluted wine of your choice (see above list of recommended wines).

3. Macerate for fourteen days; shaking the mixture frequently.

4. Strain.

5. Pour into a sterilized bottle, cap, and store in a cool location.

COMPOUND WINE OF COMFREY

A classic medicated wine recipe. Restorative Wine Bitters.

1. Take one ounce each of dried Comfrey leaf, Solomon's Seal (*Polygonatum biflorum*), if available, and Spikenard (*Aralia racemosa* or *A. californica*). Reduce them to a moderately coarse powder and add 1/2 oz. each of Chamomile flowers, Gentian, Columbo (*Frasera Carolinensis*, has a Gentian-like action, include if available), and Cardamom seeds, powdered.

2. Cover these with boiling water, and let them sit in a covered vessel for 24 hours, then add two quarts of sherry wine. Let this mixture of herbs and wine macerate for fourteen days; express and strain. Bottle, cap, and store the wine bitters in a cold place. (Modify the measurements to suit your needs.)

This classic wine-infusion Comfrey compound was used traditionally as a tonic for females to help remedy "female complaints." I might add that it also serves males to help remedy female complaints. Take a tablespoonful to a wineglassful, two to three times a day.

GRAND MARNIER DOMESTIQUÉ

> 250 ml primo-quality brandy
>
> 1 sumptuous organic orange
>
> 2/3 cup granulated sugar
>
> 1 wide mouth 1/2 gallon clear glass jar with a metal lid
> (make four holes in the lid so that string can pass through them)
>
> Some string
>
> 4 wooden toothpicks

1. Pour the brandy into the jar.

2. Pour the sugar into the brandy—*Do not stir this mixture.*

3. Push the toothpicks into the orange, one in each of four sides.

4. Affix string to the toothpicks and secure the string to the lid so that when the lid is placed onto the jar, the orange will be suspended 1 to 2 inches above the surface of the brandy (see illustration on the following page).

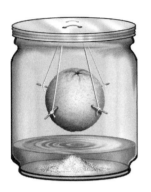

Orange Suspension Jar

5. Gently (so as not to jostle the brandy/sugar mixture) lower the orange, which is attached to the lid by hanging in its toothpick/string cradle, down into the jar and tighten the lid.

6. Let this stand wherever it is going to be completely undisturbed for 10 days.

7. Once a day, however, without lifting the jar, rotate the jar one complete rotation. (This is the touch of marnier magic; perform it with appropriate inner ceremony while holding a deep in-breath.) *Do not, at any point, jostle or shake the brandy/sugar mixture.* The alcohol will slowly vaporize. This vaporous menstruum will rise and condense on the orange peel. As it clings to the peel, it will extract the orange's volatile oils and drip back into the pool of sweet brandy below, being one of the most subtly dramatic herbal extractions you will ever witness.

8. On day 11, remove the orange and stir in any undissolved sugar.

9. Sip some Grande Marnier.

10. Sip some more Grande Marnier.

11. Bottle and store for further sipping on all special occasions.

Next time you prepare this elixir, modify it by doing things a little differently; poke some coffee beans or clove buds into the orange peel, or use a mandarin orange, work in an herb or two, use a different brandy or a different sugar, or all of the above, whatever. You'll love this one; it's totally eccentric—the Addams family would smile fondly upon its antics.

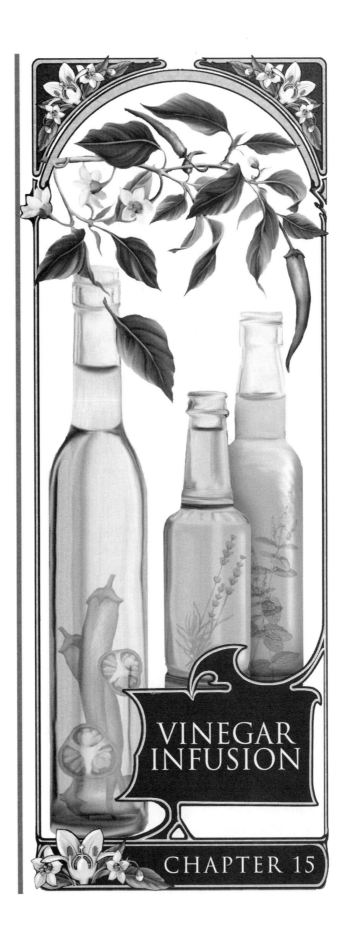

VINEGAR
INFUSION

CHAPTER 15

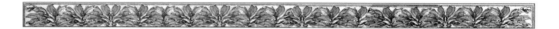

A bottle of vinegar can be found in nearly every household. It sits on a shelf ready for use in salad dressings, as taste enhancement for diverse recipes, for pickling, or as a springtime window cleaning agent; but it is hardly ever employed in modern domestic cuisine for its nutritional and medicinal properties. Vinegar's inherent abundance of nutritional components has been all but forgotten along with that of sauerkraut, yogurt, miso, and other fermented foods.

In the early nineteen hundreds, appreciation of vinegar's nutritional/medicinal properties entered the dark ages in tandem with medicinal herbs, but, unlike herbs, full appreciation of vinegar's medicinal virtues is still to be revived. When one looks closely at the inherent constituents of apple cider vinegar, its health-enhancing properties are rather astounding. Vinegar, commonly a derivative of apples or grapes (grapes being the foundation of wine vinegar), contains, in addition to sugar, starch, gluten, and gum, all the fruit's inherent mineral salts, most especially potassium, which play a major role in human metabolism, respiration, blood conditioning, and nervous system vitalization. Used topically as a facial cleanser and tonic, cosmetic vinegar infusions have a timeless reputation for being plant-wise women's favored potion for retaining the

youth and beauty of their hair and skin. All these vinegars, cosmetic, medicated, or culinary, are easily made.

An in-depth study of the medicinal properties of apple cider vinegar lies in the pages of a little book titled *Folk Medicine*, written by D.C. Jarvis, M.D. This once-renowned doctor's discussion and guide to the folk medicine practices of Vermonters illustrates common (palate-pleasing) uses of apple cider vinegar, honey, kelp, and other plant foods for sustaining health; the book documents culinary Herbalism at its folkloric best.

So many of the menstrua (oil, wine, vinegar) that were used by mankind throughout the history of Herbalism, but fell out of fashion in mainstream pharmacy because they wouldn't preserve medicinal extracts indefinitely, are nonetheless excellent for our domestic use as solvents and preservatives. These are inexpensive, nutritious, aromatic, and pleasant-tasting components we can make for ourselves at home, if so inclined. As we reestablish our experiences as medicine-making lay herbalists, it is a good idea (having a rich folkloric precedent) to embrace vinegar in the creative expansion of our contemporary solvent journeys.

The medical/pharmaceutical administrators who made the decisions to eliminate the use of vinegar (and wine) as an official menstruum in mainstream pharmacy, replacing their use with distilled alcohol and harsh solvent-preservatives, had their own good reasons for doing so. Within the medical crises intervention and heroic disease-care arena in which these doctors participate, these decisions were appropriate. But we lay herbalists are not attempting to make SWAT-drugs, and we are not assembling products designed to sit for an indeterminate amount of time in a medical dispensary (or on health food store shelves) waiting for someone to eventually come along and use them. Instead, we are making preparations that will be used in our homes and community within a year or two, and we are preparing extracts that are to be used as therapeutic agents and tonics which are formulated to promote health and prevent disease by nipping illness in the bud; these do not include highly toxic, acutely dose-specific substances. The herbs used for our purposes are nourishing, not dangerous, and in most cases yield their properties very well to a vinegar menstruum and to a wine menstruum. These two benign solvent-preservatives can adequately infuse our favorite herbs and conserve the herbal products we prepare for our domestic purposes. Bear in mind medicated vinegar has been an important player in official literature throughout medical history. The pharmacopoeias of many countries have included the Four Thieves Vinegar as an official medicine. This renowned compound is composed of vinegar infusions of a wide variety of medicinal plants — Calamus, Camphor, Cinnamon, Clove, Garlic, Nutmeg, Peppermint, Rosemary, Rue, Sage, and Wormwood, to name some that are included in this medical preparation.

These plants possess diverse components which have all been successfully (and "officially") extracted using a simple vinegar menstruum.

When deciding on a menstruum to use for your herbal extracts, keep these things in mind concerning vinegar:

• Pure, naturally fermented vinegar is non-toxic and can be tolerated by just about everyone.

• It is an excellent tonic for the entire digestive tract, and it assists one's body to regulate its acid/alkaline balance.

• It is a food high in mineral content that tastes good (dilute it or add honey to suit your taste).

• And for those who resist the use of alcohol for whatever reason, vinegar and glycerin are fine alternatives.

I encourage all who enjoy the creative process of medicine-making to experiment with the use of these out-of-fashion, currently "non-official" solvents, especially now that such excellent quality vinegars and wines are being made in the U.S. In the earlier years of the twentieth century, when the medical-pharmaceutical industry discontinued its use of medicated wines, the U.S. wasn't producing much wine of good quality, especially compared to European imports; therefore, the quality of wine was unreliable. It was also expensive and a bit of a bother to acquire, especially during the politically absurd alcohol prohibition period. But times have changed, and now the currently favored politically contrived contraband is a benign plant; no longer is government intelligence waging its domestic war on a mild menstruum. We can now buy excellent American wines made from delicious grapes grown here organically, and if you check out the vinegar section of your grocery stores you will find that the quality and diversity of this medium is likewise flourishing. This is not surprising seeing as how the fruit sources and the process of wine and vinegar production are so closely related.

A look through the marketplace meets the consumer's eye with a phenomenal array of vinegar products. One can find peculiar-shaped bottles of vinegar ranging from the acetous low-life, distilled white vinegar (made in about 48 hours in steel tanks from grain alcohol that has been heated, fermented, rapidly oxidized, and often mixed with sulfites, sugar, caramel coloring, and salt), to certified organic, raw, unpasteurized apple cider vinegars (made from the whole apple—not merely the cores and peelings) containing the natural "mother" of vinegar; or to the exotically fragrant and fruitful "balsamic" vinegars bottled with fruits of Strawberry, Blueberry, Cranberry, Pomegranate, or Raspberry; to red and white "wine vinegars" aged from 2 to 6 years in ash, cherry, or mulberry wood casks, to brown rice vinegar which is used in making the vinegared rice known as "sushi." All of these vinegars make up a fascinating community of dilute acetic acid liquids ranging from 4.2 to 6 percent acetic acid as mandated by the FDA.

HOW VINEGAR IS MADE

For those who might be interested in making some vinegar, it is an aromatic sour liquid formed by a two-step fermentation.

The first step of fermentation is accomplished when appropriate microorganisms turn sugar-containing liquids into alcohol. These base liquids can be simply a sugar and water mixture, fruit juices (Peach, Pear, Cherry, Apple, or Grape—the latter two being the most commonly used in the U.S.), sugar-containing vegetable juices, infusion of malt (barley), other grains, or rice.

The second step is accomplished by the action of the microscopic entity, *Mycoderma aceti*, which takes over and turns the alcoholic liquids (which are now hard cider, wine, beer, etc.) into a dilute acetic acid. *Mycoderma a.* is resident in all free-flowing air, and in time will find any alcoholic liquid left exposed. It also rides on the feet of vinegar flies which waste no time zeroing in on any and all alcoholic zones, most commonly the uncovered kitchen compost bucket or bowl of ultra-ripe (fermenting) fruit. *Mycoderma a.* also resides in great abundance in the naturally occurring, clear, amber-colored, thick, jellylike substance that it makes in vinegar referred to by vinegar folks as "the mother." This mother (a cloudy sediment of strand-like chains of connected protein molecules that congeal at the bottom of the bottle) can be filtered out and passed on from batch to batch as an inoculant which greatly facilitates the continuance of high-quality vinegar manufacturing.

At 75 to 90° F. the transition of alcohol to vinegar can take about four months if you're using a "mother"; but in certain circumstances this has happened from merely a few weeks to up to six months depending on the temperature during the fermentation and the length of arrival time of *Mycoderma a.*

Theoretically, one should be able to open a bottle of sweet cider, let it stand at about 70° F., and after about 5 weeks it will turn to a mild alcoholic hard cider, then to vinegar. This process can be enhanced and quickened by adding a little "mother" from a previously made batch to the fermented cider.

THE NATURE OF VINEGAR

The term vinegar is derived from the French *vin aigre*, denoting a sour wine. In the U.S., according to FDA regulations, the word vinegar (when appearing on a commercial label) without an adjective signifies the cider vinegar made from the juice of apples. Other acetous liquids may be denoted by various adjectives such as wine vinegar (grape vinegar), malt vinegar, sugar vinegar, rice vinegar, or spirit vinegar which is made directly from dilute (grain) alcohol. By further FDA regulations, all (mercantile) vinegar must contain at least 4 percent acetic acid (4 grams of acetic acid per 100 cc of volume). Viewed chemically, vinegar is a very dilute (4 to 6 percent) solution of acetic acid, containing foreign matters.

Pure (unmedicated) vinegar is known for its refrigerant qualities. It diminishes thirst, promotes the flow of saliva, and helps alleviate restlessness. It promotes the secretions of the kidneys and respiratory mucous membranes. It is well used for this purpose in managing fever, acting to diminish the frequency of the pulse and the heat of the skin. External application of vinegar helps cleanse, tone, and condition the skin. Vinegar, because of its antiseptic properties, can be sponged over the body to check perspiration odor and relieve skin inflammations, sunburn, and itching; it also reduces surface temperature of the skin in fevers. Used as a lotion, the evaporation of this liquid produces a refreshing sense of coolness on the skin; vinegar is used to sponge the surface of the skin to allay heat or with cotton cloth as a cooling discutient (a remedy that dissipates accumulations) to bruises and sprains. Used externally as an ingredient in lotions, vinegar is useful in skin conditions accompanied by dryness of the epidermis. Used as a fomentation (see Chapter Twenty-Four), vinegar's mildly stimulating nature is often beneficial for treating sprains, bruises, and bowel distress.

MEDICATED VINEGARS

Medicinal or medicated vinegars are liquid preparations intended for internal or external use and are made by macerating medicinal or culinary plants in vinegar (dilute acetic acid). This type of preparation is an eminently old one, having been in use since the days of Hippocrates, and medicinal vinegars represent one of the oldest classes of herbal Galenicals. As a menstruum, vinegar facilitates the action of stimulants for use as external applications; it augments and hastens the action of expectorants, and is most useful for preparing stimulant, astringent, and tonic gargles. *Vinegar tinctures in turn can be converted into either syrups or oxymels, for internal use* (see Chapter Twenty-Two for instruction on making syrups and oxymels).

Long before distilled spirits were known, the ancients recognized the solvent powers of vinegar, and they also realized that products made with vinegar kept for a much longer period of time (due to its antiseptic properties) than did the infusions and the decoctions prepared solely with water. Also, in time it was found that for the most part pure alkaloids, which are a highly active component in many medicinal plants, are not soluble in water, but that alkaloidal salts, which are formed upon the reaction of free based alkaloids with acids, are usually quite soluble in water. The advantage of using acidic menstrua became apparent, and experience proved the value of vinegar as a solvent in exhausting the drugs of this character, such as Goldenseal, Lobelia, Sanguinaria, and other alkaloid-containing plants.

PRESERVATION AND STORAGE

Pure vinegar is a food product that fits well in the kitchen environment, and therefore with minimal attention does well in the home pharmacy. When good, vinegar presents an agreeable penetrating odor and a pleasant acidic sour taste. When long kept, particularly if exposed to air, it can become muddy and ropy, acquire an unpleasant smell, putrefy, and lose its acidity. This may be prevented to some extent if the vinegar is boiled (pasteurized) for a few minutes, so as to coagulate and separate the gluten. The vinegar is then filtered and immediately poured into bottles and capped. This heating process possibly destroys many of the natural virtues of pure vinegar. The best way to keep one's vinegar wholesome is to keep it stored in a cool, dark location, capped, limiting its exposure to air. Medicated vinegars are kept in the same way.

In regard to the shelf life of medicinal, tonic, and culinary vinegars, my experience challenges those authorities who judge vinegar as a wimpy preservative. Just don't dilute it any further by adding water. For this reason, it is advisable to make vinegar infusions using dried plant instead of fresh plant. The water content of fresh plants can enter into the solution and dilute the vinegar to a less than 5 percent acetic acid.

I have one formula sitting on my shelf in a large amber gallon jug (Dr. John Christopher's classic Plague Formula—he used this term as a general reference to any pestilence including the flu). I assembled it more than twenty years ago. I also bottled some smaller pint jars full of this batch at the same time, then dipped the tops of all the bottles in hot wax to seal them. They've all been kicking around with me ever since. I'm mentioning this because recently we broke into one of the small flasks to see how it withstood its time exposure. Gleefully, I can report that its potency and integrity are holding up just fine. This formula consists of apple cider vinegar and a little glycerin, as co-preservatives along with some fresh pressed garlic juice and an amalgamation of nine herbal concentrates: Oak Bark, Mullein, Scullcap, Lobelia, Comfrey (before a defamation bandwagon proclaimed it toxic), Hyssop, Hydrangea, Plantain, and Wormwood. Needless to say, there are no words that can adequately describe its flavor and pizzazz, or any question why it is a strong, self-preserving, anti-plague ally.

VINEGAR INFUSION

Vinegar infusions lend themselves very well to the folk method of extraction, but are also perfectly suited for the weight/volume method (see Chapter Twelve, "Tincturing by Maceration," for details on these two methods).

To prepare medicated vinegar by infusing leaves and flowers of an herb

1. Reduce the dried herb to a moderately coarse powder.

2. Combine with pure undiluted vinegar.

3. Macerate for 10 to 14 days; shaking the mixture frequently.

4. Strain, pour into sterilized bottle, and cap.

To prepare medicated vinegar by infusing roots and barks of an herb

1. Reduce the dried herb to a moderately coarse powder.

2. Combine with pure undiluted vinegar.

3. Macerate for 10 to 14 days; shaking the mixture frequently.

4. Strain.

5. Heat the infusion to the boiling point (do not boil).

6. Filter while hot.

7. Pour into sterilized bottles and cap.

The purpose of this heating process is to coagulate any albumin which has been dissolved into the vinegar solution and remove it, for, otherwise, it can cause rapid fermentation and spoilage of the preparation. Unlike the flowers and leaves of most plants, roots and bark usually contain a large quantity of plant albumin in their tissue, and therefore usually require this added precaution.

Simple vinegar lotion recipe

This is sponged on or applied as a fomentation to soothe irritated, itching, burned, or feverish skin. Also used to cleanse the skin, check perspiration odor, and reduce the surface temperature of the skin in fever. Combine one part of vinegar with three or four parts of water.

The caustic oils of Poison Oak and Poison Ivy are fixed oils like other vegetable oils. They do not evaporate readily and therefore must be washed off of skin, clothing, and pet's fur. The simple application of pure Lavender essential oil to the affected skin is also an excellent drying, anti-inflammatory remedy for many folks.

Here is a testimonial from a grammar school teacher who, along with his associate, blissfully led their grade school munchkins through a community of Poison Oak:

"James, You asked for a follow-up on the Poison Oak remedy. Wonderful! Blisters left in 1 1/2 to 2 days, no further spreading and normalized in 4 days. Her kids went to the Dr. for theirs; it kept spreading with some relief in a week. Thanks, Tom."

Poison Oak lotion recipe

This is a recipe for a medicinal vinegar that is most useful to alleviate the discomforts associated with Poison Oak contact (I'm a West Coast native and have run into a lot of Poison Oak in my day, so I know the joy of this recipe from experience. Poison Ivy doesn't mingle with us much here in the West, however, so I have very little experience with its effect on human skin. I can only assume that this vinegar solution will also provide similar relief for those allergic to the touch of Ivy).

1. Make a strong decoction of equal parts Mugwort (*Artemisia vulgaris*) and Horsetail (*Equisetum arvense*).

2. To 2 parts of this herbal liquid, add 1 part apple cider vinegar.

3. Add 1 tablespoon of salt per cup of the above mixture of tea and vinegar. (Store it in the refrigerator.)

4. Apply externally to all affected areas. It might burn at first (which feels much better than the itching), but this soon stops.

Astringent gargle recipe

Vinegar infusion of Sage leaf (*Salvia officinalis*). Dilute 1 tablespoonful in 1/4 cup water.

Emetic vinegar recipe

Used to induce vomiting when necessary. Combine 1 oz. of Lobelia (*Lobelia inflata*) which has been ground to a moderately coarse powder with 8 ounces of vinegar. Macerate for seven days, strain, press, and filter. General dose is 1/2 oz. to 1 oz. (15 to 30 ml) per treatment.

Vinegar liniment recipe

This is used to rub onto areas of pain or soreness. Heat 1 pint apple cider vinegar, and add 1 tablespoon Cayenne red pepper.

Aromatic vinegar recipe

This is used as a mild, soothing water for bathing the forehead and temples whenever headaches and other indicators of prolonged stress arise. To 1/2 cup of alcohol, add 1 drop each of Lavender essential oil, Rosemary essential oil, Juniper essential oil, Peppermint essential oil, Cinnamon essential oil, and 2 drops each of Lemon essential oil and Clove essential oil. Shake this mixture well to thoroughly dissolve the oils in the alcohol, then add 1/2 cup of pure vinegar and mix this well. Lastly, add 1 cup of distilled water, mix this well, and let it stand for 8 days with frequent agitation. Filter the liquid and store in a tightly closed glass bottle.

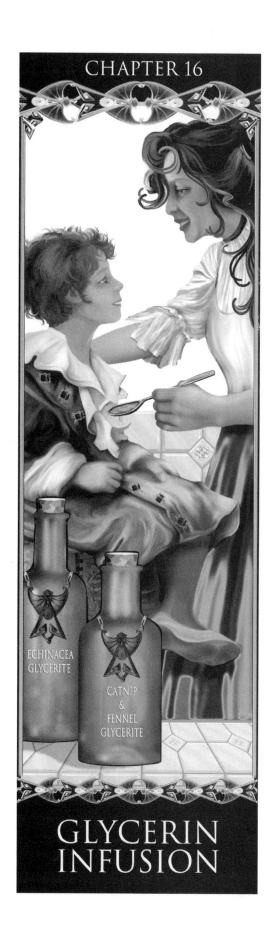

CHAPTER 16

ECHINACEA
GLYCERITE

CATNIP
&
FENNEL
GLYCERITE

GLYCERIN
INFUSION

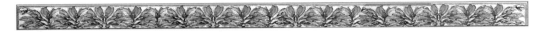

Glycerites, also known as glyco-extracts or fluid glycerates, are mixtures of medicinal substances with glycerin. The unique properties of glycerin as a menstruum provide a number of advantages. Glycerites can be easily diluted with water or alcohol without causing precipitation and are excellent to use in place of alcohol-based tinctures for children and individuals who are alcohol-intolerant. Glycerites' sweet flavor makes them especially appropriate for administering to children.

Glycerin, the sweet principle of oils, was discovered in 1789 and came into use in medicine and pharmacy around 1846. It is a liquid obtained by the hydrolysis of vegetable or animal fats or fixed oils. Glycerin can be made in several ways. One process consists of subjecting fatty bodies to the action of water at a high temperature under pressure, whereby the fats, which are *glycerides* or esters of the fatty acids, are broken up into glycerin and fatty acids. The water supplies the hydrogen and oxygen necessary to effect the change. Glycerin can be synthesized by heating trichlorpropane (a petroleum product) with water at 365° F. I recommend that you use non-synthetic vegetable glycerin. Chemically, glycerin belongs to the class of alcohols, and is sometimes termed *glycerol* or *glyceric alcohol*.

The solvent and preservative properties of glycerin (which often protect against oxidation) as well as its agreeable taste and stable consistency render it one of the most valuable liquids known to pharmacy. It may be added to finished water/alcohol extracts or used in a menstruum mixed with water, alcohol, or vinegar, or any combination of the three. Its range of solvency lies somewhere between that of water and alcohol, and it will extract a variety of constituents that makes it useful in cases where neither water nor alcohol are appropriate. It is exceptionally effective in a menstruum for herbs containing considerable tannin, as it reduces precipitation of tannins and alkaloids. However, glycerin will not dissolve or mix with resins or fixed oils, so it is not suitable as a menstruum for resinous or oily herb extracts. It will preserve volatile oils (though not indefinitely) even if it does not extract them efficiently.

Glycerin is slightly antiseptic and has anti-fermentative properties that are excellent, although inferior to those of alcohol. When diluted, glycerin is demulcent, emollient, soothing, and healing. Undiluted, it is irritant and stimulant, arousing activity. It is useful in keeping substances moist, due to its tendency to absorb water from the air, and its properties adapt it for many medicinal purposes, both external and internal. Glycerin does not evaporate at normal temperatures and produces a sensation of warmth to the skin and tongue.

At present, making glycerites is a somewhat neglected art. However, with the current popularity of alcohol-free glycerites for children's health care, this herbal delivery vehicle is coming into its own. There is still, unfortunately, only limited experience in the herbal pharmacy world from which to draw. The following processes are those that I have explored. I encourage further creative experimentation and sharing among herbal medicine-makers, so we can revive and teach this valuable extraction technique. The dawn of a glycerated herbal renaissance is at hand.

Common belief has it that the presence of 50 percent glycerin by volume will serve as a good preservative for an herbal solution. It has been my experience, however, this is not always the case when storing herbal glycerites. I have found that 60 percent to 75 percent glycerin is more reliable and suggest that, if some alcohol is tolerable, adding 10 percent to 15 percent alcohol to the 50 percent glycerin might be ideal. This is still a greatly reduced alcohol content, and the flavor will remain superior.

Bear this in mind when doing your math. Because pure (absolute) glycerin absorbs water quite readily from the air, the commercial glycerin available already contains about 5 percent water by volume. When you calculate an appropriate amount of (absolute) glycerin for its preservative action in a custom menstruum, allow for this. If you make a menstruum of 50 percent glycerin and 50 percent water figuring that 50 percent glycerin in the solution will be

an adequate preservative, remember that, in fact, this proportion will contain only approximately 45 percent (absolute) glycerin by volume and approximately 55 percent water (approximately 5 percent of which was resident in the commercial glycerin). This is why I suggest using 55–60 percent glycerin by volume in the menstruum for extracting dry plant material. When extracting fresh undried plant, the plant's juices must also be taken into consideration. If it is a very juicy plant such as fresh Dandelion, Cleavers, or Scullcap I make it a 1:2 w/v using 80–90 percent glycerin. For the relatively unjuicy fresh plants that will not dilute the menstruum to any great extent like Oregon Grape, Red Root, or Uva Ursi, one can use less glycerin. This is all part of the experimentation and sharing of experience by herbalists that needs to be attended to in order to revive this portion of our craft.

PRESERVATION AND STORAGE

Preserve all glycerites in airtight, light-resistant containers and avoid exposure to direct sunlight and excessive heat. Refrigerate when possible.

DOSAGE

Glycerites are normally more concentrated than either infusions or decoctions and therefore stronger. The dosage to be taken can be smaller. The dosage again depends on the herb at hand and the size of the person taking the glycerite. When using mild tonic herbs take up to five droppersful in a glass of water 2 to 3 times a day; for a more intense herb use anywhere from 10 to 25 drops 3 to 4 times a day.

MAKING GLYCERITES USING DRIED PLANT MATERIAL

Folk Method

See Chapter Twelve for the definition and discussion of "folk method."

1. Grind dried herb to a moderately coarse powder (mcp).

2. Place the powdered herb into a large jar that can be tightly closed.

3. If blending other solvents (water, vinegar, alcohol) with glycerin for your menstruum, be sure to mix together all the liquids of the menstruum thoroughly *in a separate container* before adding them to the powdered plant material.

4. Add prepared menstruum to powdered herb.

5. Stir the mixture well, so that all the herb is wet.

6. Add sufficient menstruum to the wet herb, so that about 1/4 inch of extra menstruum sits atop the herb; if the herb is floating, 1/4 inch below the herb.

7. Cap jar tightly★ and shake contents well.

8. Check the jar after 12 hours. If the herb has absorbed the menstruum, add a sufficient amount of menstruum to re-establish the 1/4 inch of extra liquid.

9. Shake the glycerite frequently for 14 days.

10. Decant liquid, press the remaining wet pulp, and combine these two liquids (see discussions about decanting and pressing in Chapter Twenty-Five).

11. Filter if desired (many glycerites filter very slowly).

12. Bottle, tightly cap, and label.

Dr. Edward Shook's Method★★

8 oz.	Powdered herb
2 quarts	Distilled water (plus a little extra held aside)
1/4 oz.	Potassium sulfate (vitriolated tartar)
8 oz.	Glycerin

Dissolve the potassium sulfate in water, add the powdered herb, and simmer until the liquid is reduced to 1 quart. Strain and retain this decoction and the herb. Again, add enough water to just cover the herb. Simmer this for 10 minutes. Strain and retain the liquid. Combine the two liquors, and add the glycerin, blending thoroughly. Cool the mixture, bottle in amber-colored bottles, and store in a cool place. Doing the math shows this mixture to be a little less than 20 percent glycerin; I suggest full refrigeration as an added preservative.

★ It is important to clean and wipe off the rim of the jar thoroughly before placing the lid on and tightening it down. After wiping the rim it is even advisable to place a piece of waxed paper between the rim and the lid as a gasket. This assures that you will have a tight seal preventing the loss of any menstruum that can occur due to constant shaking of the liquid contents. You will know if there has been any leakage by the discovery of narrow streams of extract appearing on the outside surface of the jar.

★★From *Advanced Treatise on Herbology*

The Weight to Volume Method

See Chapter Twelve for further discussion and details on preparing weight to volume (w/v) extracts.

Preparing the custom menstruum

• Sample measurements for making a 1:4 w/v or 25% glycerite. YIELD: ABOUT 800 ml

200 Gm	Dry herb (in moderately coarse powder)
480 ml	Glycerin (60 percent by volume of the menstruum)
320 ml	Distilled water

• Sample measurements for making a 1:5 w/v or 20% glycerite which includes 5% vinegar. YIELD: ABOUT 1000 ml

200 Gm	Dry herb (in moderately coarse powder)
600 ml	Glycerin (60 percent by volume of the menstruum)
50 ml	Vinegar (5 percent)
350 ml	Distilled water

• Sample measurements for making a 1:10 w/v or 10% glycerite which includes 15% alcohol. YIELD: ABOUT 2000 ml

200 Gm	Dry herb (in moderately coarse powder)
1000 ml	Glycerin (50 percent by volume of the menstruum)
300 ml	Ethyl alcohol (15 percent)
700 ml	Distilled water

Making the glycerite

1. Powder and weigh dried plant and place the powder into a large jar that can be tightly closed.

2. Prepare custom menstruum (see samples above). When blending other solvents (water, vinegar, alcohol) with glycerin for your menstruum, be sure to mix together all the liquids of the menstruum thoroughly *in a separate container* before adding them to the powdered plant material.

3. Add menstruum to powdered herb.

4. Stir well *making sure all of the powdered herb is wet.*

5. Cap jar tightly and shake contents well.

6. Shake glycerite frequently for 14 days.

7. Decant, press, and filter (most glycerites filter very slowly).

8. Bottle, tightly cap, and label.

The McQuade-Izard Folk Method

This process makes delightfully colored and flavorful extracts.

1. No matter what fresh herb you're using, fill your maceration container, packing it to *medium* density.

2. Dump this out and weigh it; note the weight.

3. Transfer this fresh herb to a blender.

4. Add sufficient (measured amount of) glycerin to cover the herb and blend until blender top is warm.

This process coats the fresh herb with the glycerin and to a large extent eliminates oxidation of the plant components as the blades break down cell walls.

5. Add more glycerin as needed to fully cover the herb (keep note of the amount added). Fresh plants carry their own water, so most fresh plants can be blended directly with glycerin without the addition of water. This depends, however, on the water content of the herb (make notes).

6. Pour blended marc and menstruum back into the maceration container and cap tightly.

7. Agitate twice daily for 14 days.

8. Strain, press, and store in amber-colored bottles.

With certain herbs, you may want to add more glycerin after maceration and pressing to improve preservation. Be aware that this will dilute the strength of the finished glycerite. Shelf-life will be between 1 and 3 years depending on the water content of the fresh plant used. The more water content by volume, the less preservative power the glycerin will have. Make appropriate adjustments.

The Weight to Volume (w/v) Method

Preparing the custom menstruum

• Sample measurements for making a 1:2 w/v or 50% fresh, juicy plant glycerite

400 Gm	Fresh herb (chopped)
800 ml	Glycerin (100 percent by volume of the menstruum)

• Sample measurements for making a 1:2 w/v or 50% fresh, not-so-juicy plant glycerite

400 Gm	Fresh herb (chopped)
600 ml	Glycerin (75 percent by volume of the menstruum)
200 ml	Distilled water

Making the glycerite

1. Chop the plant into small pieces and place them in a blender.

2. Prepare custom menstruum.

3. Cover the herb with menstruum and blend it like making a smoothie. (You will have to use enough of the menstruum to cover the blender blades. Use as much of the measured menstruum as you can to make the mixture churn actively in the blender. You may not be able to use all the menstruum in this blending stage.)

4. Pour the liquefied ingredients into a jar and cap tightly. *Be sure you have added all the measured menstruum to the herb during or after the blending process, so as to maintain the intended weight to volume proportion.*

5. Shake the glycerite frequently for 14 days.

6. Decant, press, and filter.

7. Bottle, tightly cap, and label.

Herbs on the "35 Herbs and a Fungus" List That Are Well Prepared As a Glycerite

Suggested percent of glycerin which is offered is a starting place for your experimentation.

	PLANT PART	WEIGHT TO VOLUME	% OF GLYCERIN IN MENSTRUUM
Burdock	fresh root	1:2	80
	dry root	1:5	60
	seed	1:5	60
Chamomile	fresh flowers	1:2	90
	dry flowers	1:4	60
Cleavers[1]	fresh whole plant	1:1.5	100
Dandelion	fresh root	1:2	80
	dry root	1:5	60
	fresh leaves and flowers	1:2	100 (this is a juicy plant)
	dried leaves	1:5	60
Echinacea	fresh root	1:2	80
	recently dried root[2]	1:5	60
Elder	fresh berries	1:2	80–90
	flowers	1:5	60
Fennel	crushed seed	1:3	60
Ginger	fresh root	1:2	100
	dry root	1:4	60
Goldenseal	fresh root	1:2	90 with 5% vinegar
	dry root and/or leaf	1:5	60 with 5% vinegar
Hawthorn	fresh leaf, flower, berries	1:2	80
	dry	1:5	60
Mugwort	dry herb	1:5	60
Mullein	fresh flowers	1:2	80
	dry	1:4	60
Nettle	fresh herb	1:2	90
	dry herb or root	1:4	60
Oat	fresh "unripe milky stage" seed	1:1.75 or 1:2	60–80
	dry plant	1:4	60
Peppermint	fresh plant	1:2	80
	dry plant	1:4	60
Scullcap	fresh herb	1:1.75 or 1:2	90
	recently dried	1:5	60
Siberian Ginseng[3]	powdered root	1:5	60 with 5% vinegar
Uva Ursi	leaf	1:5	60
Vitex	berries	1:4 or 1:5	60
Valerian	fresh root	1:1.5 or 1:2	100
	recently dried root[4]	1:5	60

1. Dried plant is not very active.

2. Good-quality echinacea root does not survive long storage.

3. It is very difficult to find authentic Siberian Gingseng in the marketplace, best to buy the authentic extract.

4. Good-quality Valerian root does not survive long storage.

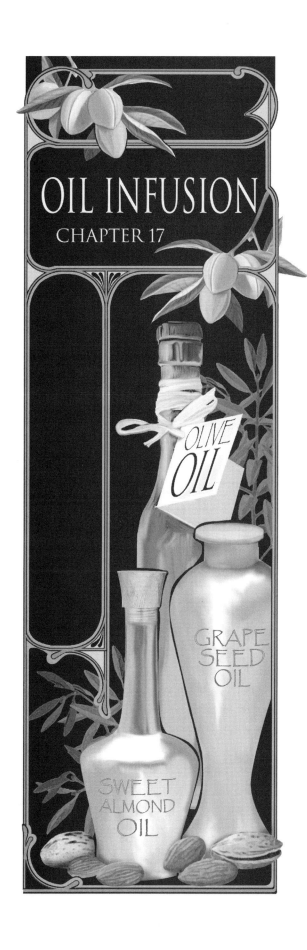

OIL INFUSION
CHAPTER 17

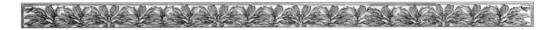

Oil infusions are an infusion of medicinal or culinary herbs in a fixed oil menstruum. Medicinal oil infusions, when applied to the skin, form a protective covering and are used to hold other therapeutic or cosmetic agents to the skin, facilitating the absorption of the herbal remedies. Oil infusions prepared for use as food carry the nutrients, flavor, and aroma of culinary herbs to the gourmet tongue, greatly enhancing the nutritional and aesthetic pleasures of the herbalist's cuisine.

Many fixed oils in themselves are well utilized as foods and as medicines. Medically, these oils are very soothing substances, and therapeutically they are most useful because of their ability to soften the keratin layer of the skin. This renders the skin pliable and tends to prevent cracking of the skin's surface.

Fixed oils are obtained from both the vegetable and the animal kingdom. They are often called fatty oils, as they are chemically the same as fats. They are more or less unctuous (smooth and greasy) to the touch, and in a liquid condition and dropped on paper, leave a permanent oily spot. Individual oils vary greatly in their point of congelation: Olive oil becomes solid at a little above 32° F., whereas Flaxseed oil can remain fluid at 4° F. below zero. Pure fixed oils have little

taste or smell. They are lighter than water and they do not evaporate easily; however, they do boil at about 600° F. and are converted into vapor at this temperature. Heated in open air, especially with the aid of a wick, fixed oils do take fire and burn with a bright and sooty flame generating much heat. These oils are quite soluble with volatile oils, but are insoluble in water. However, they are capable of being mixed (miscible) with water by the assistance of an emulsifier, forming mixtures which are called emulsions (see "Lotions & Creams," Chapter Nineteen). Fixed oils comprise most of the oils in common use, such as Olive, Almond, Sesame, Cod liver, and Castor oil (and mineral oils). They are well used as menstrua in warm to hot infusions and decoctions to abstract resins, oleoresins, and essential oils.

Some oils, such as Castor bean oil and Flaxseed (Linseed) oil, form fatty acids which act as drugs when decomposed in the intestines. These unsaturated fatty acids are slightly irritant to the mucous membrane of the alimentary canal, and as the oils decompose (hydrolyze) in the intestines, they can render a laxative effect. This can be a mild cathartic action, as when using Flaxseed oil, or it can be rather intense, as when using Castor oil. Castor oil also differs from the other oils in that it contains hydroxy fatty acids and, therefore, has slightly different solubility properties. It is soluble to a fair extent in cold 95 percent absolute alcohol, while the other oils are not. It is also miscible with such substances as Peruvian balsam, whereas the other oils are not and will separate on standing.

PRESERVATION AND STORAGE

Oils remain unchanged for a great length of time when kept in cool airtight glass containers. Rancidity in oils renders them useless in herbal pharmacy and as foods. It is extremely important to protect oils from air, light, heat, and moisture. Store all oils in a cool location (a refrigerator or freezer whenever possible) in tightly sealed, amber bottles. Fill the bottles as full as possible to eliminate the oil's prolonged contact with air during storage.

OIL INFUSIONS USING DRIED PLANTS

The "Folk Method"

1. Grind the dried herb to as fine a powder as possible.

2. Place the powdered herb in a jar that can be capped tightly and add a fixed oil of your choice (Olive, Sesame, Almond, etc.). Use enough oil to completely wet the herb.

3. Stir the mixture well.

4. Let the herb settle, then add enough oil to cover the wet herb an additional 1/4 inch. Some lighter herbs will float at first, so let there be an additional 1/4 inch below instead.

5. Many dried herbs will absorb this extra 1/4 inch of oil. Check your mixture 24 hours later, and if absorption has occurred, add enough oil to re-establish the extra measure of oil.

6. Cap the jar tightly.

7. Place it in a thick paper bag or box to keep light out, and place in the sun for 7 to 10 days (a warm to hot infusion, depending on the weather).

8. Shake or stir the mixture every couple of hours each day or at least several times a day.

9. When the infusion is completed, strain the oil from the herb and press the remaining pulp.

10. Allow the infusion to sit still indoors for several days, then decant and filter out sediment.

11. Bottle in glass containers, cap tightly, label, and store in a cool dark place.

The Digestion Method

1. Grind dried herb to a powder.

2. Add a fixed oil of your choice, in the proportion of 1 part powder by weight to 5 parts oil, or a suitable ratio depending on the nature of the powder. Quantitative ratios are not really critical for this type of preparation, for its vital energy is not really dependent on quantitative principles.

3. Place in a water bath, an electric "meat roaster vat," yogurt maker, or some other apparatus having a thermostatic control that allows you to maintain a consistent temperature of around 100° F. (Unfortunately, a crock pot's lowest range is too hot, usually about 150° F. or more. Some folks place their oils in an oven using the heat of the pilot light, but beware of this technique. There is something about an oil infusion quietly macerating in an oven that inspires others in the household to preheat the oven to 350° F. for a spontaneous baking spree.

4. Stir the mixture well, set the heat thermostat at approximately 100° F., and cover the herb/oil mixture.

5. This maceration (soaking) process using low heat is called *digestion*. Ideally, you want to continue this mild heat process for 10 days and nights at approximately 100°F., stirring it every two hours. Use a yogurt thermometer to monitor the temperature.

6. When the infusion is completed, strain the oil from the herb and press the remaining pulp. (If you strain the oil while it is still warm it flows more easily.)

7. Let sediment accumulate for a few days, decant, and filter the oil.

8. Bottle, cap tightly, label, and store in a cool dark place.

Hot Infusion Method

Taken From a Late Nineteenth Century Physio-Medical Text

1. "Infused oils may be prepared from the finely powdered herbs: Cayenne, Fucus (Bladderwrack seaweed), Lobelia, and Comfrey in proportions of 1 part herb powder by weight to 10 parts fixed oil by volume, by the process of decoction. Such infused oils may be prescribed singly or in combinations as mildly stimulating, relaxing, or toning liniments for various skeletal problems, or as the basis for stronger preparations when the therapeutic affect is reinforced by adding more powerful essential oils.

2. "The following example illustrates the method for infused oil of Cayenne, which serves as a model for all others:

Cayenne—in fine powder	100 Gm	(4 oz)
Fixed oil	1 liter	(40 oz)

3. "Mix together smoothly, place in a closed vessel over a water-bath and digest at 140°–160° F. for 4 hours. Then remove from heat, allow to cool, and leave for 12 hours for the powder to settle. Then carefully pour off the clear oil."

I include this method because I think it is interesting to see how different (expert) medicine-makers do their stuff. I would never take my oils up to this high a temperature, but these Physio-medicalists were passionate therapists and pharmacists, extremely competent in their practice—blessed be diversity.

National Formulary IV (1916) Method

YIELD ABOUT 1000 ml

The air-dried herb	100 Gm in No. 30 powder
Alcohol	100 ml 190-proof (grain) ethyl alcohol
Ammonia water★	2 ml
Sesame oil	1000 ml

1. Moisten the herb with the alcohol and ammonia water (already mixed together).

2. Macerate for six hours in a covered glass or enameled steel vessel.

3. Add the sesame oil.

4. Using a water bath, warm this mixture at a temperature between 120° and 140° F. in an open vessel, stirring frequently until the alcohol and ammonia water are dissipated.

5. Then transfer the mixture to a strainer, express the residue, and filter the strained oil.

★ Ammonia water (USP Dilute Solution of Ammonia) is prepared by mixing 9-10 Gm of ammonia (NH_3) into 100 cc of distilled water. This solution deteriorates rapidly in open containers.

OIL INFUSIONS USING FRESH PLANTS

The "Herb School Method"

1. (Optional) Wilt the fresh herb for 12 hours (do not dry it).

2. Chop the freshly cut or wilted herb to a fine pulp or grind plant in a metal Corona grain mill, or in some other suitable instrument, and place the resultant mash into a "meat roaster vat," yogurt maker, or some other apparatus with a thermostatic control that allows you to maintain a consistent 100° F. temperature.

3. Add a fixed oil of your choice, enough to make your mixture thick-juicy-wet (Olive or Sesame oil are recommended, Sweet Almond oil will be used for skin care).

4. Stir the mixture well and smell it (make an olfactory note of the nature and quality of the aroma).

5. Set the heat thermostat at 100° F. and cover the herb/oil mixture. With some plants, I leave them uncovered for the first couple of days to allow moisture to evaporate. Ideally, you want to digest this oil infusion for 10 days and nights at 100° F., stirring and smelling it every 2 hours. Use a yogurt thermometer to monitor the temperature.

6. If this fresh plant oil begins to ferment (a change in its aroma will alert you), raise the temperature to 150° F., immediately let it fall back to 100° F., and continue the procedure. (This usually eliminates the opportunistic activities of the fermentation-inducing organisms.)

7. When the infusion is completed, strain the oil from the herb (this is accomplished more easily when the oil is still warm) and press the remaining pulp.

8. *Now:* At this point we have created a problem that needs to be dealt with. The juices of the undried herb introduced water into the infusion. The presence of water in a fatty oil, as mentioned before, favors fermentation and rancidity, which will ruin your medicinal oil. *All the water must be removed before permanent storage.*

9. *So:* Allow your oil infusion to sit in a clear glass jar undisturbed for 4 or 5 days.

10. The water and other impurities (gunk) will settle to the bottom, at which point you can decant (gently pour off) the oil or draw it off with a basting syringe and then discard the water/gunk portion.

11. It is advisable to let this decanted oil sit undisturbed for a few more days and check it for remaining water impurities.

12. When you are satisfied that the oil is free of all water, bottle, cap tightly, label, and store it in a cool dark place.

Physio-Medicalist Method for Making Fresh Plant Cold Oil Infusion

According to William Cook, physio-medical physician and herbal pharmacist, "Just as fresh plant tinctures are in many cases better than their dry plant counterparts, so lotions, ointments, and other forms of surface medication based upon fresh plant oil infusions may be preferred to dry plant preparations."…"Because of its greater oleaginous property, Olive oil is preferred as the basis for these, whereas infused oils intended for liniments or rubbing oils are better prepared from rape-seed oil which is less greasy….Where it is desired to avoid the use of heat in preparing the infused oil, and this especially applies to preparations from flowers the following method is used":

1. Fill a canning jar with alternate layers of cotton-wool and flowers, each layer not exceeding 1/4 inch.

2. Layer these lightly and do not compress them, so that inter-spaces are left.

3. Fill up the jar with Olive oil.

4. Seal the jar with cap and screw lid.

5. Set aside in a cool dark place for one month.

6. Remove the contents of the jar, keeping the layers of cotton-wool and flowers together and intact as far as possible.

7. Place in a press and press out the oil by slow steady pressure. This removes the plant material and cotton-wool.

8. Filter the oil infusion if necessary to remove particles and dust.

9. Store in brown glass bottles.

As a precaution, I suggest that you refer back to method 1, The "Herb School Method," and proceed with steps 8 through 12.

Herbs on the "35 Herbs and a Fungus" List That Are Well Prepared As Oil Infusions

DRY PLANT OIL INFUSIONS

Burdock root

Calendula

Cayenne

Comfrey leaf and root

Elder flower

Ginger

Golden seal leaf and rhizome

Marshmallow root

Mullein leaf

Nettle leaf

Plantain

Yarrow

FRESH PLANT OIL INFUSIONS

Mullein flowers

St. John's Wort flowering tops, especially in the flower bud stage

Garlic★

Arnica★★

★ Garlic is included in this list because it works so well when blended in equal parts with Mullein flower and Calendula flower oils for making an earache remedy. One or 2 drops of this blend are dropped into the ear canal and the ear is plugged with a small cotton ball. Please note that I am recommending here the use of an oil infusion of Garlic, not Garlic juice.

★★ Arnica is included in this list because it works so well when blended in equal parts with Calendula and St. John's Wort oils to make an excellent application for soothing traumatic injuries (from very little traumas to major ones). Rub the blend of oils directly onto the injured parts, especially bumped, bruised, and/or crushed parts. If the injury includes an open wound, rub the oil compound around it; it is not advisable to put Arnica directly on an open wound. Arnica is equally well prepared as a dry plant oil.

CHAPTER 18

SALVE

LIP BALM

ear
oil

LIP
BALM

MacBroach's
OINTMENT

LIP BALM

LIP BALM

OINTMENT,
SALVES & BALMS

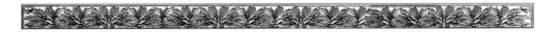

Salves (also called ointments or unguents) are semi-solid fatty herbal mixtures normally prepared as external healing mixtures. They soften when applied to the skin, and provide a healing, emollient, protective, nourishing, or counter-irritant effect. Salves can vary in consistency from greasy to thick and hard, depending on the base used, the elements mixed together, and the purpose intended for its production. A balm is simply a salve that contains a relatively high amount of volatile oils. Upon application it delivers a notably intense cloud of aromatic vapors.

The base for most salves is a mixture of a wax and a fixed oil, usually mixed or infused with medicinal plant substances (see Chapter Seventeen, "Oil Infusions"). The oil enhances the absorption of the medicinal substances into the skin, and the wax gives firmness to the finished salve for ease of application. I prefer to make my salves with vegetable oils, although some people use animal fats. Often, essential oils and/or other solid or liquid materials are incorporated during the salve-making process.

Body heat melts the wax, and the oil fosters quick absorption of the plant's medicinal constituents into the skin. Generally, it is best to massage the salve into the skin. With counter-irritant salves high in

Cayenne, or salves that incorporate stimulating or warming essential oils (like Ginger, Peppermint, or Camphor), massage is not normally required, unless, of course, it feels good, in which case rub with gusto.

PRESERVATION AND STORAGE

Salves are well stored in dark-colored or opaque glass, tightly capped jars that have openings sufficiently large to allow easy access to the semi-solid ingredients. Salves are best kept in cool locations. They don't preserve as well in locations where they are subjected to continual melting and re-cooling (like in automobile glove compartments and similar environments). In some instances the presence of benzoin as a preservative in salves can cause irritation on tender and already irritated skins.

DOSAGE

Use as much salve as needed, but it can be bothersome to leave too much on the skin surface unless it is to be covered.

GENERAL NOTES

• Other ingredients such as vitamin E, honey, or essential oils, etc., can be added and stirred into a salve mixture as a very last step before pouring the salve into its final storage container(s).

• The best way to add essential oils to a salve is to drop them into the container *just prior* to pouring in the warm salve mixture.

• Some of the ingredients (other than the infused herbs and essential oils) added to the salve mixture can separate out and settle to the bottom of the container during the sitting and cooling period. While the salve is sitting in the final storage container(s), still a little warm, becoming firm, but not quite hardened (you'll know the right moment), stir the entire mixture (especially the bottom portion) briskly with a chopstick. This will suspend all the ingredients throughout the salve base, which will now quickly harden and retain the added ingredients in a suspended condition. But now the top surface will look weird. If you care about this, place the uncapped jars of salve in a hot oven for a few moments. This will melt the very top surface of the salve rendering it flat, smooth and, to some folks, more visually appealing. Or melt the tops by heating them with the hot air of a hair dryer. I used to use a hand-held propane torch (available in any hardware store) for this job when preparing large quantities of salves for my small cottage industry. Let the surfaces harden, then cap, and store them in a cool location.

★ The volume of herb will vary greatly depending on its density; 1 ounce of powdered root or seed will usually present considerably less volume than 1 ounce of powdered leaf or flowers. It is important that the final proportion of herb to oil is such that it renders the herb quite wet with oil. It is also recommended that you powder the herb to a moderately coarse powder whenever possible to expose more surface area to the oil menstruum.

TO MAKE A SIMPLE SALVE STARTING WITH DRIED HERB(S), FIXED OIL, AND BEESWAX

1. To each cup of fixed oil (Olive oil, Sesame oil, Almond oil, etc.) stir in approximately 1 to 2 oz.★ of dry herb or a formulated combination of dried herbs.

2. Place this mixture in an uncovered container. Put it into an oven leaving the oven door slightly open or place it over a burner using a flame shield to disperse the direct heat. Heat the mixture at a low heat (preferably between 100 and 140° F.) for 3 to 5 hours. Check the temperature of the mixture periodically, each time stirring it thoroughly.

3. Line a large strainer with a cotton muslin cloth.

4. Remove the mixture and, while it is still warm and flowing easily, pour it into the strainer to separate the spent herbs from the oil infusion. Let this sit until well-drained, press out remaining oil if you want to, and discard the marc.

5. Measure the amount of infused oil you have at this point and place it in a suitable container over low heat.

6. Add shaved beeswax (approximately 1 oz. of wax per cup of oil) to the oil infusion and proceed as outlined in steps 4 through 10 on the following page.

There is no other wax as precious and excellent as that which the bees make for us. The high chemistry of its fine texture, subtle aroma, and soft golden hues is yet another mark of perfection inherent to the varied skills of these master herbalists. Send the apiarian workers and their fecund queens your gratitude while making salves, lotions, and creams. In nature's way, they'll appreciate your regard.

TO MAKE A SIMPLE SALVE FROM A
PREVIOUSLY PREPARED HERBAL OIL INFUSION

1. Measure 1 cup of a previously prepared herbal oil infusion or 1 cup of a formulated combination of two or more oil infusions.

2. Set aside a small amount of the same oil or oil blend which can be added later, if necessary, to alter the consistency of the salve (see step 8).

3. Pour the measured oil into a stainless steel, earthenware, unchipped enamel, or glassware container that can be heated.

4. Add 1 ounce of beeswax that has been shaved or grated into small pieces. Set aside a small amount of beeswax that can be added later if you decide to alter the consistency of your salve (see step 8).

5. Warm this oil infusion and beeswax mixture over low heat until the wax is fully melted.

6. Remove the mixture from the heat and dip a metal spoon (or like instrument) into the warm mixture.

7. Place this spoon into a freezer, a refrigerator, or the coldest spot available, so that the salve sample will cool quickly.

8. When cool, the salve will have hardened on the spoon, allowing you to test its firmness without waiting for the entire pan of salve to harden. If the sample on the spoon is too soft for your purposes, add a little more wax to the pan of warm salve; if the sample is too hard, add a little more of the oil infusion.

9. Repeat the teaspoon test until your salve consistency is perfectly suited to your purposes.

10. Pour the liquid salve from the pan into appropriate containers, and let it cool and harden.

VEGETABLE LARD VEGAN SALVE

Pure commercial vegetable lard is a sterile medium composed of hydrogenated soybean and palm oils. Vegetable lard hardens at room temperature, making it acceptable when a salve is needed quickly. Lard has the immediate advantage of requiring no beeswax for hardening. Using the lard as a catalyst to draw out the value of fresh cut or dried herbs is quite appropriate for immediate use, since with no lengthy storage time spoilage will not be a factor. Actually, hydrogenated oils, although considered by many nutritionists to be unwholesome food for many reasons, are less likely to go rancid than unhydrogenated vegetable oils. That works for us here.

1. Gather either freshly cut or dried herbs. Have the fresh herbs chopped and ready. It is okay if they wilt. Use approximately 1 cup chopped fresh herb to 1 cup vegetable lard. Crush or powder the dry herbs as much as possible. Use approximately 1/2 cup powdered dry herb to 1 cup lard.

2. Melt the lard in a saucepan over low heat. Leave the pot uncovered throughout the preparation, so the lard will not overheat and some of the fresh herb's water content can evaporate.

3. As soon as the lard is melted, carefully stir in the herbs.

4. Allow the herbs to steep in the lard over low heat (deep-frying them is a big mistake).

5. Stir the herbs periodically to determine when they have surrendered their properties to the oil, approximately 1 hour.

6. When satisfied that the decoction is completed, remove the pot from the heat and pour the contents into a cotton-muslin lined wire strainer.

7. Strain out the liquid salve, pour into jar, cap, and let it cool.

Be careful when heating lard; it can ignite when it gets very hot.

PETROLEUM JELLY AROMATIC SALVE (A BALM)

Do not use plastic containers to store any medium that contains volatile oils; the oils will eat the plastic over time.

Clear, unmedicated petroleum jelly is a sterile inorganic medium that, when applied, is not absorbed into the skin. It can therefore act merely as a carrier for volatile oils. Commercial petroleum jelly (Vaseline® is a brand name) is easily attained. This is an excellent substance to use for quickly preparing an essential oil carrier that can be applied into the nostrils in a small amount. Antiseptic, decongestive essential oils can be inhaled this way during the day to relieve nasal and upper respiratory congestion.

Some appropriate essential oils to use for antiseptic and decongestant properties are Eucalyptus, Rosemary, Pine, Peppermint, Cypress, and Lavender.

Note:

• Have paper towels ready—this stuff is sticky.

• A "square-handled" chopstick is a very handy tool for manipulating this medium.

• Two level tablespoonsful of petroleum jelly fill a small 1 fl. oz. (30 ml) salve jar perfectly.

• 30–50 drops of any combination of the above essential oils is a good amount to add to each 1 fl. oz. of petroleum jelly.

• Plan to spend some time cleaning up; this petroleum jelly stuff is resilient. (I suggest using paper towels initially, then soap and hot water.)

To Prepare an Aromatic Medicated Vehicle

1. Purchase a jar of unmedicated petroleum jelly. This is readily available in drug stores in 1.75 oz. (49 Gm), 3.75 oz. (106 Gm), 13 oz. (368 Gm) and 15 oz. (425 Gm) sizes.

2. Melt the petroleum jelly over a very low heat. Do not overheat it.

3. Just as the jelly turns liquid, move it away from the flame.

4. Add the drops of volatile oils to the liquid and stir them in quickly. For starters, I suggest using 8–12 drops of each single essential oil (or 30–50 drops total) per 30 Gm of jelly (adjust this + or − as you see fit). Use up to 4 different essential oils per 30 Gm.

5. Immediately pour the warm salve into a glass container(s).

6. Cap immediately so volatile oils do not escape salve as it cools.

ETHYL-OIL SALVE

This procedure renders a most superior salve from the dried resinous, golden-orange flowers of the *Calendula officinalis* in particular, and/or from any other dried plant which has primarily alcohol-soluble properties that are not particularly oil-soluble (i.e., Arnica, Goldenseal, Gumweed, Chaparral).

1. Weigh out dried powdered herb (let's say 120 Gm).

2. Measure an equal amount by volume of 190-proof ethyl alcohol (that will be 120 ml).

3. Mix the herb with the alcohol and stir the mixture until all of the herb is moist.

4. Place this in a tightly sealed container and let it macerate for 24 hours.

5. Measure out 6 parts by volume of vegetable oil (that will be 720 ml).

6. Pour the oil into a blender and add the moist herb.

7. Blend this at a medium speed until the blender basket feels warm.

8. Strain by pouring into a muslin cloth-lined strainer and press.

9. Pour the liquid into a double boiler and heat over a low flame for a few hours until all the alcohol has evaporated (do not burn the oil). Check to see if any alcohol is still present by carefully placing a lighted match to the surface of the oil.

10. Bottle the oil in tightly capped containers and store in a cool place for future use, or add sufficient beeswax to transform it into a salve as outlined in steps 4 through 10 on page 204.

Herbs on the "35 Herbs and a Fungus" List That Are Well Prepared As Salves

Burdock root

Calendula

Cayenne

Comfrey leaf and/or root

Elder flower

Ginger

Goldenseal leaf and rhizome

Marshmallow root

Mullein leaf

Nettle leaf

Plantain

St. John's Wort

Yarrow

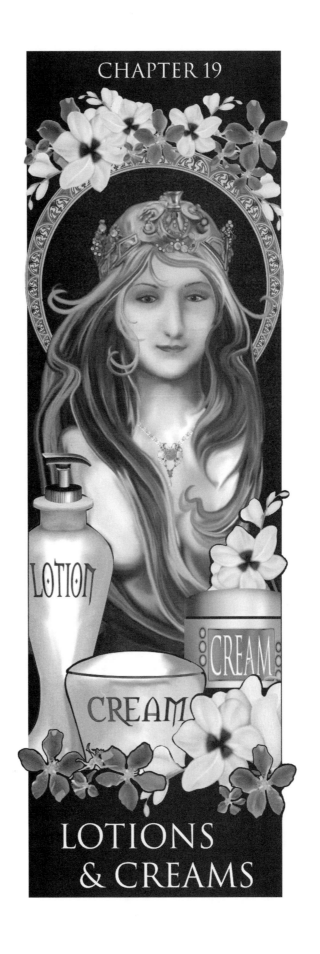

CHAPTER 19

LOTION

CREAM

CREAM

LOTIONS
& CREAMS

Lotions are water preparations containing insoluble materials used for external application that requires no friction. They are less intense than liniments, and because they are wetter, they are more sensual in their effect on the skin than salves. Lotions also require less rubbing in their application than salves, and they tend to leave a smaller amount of residue on the skin. The term *lotion* has derived from the Latin verb *lavare*, meaning *to wash*.

Medicinal lotions usually contain antiseptic or germicidal substances used to treat skin maladies, or they contain substances cooling and soothing to irritated skin, and healing to broken or bruised skin. Some lotions are a blend of liquid solutions, while others are either emulsions (a dispersion of droplets of a liquid in a second liquid with which it is insoluble) or suspensions (for our purposes, a finely divided solid dispersed in a liquid—the solid settles out more or less rapidly). The emulsions and suspensions frequently contain insoluble bodies that should be in a condition to diffuse easily when the liquid is shaken.

Cosmetic lotions normally contain nourishing, softening, moisturizing, and aromatic substances. The use of vegetable oils in cosmetic preparations, such as creams, hand lotions, and cold creams, for dry skin is very extensive. In cosmetic lotions and creams used for nourishment, Olive oil seems to be preferred, while expressed Almond oil, Sesame oil, Jojoba oil, Cocao butter, and Coconut oil follow respectively. These fixed oils are insoluble (immiscible) in water, but are capable of being mixed with water by the assistance of an emulsifier, forming an emulsion. Natural (non-chemical) emulsifiers most often employed are beeswax, deodorized hydrous lanolin, vegetable glycerin, and lecithin.

EMULSIFYING AGENTS

As defined above, an emulsion is the dispersion of droplets of a liquid in a second liquid with which it is immiscible. This can usually be accomplished by merely mixing the two liquids in a roomy container and agitating them vigorously. However, in order to stabilize this emulsion, a third agent is generally necessary; this is called an *emulsifying agent* or an *emulsifier*. In addition to making the suspension of the oil in the water medium more permanent, this emulsifying agent also works to allow a far more concentrated emulsion. For our purposes in making lotions and creams this means we can get a much higher proportion of oil to disperse in the water. Many medicinal and cosmetic herbal agents are taken into the body through the skin's oil components. The natural emulsifying agents, beeswax, hydrous lanolin, glycerin, and lecithin, do not interfere with this skin penetration as chemical emulsifiers are believed by some to do.

As an emulsifier, beeswax will also thicken and harden a cream or lotion to some extent; lanolin (extracted from sheep wool) is protective and moisturizing to the skin and tends slightly to thicken a lotion, but is not as reliable as beeswax for this action; glycerin has been discussed a great deal in this handbook already, so it is sufficient to say that as an emulsifier it is a mild preservative and is also an excellent moisturizing agent for the skin; lecithin is a smooth and slippery emulsifier and lends these qualities to a lotion. Avoid using too high a percent of either glycerin, lanolin, or lecithin, for they can make a lotion somewhat sticky; a half to three-quarters of a teaspoon of any one or a combination of these per 8 oz. cup of lotion is sufficient. Lotions and creams tend to thicken a bit as they age.

COLORING AGENTS

Lotions and creams (and salves and lip balms, etc.) can be colored by the addition of various herbal oil infusions. First make a highly saturated oil infusion (see Chapter Seventeen, "Oil Infusion") of a specific coloring plant, then incorporate this pigmented oil as part of the fixed oil ingredient of a recipe (see inclusion of the Alkanet and Calendula oils in the Rose Cream recipe, page 216). Depending on the amount used, an oil infusion of Alkanet root (*Alkanna tinctoria*) gives a soft pink to deep red color; an oil infusion of dried Turmeric (*Curcuma aromatica*) or Calendula petals renders a bright-hued yellow; and many green plants,

especially an oil infusion of dried Nettle, or Plantain, or Comfrey leaf lend a delightful green color.

NUTRITIONAL/MEDICINAL AGENTS

Lotions and creams can be enriched by the addition of other herbal agents. Bees, while being notorious emissaries of dermal inflammation, also create for us some of our skin's most extraordinary accessories: royal jelly, propolis, honey, and pollen. The apian chemistries of these accomplices blend magically with the water and oil portions of lotions and creams carrying with them an enormous array of vitamins, minerals, and enzymes that nourish our body and enhance our wellness. Herbal tinctures and/or liquid concentrates including Aloe vera juice and aromatic hydrosols or floral waters (see Chapter Ten, "Distillation of Hydrosols") can be included in a lotion as part of the water content, bringing with them a host of nutritional and therapeutic actions. Your whimsical imagination (and accumulating experience) can arrange and rearrange these ingredients into unique formulas that suit your personal needs and creative inspiration.

PRESERVATION AND STORAGE

As an initial step to preserve your lotions and creams, you should sterilize all the equipment you use to manufacture them, and sterilize all the containers (including the lids) you use to store the products. Avoid using your fingers to apply a lotion or cream, for fingertips readily inoculate the emulsion with microorganisms that will spoil the lotion as they joyfully procreate at rates even faster than the speed of human reproduction. Instead, pour your lotions into a plastic squeeze bottle or a bottle having a pump dispenser that permits the accurate dispersing of the liquid on targeted areas in convenient quantities. This eliminates the need to touch the lotion with your fertile fingers. Use a cosmetic spatula or some other small instrument to scoop and apply more viscous creams. Whenever you use a jar or a bottle as a holding and dispensing container, wipe off the lid after each and every use. Like regular flossing of teeth, this action greatly inhibits the land-squatting activities of microorganisms by surprising and temporarily disorganizing them.

You can incorporate preservative agents as a portion of the ingredients. Essential oils are anti-bacterial and anti-fungal and are probably the most easily incorporated, but when including them in a formula you will need to take into account their properties and aromas. Lavender and Benzoin are relatively inexpensive essential oils, and they are quite effective; Rose is not inexpensive, but effective and exquisite. Tea Tree is effective and inexpensive—I think it stinks (olfactorily speaking), though some folks like its scent, but then some folks don't mind jogging in clouds of exhaust fumes.

Adding vitamin E oil for an antioxidant to the oil portion of a recipe also provides a concentrated restorative food for the skin. A couple of 200 IU capsules expressed into 8 ounces of the lotion will do quite well.

And, of course, refrigeration is one of your most reliable preservatives.

A Liquid Lotion Base for Medicinal or Cosmetic Purposes

This preparation is gently astringent, anti-inflammatory, and moisturizing to the skin. It is a toning agent that can be used after skin cleansing for sensitive, dry, weather-damaged, and mature skin. It is especially soothing and healing for chapped or dry skin, eczema, or psoriasis. The lotion can be used as is for the inherent actions listed above. It also provides a general base to which a variety of other herbal agents can be added for treating specific conditions. Suggested herbal agents are listed following this base lotion recipe.

1. Mix together 600 ml (20 fl. oz.) of Rosewater (Rose hydrosol) and 45 ml (1 1/2 fl. oz.) of glycerin.

2. 60 ml (2 fl. oz.) of absolute alcohol can be added to this as a preservative. This is optional and only necessary if one intends to take this lotion on the road where it will be stored in varying temperatures. If refrigeration is available, or if one adds any of the following alcohol-containing tinctures to the base, this step is probably unnecessary.

Vulnerary, Anti-inflammatory Lotion

Add Arnica tincture 60 ml (2 fl. oz.) to create a *vulnerary, anti-inflammatory lotion* for washing sprains and bruises; for providing relief of rheumatic pain and the pain and inflammation of phlebitis, or whenever there is pain and inflammation of the skin. (*It is considered best, however, not to use Arnica directly on open wounds.*)

Anti-inflammatory, Vulnerary, and Anti-fungal Lotion

Add Calendula tincture 60 ml (2 fl. oz.) to create an anti-inflammatory, vulnerary, anti-fungal lotion useful for relieving inflammation of the skin. (*This can be used on an open wound.*)

Antiseptic Lotion

Add Goldenseal tincture 7 to 15 ml (1/4 to 1/2 fl. oz.) and Myrrh tincture 30 ml (1 fl. oz.) for an antiseptic lotion.

Vulnerary, Astringent, and Demulcent Wash

Add Comfrey 60 ml (2 fl. oz.) tincture as a *vulnerary, astringent,* and *demulcent* wash to assist the healing of external ulcers, for washing wounds and fractures, varicose veins, and ulcers.

Other Lotions

Any other appropriate tincture or blend of tinctures, add 60 ml (2 fl. oz.).

An Emulsion Type Lotion Base for Medicinal or Cosmetic Purposes

Start out by using the following simple ingredients to experiment with as you learn to blend water with oil. Once you have developed a familiarity and skill with this basic technique, begin incorporating exotic essential oils and other precious ingredients. (Some excellent recipes for cosmetic lotions and other skin care products may be found in *Aromatherapy—A Complete Guide to the Healing Art*, by Kathy Keville and Mindy Green.)

Equipment

Make sure all equipment is sterilized.

Kitchen blender

Plastic spatula

Chopstick

Small funnel

Glass measuring cup (1 cup size)

Metal saucepan (large enough for the measuring cup to sit in)

Grater (for shaving beeswax)

Small glass jar container(s)

Paper towels or tissues

Ingredients

3/4 cup	fixed oil
1 cup	distilled water (or floral water)
1/2 oz.	beeswax (shaved)

1. Place lid on blender and remove its center ring; set a wide mouth funnel into the ring opening.

2. Pour the water into the blender and set it aside. (There must be enough water used to cover the blades, so they can engage the liquid sufficiently to generate this emulsion.)

3. Put the oil into a measuring cup, and add the shaved beeswax to it.

4. Set this into the saucepan of water. The water surface should reach up to or a little above the level of the oil in the cup, making a water bath.

5. Place the pan on a low heat and warm the oil just long enough for the beeswax to melt.

6. Remove the measuring cup containing the oil and beeswax from the pan.

7. Let the oil/wax mixture cool a few minutes just until you see a faint rim of hardened wax forming on the side of the measuring cup.

8. Turn the blender on high speed and very slowly add the oil/wax until all the oil has been poured into the mixture. (Some lotion-makers start with a lower setting, and when the blender motor begins to bog down, turn it up to the next higher speed, continuing this until the high speed is reached—it's a matter of getting to know your machine.)

9. When all is going well, the emulsion will begin to harden after about two-thirds to three-quarters of the oil/wax has been added to the water.

10. You can remove the entire blender lid at this point and use the chopstick to carefully stir the top edges of the lotion as you pour the remainder of the oil (be mindful of the currently invisible whirling blades).

11. You now have a silky smooth lotion; you can turn off the blender.

12. If you choose to add essential oils [30 to 50 drops for this recipe/15 to 25 drops per 250 ml (8 oz. cup) of lotion], turn on the blender just long enough to incorporate the oils; *do not overblend the lotion.*

13. Pour the lotion into containers, using the spatula to get all of it.

14. Store in the refrigerator, for at this point, aside form the essential oils, you have not incorporated any preservatives.

A good emulsion is a product of the combination of the proper temperature of an oil/wax mixture and the uniformity of the flow of oil as it is poured into the churning waters below. This is not difficult to accomplish, but unsuccessful attempts have been recorded, predominantly by those who have successfully performed this procedure hundreds of times, but are presently demonstrating the technique in front of many others. Dignity is such a fragile commodity.

An Elegant Rose Cream

A cream is made in the exact same fashion as a lotion, requiring the same tools as listed above. The consistency of a cream ends up being thicker, due to employing a little more wax and a little less liquid. Sometimes when making a cream all the water will not blend with the oil, so it needs to be removed by pouring it off or by touching it with an absorbent tissue; when preparing a lotion this is seldom required.

Ingredients *I will not give approximate metric equivalents for these measurements. I've used these, they work well, and I think their precision is important.*

10 Gm	beeswax
1 1/4 cup	rosewater
1 1/2 ml	Rose essential oil
1 tsp.	glycerin
3/4 cup	almond oil (which includes 1 tablespoon Alkanet infused oil, 1 tablespoon Calendula infused oil)

1. Pour Rosewater and glycerin into blender.

2. Put the blender lid on (remove the center ring from the lid, so oils can be poured into the blender later), and set aside.

3. Grate the beeswax.

4. Place the Almond oil mixture and grated beeswax into the glass measuring cup.

5. Place the glass cup into a metal pot and fill the pot with water up to the level of the oil in the cup, making a water bath.

6. Heat the oil just until the wax is completely melted.

7. Remove from the heat and set aside.

8. Let this cool a few minutes, just until you see a faint rim of wax hardened on the side of the measuring cup.

9. Turn the blender on low speed and pour oil/wax mixture *very slowly* into the rosewater/glycerin mixture—pour a slow steady stream using a funnel or the chopstick as a guiding rod (see *"Guiding Rod"* under *"Decanting,"* Chapter Twenty-Five).

10. When the blender motor begins to bog down, turn it up to the next higher speed. Continue this until you reach the high speed, until all the oil has been poured into the mixture.

11. While the blender is still running remove the lid.

12. If you see any liquid in the corners of the blender, scrape the sides down with the spatula until all the liquid is incorporated and blended together (be aware of the blender blade).

13. The cream will become either too stiff to take any more oil or all the water will have been fully blended with the oil. If any water remains unblended, pour it off or blot it with a clean absorbent paper tissue.

14. You now have a luscious thick cream.

15. Add the Rose essential oil and blend it in for 10 seconds. *Do not overblend the cream.*

16. Scoop the cream into containers and refrigerate.

17. Be sure to wipe the lid after each use!

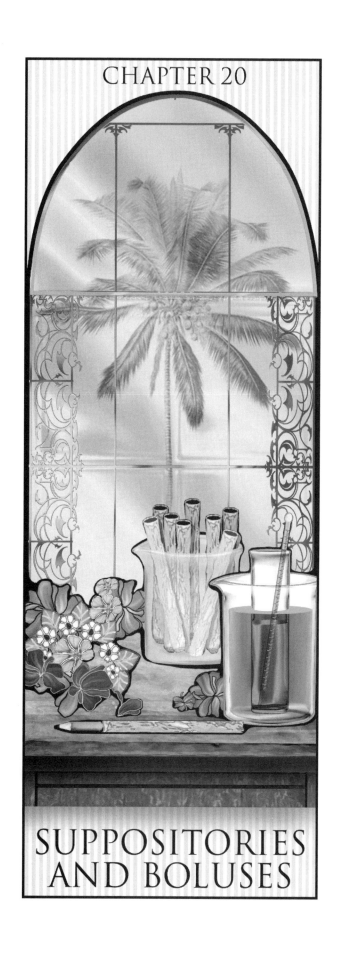

CHAPTER 20

SUPPOSITORIES
AND BOLUSES

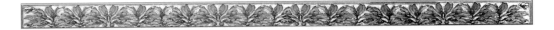

Recorded history reveals that herbalists and physicians of ancient India and Egypt used suppositories for local and systemic affect. "Suppository" is defined as something that is "placed underneath," designed to penetrate and dissolve in a body cavity other than the mouth. In this country, during most of the 1800s, suppositories were prescribed mainly for local problems. However, as the fundamental anatomy and physiology of the rectum have become more clearly understood by Western science, it has become apparent that herbs can be absorbed from the lower regions of the rectum and then can enter the general circulation, thus becoming systemic. We know now that rectal insertion can be an excellent method for administering herbs to infants, young children, and adults on correct occasions.

According to the Greeks a bolus was a "lump" or a "clod." Today it is defined as "a rounded mass of anything," a large pill or tablet, and in some lexicons it is defined as "a large pill for a horse." Somewhere along the way, from the time when a bolus was considered by the Greeks merely a lump and a clod, it has become a country cousin to the more sophisticated-sounding "suppository." Among herbalists the term most commonly used is "herbal bolus." So today, for all practical purposes, boluses and sup-positories are considered to be the same thing. Whatever you choose to call this vehicle, it is a single dosage preparation, intended primarily for insertion into the vaginal or rectal cavity for local or systemic action.

The primary advantage of using a bolus is that it is a slippery little vehicle that gets in there and deposits the goods forthright. The "goods" are therapeutic and tonic herbs, and "there" are those inner body parts that, when signaling for help, are soothed and nourished by an herb being placed right up against them, or at least as close to them as physically possible. A bolus can be inserted directly into the vagina to soothe infections and treat inflammation of the cervix and other inner vaginal tissues, or it can be inserted into the rectum to soothe and tone mildly or highly disturbed prostate glands in males, or to soothe and shrink hemorrhoids and cysts in anyone. Boluses are also employed to deliver herbs directly to rectal mucous membranes which readily absorb them into the bloodstream. This can elicit the same systemic effect as herbs that have been taken orally. In line with this, it is important to note that a bolus is an excellent means for administering fever-reducing and other soothing and nourishing herbs to infants and young children who can't or won't take them orally. (A number of piqued children opt for the oral method the next time around.)

While we're in this discussion, I'll insert the concept that enemas and vaginal douches are extensions of the bolus. Designed to deliver a single liquid dosage, they are an equally efficient delivery system to administer herbs "underneath" for local and systemic action.

Medicinal herbs used in boluses can be strong astringents, such as White Oak bark, used to contract, firm, and strengthen tissues and to reduce secretions and discharge; demulcent and mild astringents such as Comfrey root or Marshmallow root used to relax, soothe, protect, and heal tissues; antimicrobial tonics like Goldenseal, Echinacea, and Chaparral, used to prevent and allay infection while toning body tissues; and/or distinct tonic herbs such as Saw Palmetto, which is often used with Echinacea to soothe and tone an infected or otherwise disturbed prostate gland.

These active herbal agents are suspended in a solid base designed to melt at body temperature or in a base that will dissolve and disperse when in contact with body tissues. The two main types of bases used for making boluses are cocoa butter and a gelatin-glycerin mix. The cocoa butter is most appropriately used when dry herbal preparations are to be administered and the gelatin-glycerin mix is well used when one wishes to combine liquid preparations with a base. It is worth noting that the glycerin will extract moisture from tissue. Therefore, please note that if it is *used frequently*, it can cause a drying of the mucosal membranes, possibly provoking mild inflammation.

THE FORMING MOLD

Enthusiasm about preparing herbal boluses (hey, some folks get excited about collecting old hub caps) can prompt an all-pervasive search for bolus-forming molds. From thimbles to fountain pen lids, you may find yourself haunting supermarkets, hardware stores, flea markets, garage sales, closets, kitchen drawers, kids' (those you're not even related to) toy boxes, the car's glove compartment, etc., for potential molds. If you do find yourself involved in this odd quest, I suggest you keep it a private pursuit; go about your search telling no one what you are looking for or why you want it….It's simpler that way and avoids a lot of talk.

I have found numerous potential devices that I won't bother to list. Suffice it to say, some of them panned out, most didn't, but I've learned to enjoy the hunt. All in all, my initial technique, which is rather standard knowledge, remained the simplest and probably the overall best. Meanwhile I've moved on to other challenges, but the exhilaration of the hunt lingers, and my eyes remain alert for "the perfect bolus-shaping mold." It's not like bolus consciousness is my main event, you realize. I seek the burning bush and contemplate the sound of one hand clapping too, like all the other deep and spiritual guys.

Therefore, a quick and efficient method for making a shaping mold:

1. Roll aluminum foil tightly around a fat pencil, a magic marker, the handle of a large wooden spoon, whatever, depending on the diameter of the bolus you want. The width of your small finger is a good size approximation.

2. Leave a substantial portion of the pencil (or whatever shape-giving device you use)

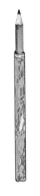

Foil Wrapped Snuggly
Around the Pencil

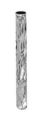

A Completed Form

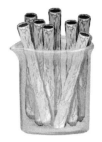

Tubes Standing Up in a
Narrow Container

sticking out of one end of the foil wrap, so that once you are finished rolling it up you can still grasp it and pull it out of the newly formed tube. Indulge heavily in abundance by wrapping the foil around the implement a number of times to supply a sturdy wall to work with.

3. Close off one end of the tube by twisting or crimping the foil and remove the implement.

4. Find a container that will support this tube (or a number of these tubes) and can hold it (them) securely upright once it has been filled with the warm liquid mixture.

SIZE AND SHAPE

Rectal suppositories should weigh around 2–3 Gm each, smaller sizes being made for infants. Vaginal suppositories should weigh in at about 4 to 5 Gm each.

Rectal suppositories are retained more easily when they have been shaped to taper at both ends, the taper being greater at one end (the front or lead end). Vaginal suppositories are best shaped into a globular form or oviform (egg-shaped).

METHODS OF PREPARATION

There are two types of boluses or suppositories that I will discuss in this chapter. The first is made by using cocoa butter as a base, and the other is a product of a glycerated-gelatin base.

COCOA BUTTER

Cocoa butter, *Oleum Theobromatis* (also spelled Cacao butter), is a non-irritating, yellowish-white fat derived from the nut of the chocolate tree (*Theobroma cacao*). It is probably the best general base for boluses and suppositories. It is hard and wax-like at ordinary temperatures, but melts at 86 to 95° F. (30 to 35° C.). It can be incorporated with powdered herbs, small portions of aqueous substances, or with oils, and it does not become rancid. The cocoa butter melts from the natural temperature of the body and releases the herbs.

It is suggested that boluses be inserted at night prior to going to bed, so the person is lying horizontally, a more retentive position than standing up. The use of protective accoutrements is suggested to deal with any leakage that might occur.

Cocoa butter begins to liquefy to a semi-solid when warmed to around 86° F. (30° C.) and it usually melts at 93 to 95° F. (34 to 35° C.), which is slightly below normal human body temperature. However, in certain circumstances, if the cocoa butter has been heated to about 97° F. (36° C.) and then quickly cooled in a chilled suppository mold, it solidifies into a less stable form which will then melt at about 73 to 75° F. (23 to 24° C.), rendering it difficult to handle and insert. A bolus in this state might not make it intact into the intended orifice. So it is worth knowing that for best overall results one should avoid overheating cocoa butter. This is best done by melting (liquefying) cocoa butter slowly with low heat (using a double boiler apparatus or a small glass beaker placed into a larger container which is half filled with warm water) and pour the liquefied cocoa butter into molds that are room temperature.

MAKING THE COCOA BUTTER BASE SUPPOSITORY

When using cocoa butter as the base, there are two basic methods for making boluses, the *Cold Process* and the *Warm Fusion Process*. The latter employs heating and the use of pre-shaped molds in which to cool and solidify the liquid; the former requires neither heat nor molds.

In the warm process, the powdered herb(s) is added to the melted base, poured into a mold, and allowed to cool. In the cold process, the herbal powder is incorporated with the unmelted base and the resulting mass is shaped by hand. As to which method is best, I'd say it pretty much comes down to which one you enjoy doing more.

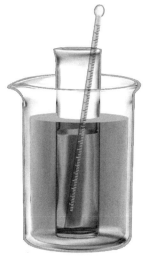

Glass Beakers Set Up
with Thermometer

Warm Infusion Process

The following warm fusion procedure takes into account that cocoa butter base herbal boluses, when they are not overheated and not too rapidly cooled, remain more stable and retain their ideal melting point of around 90 to 95° F.

1. Grind your herbal ingredients into as fine a powder as possible. Use the electric coffee bean grinder to grind the herbs and then run the ground herbs through a fine sieve to ensure that they are finely powdered. Weigh and make note of the amount of your herb powder for future reference.

2. Reduce the cocoa butter to small pieces by grating or shaving it. Avoid using large particles; they melt slowly and mess with the low temperature melting process. Weigh and note the amount for future reference.

3. Place the herbs and the cocoa butter into the top portion of a double boiler or into a small glass beaker and mix them lightly with a stirring rod or a thermometer. (You're going to be using the thermometer to help monitor the temperature soon anyway.)

4. The amount of herb you use in relation to the amount of binder will depend on the nature of the herb. You will have to work with this. Make notes. Try to get as much herb into the mixture as you can while allowing enough base material to easily bind and hold it all together.

NOTE: Using glass beakers allows you to observe the mixture better, and most importantly, the thin walls reduce the chance of overheating. Metal pots and double boilers work fine, but they offer more of a challenge when it comes to heat control.

5. When using a *double boiler*, place the top of the boiler containing the mixture of ingredients into the bottom, which contains water that has been brought to a boil and removed from the fire. While stirring, let this heat melt the cocoa butter. When using *glass beakers*, place the smaller beaker full of the ingredients within a larger beaker of hot water. Stir the mixture with the thermometer and watch the temperature. The mass will soften at about 89° F. (32° C.) and should be kept at or below 92° F. (33° C.).

6. When the mixture reaches 92°, separate the beakers or pots. Stir until the mixture of powdered herbs and cocoa butter appears to be uniformly blended and fully melted.

7. Pour the thick mixture into a mold that is *room temperature*. When using the narrow tube of aluminum foil described above or any other narrow-shaped device as a forming mold, a very small plastic funnel will be of great assistance for this step. After a couple of minutes, the mixture will become somewhat firm.

8. Place the mold full of the bolus mixture into a freezer for about 2 minutes.

9. After this brief cooling, remove the bolus from the mold.

10. *Cut* the boluses into desired lengths, *shape* them as you will, and *store* them in the refrigerator in a small jar which is labeled. (If you don't label the jar, inevitably someone will bite off a piece of one of the boluses thinking it is candy. Actually, about the only difference between a cocoa butter bolus and a piece of candy, aside from its social status, is the addition of a sweetener, and of course the orifice of insertion.)

11. If something doesn't work out, re-melt the mixture, and do it again.

In spite of the above precautions, I should assure that this warm process is fairly low-pressure medicine-making. It is while percolating tinctures and making lotions that the brow and palms tend to get a little sweaty. The key here is to melt the cocoa/herb mixture at a minimum temperature and use a room temperature mold into which you pour the warm mixture. If you use a previously cooled mold, it causes a super-cooling of the cocoa butter and the resultant crystallization (rehardening) makes for a lower melting point. If you do overheat the mixture, complete the project, and then let this batch of boluses age in the refrigerator for a month. Upon aging, they (both the overheated and the super-cooled boluses) eventually recoup their normal melting point characteristics.

I praise the medical pharmacists who figured out the intimate dynamics of this cocoa chemistry and all the other excellent medicine-making knowledge they have amassed throughout the years. The members of this inspired profession avidly pursued this kind of pharmaceutical investigation in the 1930s, '40s, and '50s while most herbalists (and herbal lay-pharmacy) in the U.S. had withdrawn into a deep slumber. But, one by one, we lay-pharmacists are returning to the medicine-making arena; like recently kissed enchanted frogs, who have awakened to their original nature, we are emerging from some strange cultural spell, and can now contribute our peerless perspective to the evolving art and science of herbal pharmacy. One acquires deep green insight and unique capabilities being a frog for a while.

Cold Process

Cocoa butter and other fat bases that do not require melting in order to mix with powdered herbs can be made into bolus suppositories by a cold method.

So far, the best tools I've found for this method are a dinner plate and two 1 1/4-inch *stainless steel* putty knives (you can find these in the paint section of a hardware store). One putty knife is used to knead and blend the cocoa butter and herbs together, and the other one is used to intermittently scrape off the first one. You'll also want some paper towels close by.

1. Powder the herb(s) you plan to use. If you are using more than one herb, powder and blend them at this stage.

2. Grate or shave with a putty knife an appropriate quantity of cocoa butter onto a glass or ceramic dinner plate.

3. Mix the powdered herb with the shaved cocoa butter base and then work them into a plastic mass with the aid of the putty knife. A more even distribution of the herb is obtained if it is first mixed with only a portion of the cocoa butter base, then the remainder of the base can be worked in gradually.

4. Add essential oils during this blending process if your formula calls for them.

5. Knead the entire mass with the putty knife until the herbs (and essential oils, if you've added any) are well dispersed. If you took the suggestion in the margin, have another cookie.

6. Wash your hands well, and, with your fingers, form the mass into appropriately sized and shaped boluses. The necessary skill is easy to acquire. Weigh the first bolus to get a sense of the size you want to make (see size and shape, above). If you find that the skin temperature of your fingers exceeds the melting point of cocoa butter, you can keep your hands cool by dipping them in ice water, or by holding on to the glass of ice cold milk you're having with your cookies.

7. Place boluses into a small jar, cap it, label it, and store it in the refrigerator.

This Cold Process is a lot like making chocolate chip cookie dough from scratch, which you might even want to start now for, inevitably, smelling and handling all this cocoa butter will lead you into some form of chocolate frenzy.

Coconut Oil Base Substitute

Some folks use coconut oil (derived from the fruit of the Coconut palm, *Cocos nucifera*) in place of cocoa butter as a base for making boluses. Rosemary Gladstar, in her book *Herbal Healing for Women*, gives the following recipe for such an event:

"Melt coconut oil in a saucepan over low heat. When the oil is completely melted, remove it from the heat and stir in the powdered herb mixture. Add enough herbs to make a thick paste. When you have added enough powder so that the oil is thick, yet still pliable enough to work, add (*essential oils*). Quickly roll into boluses the size and shape of your small finger. They will look like herbal tootsie rolls."

Making the Glycerinated Gelatin Base Suppository

This mixture of gelatin and glycerin creates a base that readily incorporates liquid extracts such as herbal infusions, decoctions, concentrates, tinctures, fluid extracts, and essential oils into a suppository form. Gelatin is found in the "jello" section of the grocery store, and glycerin can be purchased in health food stores, herb stores, and drug stores.

I'll give you a basic recipe and method for making this type of bolus, but you will, I'm sure, quickly modify it in your own fashion.

1. Into a small glass or stainless steel saucepan, pour 1 oz. (30 ml) of herbal tincture, fluid extract, strong herbal concentrate, or whatever form of liquid single herb or herbal formula you wish to use. You certainly can incorporate finely powdered herbs in this base as well.

2. Add 1 oz. (30 ml) of pure vegetable glycerin.

3. Add 2 oz. (60 ml) of distilled water.

4. Stir these ingredients together until they are well mixed.

5. Open 1 envelope of unflavored gelatin and pour it into the liquid mixture. (The box of gelatin I buy holds 4 envelopes of pure granulated gelatin, each containing 7 Gm.)

6. Place this combination on the stove burner over a low flame.

7. Stir continuously until the gelatin is *completely dissolved*.

8. Remove the mixture from the stove and pour it into molds.

9. Let it cool a bit and then put it into the refrigerator to solidify.

An excellent suppository to prepare for treating hemorrhoids incorporates 25 ml of Witch Hazel (*Hamamelis virginiana*) tincture and 5 ml of Horse Chestnut (*Aesculus hippocastanum*) or California Buckeye (*Aesculus californica*) tincture in the above recipe.

A Crude Process

This is a short story about making a bolus by what I call the Greek Method. This method is a procedure I bumbled upon, while not having a clue what I was doing, during my first impromptu attempt to make a herbal bolus.

I assembled a pile of powdered herb on a glass dinner plate. I then liquefied some cocoa butter and poured this, a little at a time, onto the pile of powder. Then I kneaded the powder and cocoa butter together with a small metal cookie spatula until they were blended. I added more liquid cocoa butter as I proceeded until I had a well-formed mass (certainly, what I perceived to be a "lump" or a "clod"). When it felt "right" (and this is totally up to one's speculation), I used a second cookie spatula to scrape off the stuff that had hardened and was clinging to the first spatula. I then scraped up the other hardened stuff that had spread all over the plate and on the countertop. I gathered all of these scrapings into a pile, and began to press, mold, and form portions of the pile with my fingers into various shapes and sizes that seemed appropriate for the dynamics of orifice insertion.

This worked for me at the time, and I was happy with the results. Yes, the manufacturing process was crude, and some less aware of the intent behind the task might have judged it merely as making a mess in the kitchen. But my vision was clear and my determination was heated. Even during the moments when I was feeling a little dorky, as I do when first walking around in a brand new pair of shoes, I was also experiencing a feeling of contentedness. And although I was obviously flailing about in the unknown, flickers of discovery and a measure of success flared in my novice medicine-maker's humble demeanor, and I found myself enjoying the initial stages of my medicine show.

The point of this tender disclosure is not to recommend this method of production, but simply to convey a suggestion about medicine-making (and, what the heck, about life in general), which is: When you get an idea of what you want, plunge in and do it! Take a risk. You may only semi-succeed, or you may blow it entirely, but so what? The materials of Herbalism are inexpensive (actually the cost of cocoa butter is a bit outrageous). Most likely you'll ultimately create a successful experience far beyond your initial dream. It's an adventure, and it's fun. If it's not, you should probably forget about the whole thing anyway and do something else. And you're guaranteed to learn something of value (make notes), and it might make a poignant story you can divulge someday when you write your book.

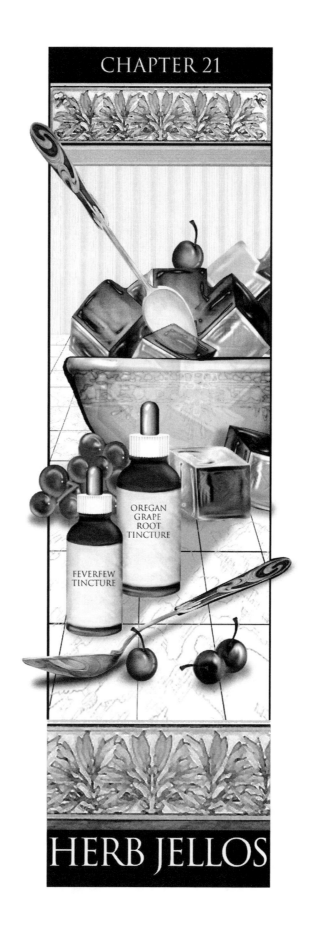

CHAPTER 21

FEVERFEW
TINCTURE

OREGAN
GRAPE
ROOT
TINCTURE

HERB JELLOS

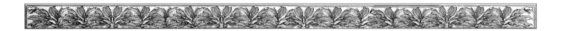

One afternoon, as I was manipulating the makings of glycerated-gelatin suppositories, getting my procedures clear for writing Chapter Twenty, I discovered (actually crashed into) an interesting new(?) herbal vehicle—a medicinal herbal jello.

As a result of this impact and the events that followed, I have reason to suspect that tonic and therapeutic herbal jellos offer notable potential for assisting herbalists and parents to increase child and "ill-tempered adult" patient compliance.

This discovery stemmed from a blunder of mine that involved a particularly precious tincture of primo-wildcrafted Oregon Grape root (OGR). The simple pharmaceutical event was supposed to culminate in a manifestation of many, perfectly molded glycerated-gelatin suppositories, but instead, ended up as an unintended mass of OGR jello. Momentarily deranged by my frustration and self-pity (I was racing toward a publishing deadline at the time), I lost control. In my mindless anguish, I took a spoon to it all, slashing and scooping at it blindly as I cried out, "Why me!? Why now!? Why all that glycerin!? Why my finest OGR tincture!?"

Immediately following the gelatal carnage, as I stood at the kitchen counter, bewildered, remorseful, emotionally spent, questioning the meaning of life and the purpose of man's toil on earth, gazing aimlessly at the sordid glycerated remains, the empty tincture bottle laying on its side, the soiled beakers, I ate a spoonful of the still quivering blunder…and behold…I was instantly uplifted! It was fun, like eating jello always is (even for those cranky adults who won't admit it). And it tasted…"all right!" which OGR tincture never does. Right, kids?

I discovered that jellofied herb effortlessly jiggles and diffuses ghastly flavors, distracting one's taste buds from the roots of bitterness, and the glycerin follows up smoothly with a pleasantly sweet aftertaste. I liked it! I ate another scoop. The herbalized jello played in my mouth. I slurped another scoop, then another. My face smiled big; the universe, amused by my blunderability had given me an answer to my questions…*herb jello* (*Botanica wiggleus; Gelatinaceae* family)! What an idea! (Individuals requiring a more sophisticated air of credibility in their future discussions concerning this important new clinical vehicle can use the currently more fashionable European-flavored term "phytojel.") Such a joyous footnote this will be scribed in the herb section of the Akashic records and in the future archives of twenty-first century

American phyto-folklore. Herbal pharmacy of the new millennium will have a wiggle.

Not long thereafter, creativity ablaze, I boarded my bike and sped to the local grocery store, where I bought myself a couple packs of lime-flavored Jell-O® (what can I say, lime is green). I flirted with the idea of getting the sugar-free type Jell-O, but its label said "aspertame" on the ingredients list, so I reconsidered and bought the ones that said "sugar" instead. In my belief system, aspertame makes white sugar the good guy. And, with all that good herb that's going to be taken, a little sugar isn't going to hurt anyone.

Upon returning home, I opened my box of lime Jell-O, immediately poured a little bit of the green powder into my palm, and proceeded to lick it, mm-*mm*! You've gotta do that; every kid does. Then I poured the rest of the powder onto a scale and weighed it. I wanted only to use 1/4 of the Jell-O to experiment with. I weighed out 22 Gm (the 3 oz box said 85 Gm, but I got 86 Gm + my approximately 2 Gm compulsive lick).

Possibly, we've turned a significant corner here in herbal kinderland. Try out the idea of using herb jellos; have fun with it, and let me know what recipes and results you come up with. I can be reached at: JG, P.O. Box 39, Forestville, CA 95436.

Kindernote: Leave an herb jello uncovered in the refrigerator for a couple weeks and you've got yourself a phyto gummy bear to chew.

HERB JELLO

1/4 box	lime Jell-O (I did cherry Jell-O next) = approximately 22 Gm
1/4 cup	boiling water (60 ml)
1 oz.	tincture (I used Feverfew for my first intentional herb jello) (30 ml or 1/8 cup)
1 oz.	cold water (30 ml or 1/8 cup)

1. Put the jello powder into a small rectangular shaped baking tin. (I used a small loaf tin that measured 2 1/2 inches by 4 1/2 inches. Using this squared-off shape makes it easy to divide the herb jello into equal-sized pieces in order to give relatively equal-sized doses.)

2. Pour the boiling water onto the jello powder and *stir well* for 2 to 3 minutes, *making sure that the gelatin is completely dissolved.*

3. Add the tincture and stir this well.

4. Then add the cold water and stir well.

5. Pour this mixture into the pan and/or into any other molds you wish to use. I bought some candy molds of various forms (shells, cars, cigars, Christmas trees, etc.) that make kid-approved shapes for eating. (The research that remains for us is to discover the jello flavors that work best with each uniquely flavored herb or herbal blend. This is why I use only 1/4 of the pack, or less, at a time.)

6. Once the herb jello has hardened, cut it into 6 equal portions, each one delivering about a 5 ml dose of tincture.

The Feverfew jello turned out tasting "all right." At least it is the best-tasting, most palatable dose of Feverfew I've taken so far, and taste-wise, Feverfew is one of the herbs most folks applaud the least.

This water-gelatin vehicle scoots the herbal flavors quickly past the taste buds and on down to the stomach with a minimal amount of gustatative resistance; yet in passing, it makes its moves on the mouth long enough for the tongue to party whimsically with the gelatin portion.

Following this, I made a cherry St. John's Wort jello and called it "cherry up." Next, I assembled a relaxing nervine jello using Valerian and California Poppy with lemon Jell-O and called it "mellow yellow jello" (naming your herb jello is optional).

I feel a great potential here for parents, grumps, and wee ones. One can experiment with all types of flavored Jell-O® brand jellos in order to find those that cohabit harmoniously in a jelly-body with otherwise strange and frightful tasting herbal extracts, like Feverfew, Oregon Grape, Yarrow, and Mugwort. If you prefer to use no sugar at all, you can use the glycerated-gelatin recipes for making suppositories that are given in Chapter Twenty. That is what I did involuntarily the first time. Glycerin is a non-sugar sweetener. Or one can experiment with using Stevia, which has been infused into the water that is used to dissolve an unsweetened gelatin. Stevia (*Stevia rebaudiana*) is an herb that has come to us from its native land Paraguay. It tastes sweeter than sugar, but by FDA (the Federal Denial Attendants) pronouncement, cannot be called a sweetener (this edict is probably another side effect of the aspertame industry). Use Hains® brand vegetarian jello or a flavored pectin if you prefer a vegetarian variety.

You can incorporate herbal infusions, decoctions, tinctures—any and all forms of loathsome tasting herbal liquids children and ill-tempered adults often refuse to take or complain about so incessantly it's hardly worth the effort trying to help them. Of course, all the naturally good-tasting herbal teas, glycerites, and tinctures like Lemon Balm, Mint, Chamomile, and Fennel are also garnished with fun when transformed into a phytojel.

Adults (senior kids) can take a bit of dessert before meals as a digestive aid, using an herb jello incorporating Peppermint, Chamomile, Lemon Balm, Ginger, or any of the other carminatives. Merely the name "Lemon Balm-lemon-lime jello" shimmies with vibrations of gastric approval and upliftment.

I'm planning to prepare a Meadowsweet jello which will be a consoling herbal therapeutic treat for any child who is experiencing diarrhea. The jello portion will proceed to make his or her insides feel soothed and happy, and the Meadowsweet will supply its gently efficient internal action to help balance out the child's troubled intestine. Catnip and Fennel is an herbal blend I strongly recommend having on hand in all households inhabited by babies and young children. It is an excellent compound to use for soothing children's colicky digestive systems and for allaying children's fevers, especially during childhood fever diseases such measles, mumps, chickenpox, etc. The name "Catnip-Fennel-jello" carries an inherent giggle and just sounds like a good time. The babe will love it as a medicinal treat, and a touch of party. (If the child's fever is prolonged and quite troublesome, the insertion of a homecrafted Meadowsweet, Yarrow suppository will be quite helpful.)

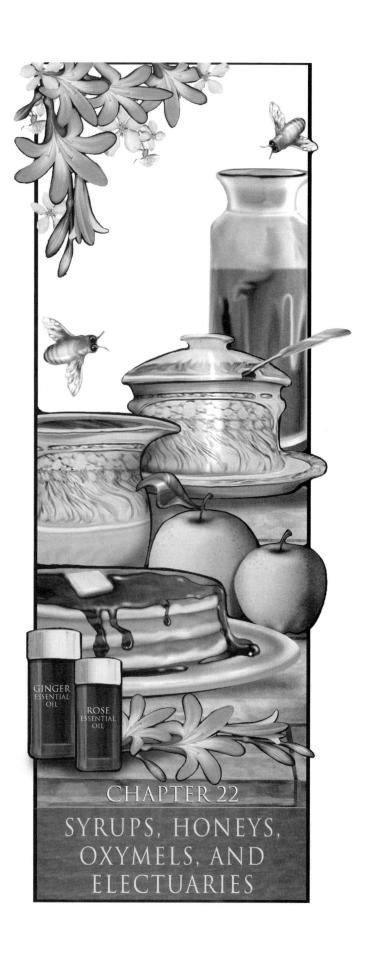

CHAPTER 22

SYRUPS, HONEYS, OXYMELS, AND ELECTUARIES

HERBAL SYRUPS

When an herbalist concocts an admittedly unpleasant-tasting herbal tincture or tea blend that he or she feels will do a sick child a world of good, and the ailing little person still has enough reason, will, and determination to wholeheartedly reject the favor, a sweet syrup often settles the dispute. Syrup is a traditional way to make herbal preparations (especially bitter sore throat and cough mixtures) more palatable for children and for other folks who aren't ready to hear that bitter is good.

Syrups are an old and favored form of administering herbal medication to be taken internally. This popularity is due to a variety of reasons. Aesthetically, syrups' sweet flavors are highly palatable and they offer a pleasing appearance; concurrently, syrup has a nutrient value as a carbohydrate (in spite of popular opinion, sugar is not a nutritional problem, whereas manic consumption of sugar is a problem), and the sugar used in making syrups can be an eminently effective preservative in place of alcohol or refrigeration for otherwise unstable herbal solutions.

When using sugar as the preservative, the adequate concentration of white sugar (sucrose) in a syrup is a crucially important factor in its keeping quality. (Sucrose is the official chemical name used for common white sugar in pharmacy texts.)

Sugar is a carbohydrate. When present in a water solution, diluted sugar provides a nutrient source which vigorously supports the growth of micro-organisms, especially yeast and molds. *However, the ability of these organisms to grow is decreased as the concentration of sucrose is increased.* Therefore, a simple sugar syrup needs to approach saturation in order to succeed as an effective preservative agent. One does not want to attain true saturation, however, because any slight cooling might start a crystallization process within the syrup body which can lead to complications. Large crystals form, which are difficult to re-dissolve, and the formation of these crystals leaves behind a solution with insufficient sugar concentration, that will support microorganism growth. The concentration of sugar in a syrup must be sufficient to render the solution so saturated with pure sugar (sucrose) that there is no longer enough water available to provide the environment required for microorganisms to proliferate. This is similar to drying herbs for preservation so that not enough water is available in the dried vegetable materials to provide a proper environment for bacteria and mold to proliferate and cause deterioration.

The use of sugar as a preservative for making permanent herbal preparations was quite popular and certainly practical in times when refrigeration was not a common household luxury. One winter, while I was immersed in writing this chapter, Sonoma County, California, hosted an uncompromising windstorm that felled nearby trees, demolishing numerous power lines. This supplied me with two electricity-free (void) days to deepen my appreciation for non-electric light and heat-giving devices not dependent on electric power. As my refrigerator and freezer slowly lost their cool, my appreciation deepened as well for stored food products that don't rely on electrical power for their preservation. Experiencing (yet again) the obvious vulnerability of my dependence on electrical power, my extemporaneously expanding appreciation soon embraced all the methods I was aware of that preserve herbal extracts that do not rely on electricity-fed devices, or on the over-taxed liquids supplied by the alcohol industry. Therefore, I have decided to discuss here not only the making of syrups that are best kept in the refrigerator but also a method for making a syrup that, in line with "the technology of independence," when prepared properly, can survive entirely off the grid.

Syrups are defined as saturated solutions of sugar in pure water or in other aqueous liquids; sugar is the preservative component. Syrups sometimes contain vinegar, honey, glycerin, and occasionally a small quantity of alcohol. In pharmacy, when distilled water alone is used in the nearly saturated solution with sugar, the distinctive term *simple syrup* is applied. When the solution contains various aromatic or pleasantly tasting substances it is called a *flavored syrup*, and when the sugar solution contains soluble princi-ples from various medicinal plants used as therapeutic agents it is called a *medicated syrup*. Medicinally, syrups can be divided into two general groups. The flavoring group composed of those syrups prepared solely for their agreeable flavor are used chiefly as vehicles for carrying and improving the taste of other preparations of medicinal agents (i.e., Peppermint, Blackberry fruit, or Cherry syrups). The second group, medicated syrups, are prepared to access their intrinsic medicinal ingredients and are used as therapeutic agents (i.e., Garlic, Marshmallow, Horehound, Black Cohosh, and Senna syrups).

CONTAINERS FOR SYRUPS

Mixing (agitating) containers, storage containers, and any funnels or other implements used to help fill the containers must be dry to avoid dilution of the syrup, and they must be very clean in order to avoid contamination of the syrup by fermentation organisms that frequent imperfectly cleaned bottles. It is best to use small storage bottles so that a large quantity of syrup will not be exposed to the air each time the container is opened.

SYRUP DOSAGE

Standard dose for taking a syrup is approximately 1 teaspoonful as needed, or as some therapeutic literature decrees, *ad libitum*.

SYRUP PRESERVATION AND STORAGE

All syrups do better if, before bottling, they are first strained through clean cotton flannel or muslin cloth that has been previously moistened and wrung out. This removes any particles of dust and dirt that might find their way into the syrup.

Finished syrups will keep unaltered for a

"Sugar is the cleavage of the culinary arts, chocolate the plunging neckline."
—T. Elder Sachs

long time if properly prepared. They are best preserved in sterile, tightly capped bottles and stored in a cool place where the temperature is uniform. It is important that, before filling, the storage bottles be clean (immersed in boiling water for a period of time), and dry to avoid dilution and possible contamination of the syrup by fermentation organisms that frequent imperfectly cleaned bottles. It is best if these storage bottles are fairly small, so that a large quantity of syrup will not be exposed to the air each time the container is opened.

Syrups, properly prepared, usually are stored at room temperature. But for those syrups that don't keep well, at a risk of causing some crystallization due to supercooling the saturated solution, their original quality is maintained for a longer time if they are kept in a refrigerator. Air and heat are far more detrimental to the stability of sugar solutions than diffused light, but direct sunlight should always be avoided because of the heat transmitted by the sun's rays.

Other agents can be added to the syrup, to help prevent fermentation:

Essential oils, which of course greatly modify the taste, aroma, and other properties of the preparation.

Brandy, which is much used with aromatics, or a small proportion of pure ethyl alcohol can be added to syrups to serve as a preservative as well as a solvent for the addition of alcohol-soluble ingredients, such as essential oils. Some folks speculate that the alcohol concentrates in the vapors above the syrup and from this strategic location prevents the growth of surface molds.

Glycerin can be used in syrups as an agent to help retard fermentation. It is effective if the concentration is sufficient, 30 percent or more. It has a sweet taste, but its sweetness is not as pleasing as sucrose. Glycerin is a solvent for tannins, and as such acts as a preservative against precipitation of extracted vegetable matter.

Honey is a health-promoting substance that supplies a delightful flavor and provides excellent preservative activity.

Syrups that go off and ferment are best composted. Once a syrup has undergone fermentation it is no longer fit for use. Even if an attempt is made to restore it by boiling, it is quite likely to spoil again soon, due to the decreased proportion of sugar remaining in solution.

WATER FOR MAKING SYRUP

The best water to use for making syrups is recently boiled distilled water. Using this menstruum ensures that the syrup is free from mineral matter and from spores that might cause fermentation in the presence of sugar. In the preparation of some syrups and oxymels, however, vinegar is often used in preference to water or alcohol (see garlic syrup and oxymel recipes, page 246).

SUGAR FOR SYRUPS

The best kind of sugar to use in the preparation of syrup is very dry, refined white sugar in a crushed, powdered, or granulated form. This is a chemically pure sugar produced by sugar refineries. It requires no further preparation. Pure white sugar is best used in the preparation of an independently permanent (off-grid) syrup due to the fact that the sugar (sucrose) to water ratio is critical for the resulting syrup to provide adequate preserving properties. For this class of preparation, the use of damp sugar should be avoided, as it can disturb this crucial water/sugar proportion.

If raw, unrefined, or brown sugar is to be relied on as a preservative, it is necessary to simmer the syrup; then skim or strain off the froth (in certain pharmacy texts you find the more scornful term "scum" applied here), which contains vegetable "impurities" (the organic ballast products of Nature seem to perturb pharmacists). If impurities are obviously diffused in the liquid, which will not readily rise as froth, it is useful to add, before applying heat, a little egg white, previously beaten up with water, which by coagulating at the boiling temperature forms a clot, enclosing the impurities, and facilitating their removal. (Gotcha!)

Dissolving sugar in water can be accomplished by either cold or hot process.

DISSOLVING SUGAR BY COLD PROCESS

This process is used to dissolve sugar in distilled water to make a simple syrup; or to dissolve sugar in a medicated liquid (infusion, decoction, concentrate) to make a medicated syrup, or in fruit juice to make a flavoring syrup by agitation without the use of heat. Sufficient agitation is accomplished by shaking the container vigorously from time to time.

1. Place the properly weighed white sugar in a sterilized bottle that is one and a half to two times as large as the required volume of syrup (this allows for active agitation of the mixture and more rapid solution).

2. Add a properly measured amount of purified water.

3. Securely cap the bottle.

4. Hasten solution by vigorous agitation of the bottle until the sugar is dissolved. The syrup will be crystal clear when the sugar is completely dissolved.

5. Finally, the syrup should be strained through a piece of cotton flannel or muslin placed over the orifice of a large funnel directing the syrup into a very clean, completely dry bottle.

DISSOLVING SUGAR BY WARM PROCESS

In the case of some syrups, where the thick or cohesive character of the solvent impedes rapid solution of the sugar, or when the syrup is wanted in a hurry, a moderate heat can be employed to facilitate solution. This is done as follows:

1. Put the accurately weighed white sugar and properly measured liquid (plain distilled water, infusion, decoction, concentrate) into a strong sterilized bottle that is one and a half to two times as large as the required volume of syrup.

2. Securely cap the bottle.

3. Place it in a water bath and keep it at a temperature of about 120° to 125° F.

4. Frequently agitate the mixture until perfect solution is consummated. Loss of any volatile principles is avoided by keeping the bottle tightly capped throughout and after the preparation process.

MAKING A PERMANENT SIMPLE SYRUP THAT REQUIRES NO REFRIGERATION TO PRESERVE

A simple syrup is a very simple preparation, but it has to be made with care and precision using sterilized equipment along with proper concentration of the sugar in pure (distilled) water. These factors are crucial for a self-preserving product with minimum possibilities of crystallization because the solution is too concentrated, or not concentrated enough so that yeast, molds, and bacteria develop.

It has been found that 85 Gm of white sugar (sucrose) to 47 ml of pure water is the ideal proportion to render a perfectly concentrated solution (syrup) that is self-preserving. This will render approximately a 64 percent strength of sugar by weight in the syrup. As mentioned, less sugar allows enough water activity to promote bacterial growth, and too much sugar concentration will soon crystallize and precipitate out of solution. This removes too much sugar from the solution, thereby making available sufficient water to allow bacterial growth and consequent fermentation.

1. Weigh out 85 Gm of white sugar. (This is an adequate amount to experiment with at first.)

2. Place it in a sterilized, dry jar (one of those slender 10 oz. jam or jelly jars is a good one to use).

3. Pour onto the sugar 47 ml of distilled water (see "*Meniscus*," Chapter Twenty-Five).

4. Cap the jar tightly and agitate it vigorously.

5. Continue agitating it intermittently throughout the day until the solution is clear.

6. Filter the syrup through a very clean flannel or cotton muslin cloth.

7. Store in a cool location.

8. Check the syrup during the next two or three months to see how it's doing.

This nearly saturated sugar solution is supposed to be anti-fermentative, and I have found it to be so; however, be forewarned, it is not anti-ant. Legions of festive six-leggeds will arrive overnight to celebrate each mislaid drop of this seductively saccharine elixir.

MAKING FLAVORING SYRUPS

Cherry Flavoring Syrup

This makes a brilliant red syrup that is an excellent vehicle for administering bitter preparations. It has a pleasant taste. This syrup is acidic due to the malic acid content of the Cherries.

1. Measure out 50 ml of pure Cherry juice. I dilute and use a Bernard Jensen's black cherry concentrate purchased from a health food store (years ago).

2. Weigh out 85 Gm of sugar.

3. Mix, and with assistance of a warm water bath, dissolve the sugar in the Cherry juice.

4. A small quantity of alcohol (brandy is best) can be added to help preserve this syrup.

Raspberry Ferment Syrup

Here's an interesting angle on making a fresh berry syrup appropriate to contrive when the electrical wires that service your home have been demolished and everything else in the refrigerator is also fermenting.

1. Reduce fresh Raspberries to a pulp and let them rest for 3 days.

2. Separate the juice by pressing, and set it aside until it has completely fermented and become clear.

3. Filter the fermented juice.

4. To 3 parts (90 ml or 3 fl. oz.) of the fermented liquid, add 5 parts (150 Gm or 5 oz.) of white sugar.

5. Heat the mixture until the sugar is dissolved and just brought to a boiling point.

6. Bottle in clean bottles, cap, and store in a cool place.

Blackberry Fruit Flavoring Syrup

This is a flavoring syrup having slight astringency.

1. Pick and clean ripe Blackberries.

2. Strongly express the juice.

3. Mix 5 parts sugar with 3 parts juice.

4. Heat the mixture until the sugar is dissolved and just brought to a boiling point.

5. Strain and put hot syrup into sterilized bottles.

6. Cap tightly and store in a cool location.

The manufacture of syrup is considered from two points of view: first, the method by which the sugar and flavoring is dissolved in the solvent as discussed above, and second, the method by which the medicinal constituent is blended with the sugar and/or flavored syrup as illustrated by the examples below.

There are several methods in which a medicinal constituent(s) is blended with a syrup. These methods can vary with each different medicinal agent, and like making any type of herbal preparation, skill comes from experience complemented by the taking of notes. There are numerous flavored and medicated syrups useful in herbal pharmacy. The following examples will illustrate some basic methods for blending constituents with a syrup.

MEDICATING SYRUPS

Medicating a Simple or Flavored Syrup

A simple syrup can be prepared as directed previously and stored in a cool location, ready for use as a carrying agent. Merely blend a tincture or finely powdered herb into a measured portion of the syrup and administer whenever needed.

A Simply Made Herbal Syrup

1. Begin with an herbal decoction or infusion that has been concentrated to about a half to a third volume (see "*Concentrates*," Chapter Twenty-Five).

2. To 500 ml (1 pint) of this concentrate, add about 30 to 60 ml (1 to 2 ounces) of honey and 30 to 60 ml (1 to 2 ounces) of vegetable glycerin. Alter these amounts depending on the consistency you desire.

3. Tinctures can be added to this syrup by adding 1 part of tincture to 3 parts of syrup.

4. Even though the honey and glycerin (and the tincture's alcohol) will act to preserve this syrup, store it in the refrigerator whenever possible.

An Embellished Syrup Made from Dried Herbs

1. Weigh out 60 Gm (2 oz.) of the dry herb or herbal mixture and measure 1 liter (1 quart) of distilled water.

2. Mix and stir together the herb and water, then let this mixture soak for a few hours if you have the time.

3. Place over a low heat and simmer the mixture slowly until the liquid is reduced to about 1/2 original volume (approximately 500 ml or 1 pint).

4. Remove from heat, strain, and press the herbs.

5. Measure the retrieved liquid and pour it back into the pot.

6. Add sweetener to the decoction at the ratio of 2:1 (2 cups sweetener to 1 cup of liquid).

As sweeteners and preservatives, use any one or a blend of honey, white or brown sugar, maple syrup, rice syrup, or vegetable glycerin. This 2:1 proportion will create a very sweet syrup. Use less sweetening if desired when refrigeration is accessible.

7. Warm the decoction and sweetener(s) and mix them until the sweetener is completely dissolved.

8. If you want to thicken the syrup further, simmer it over a moderate heat for 20 to 30 minutes or until you attain the desired consistency. If using raw honey, this last step will destroy its active enzymes. To avoid this, merely warm the syrup adequately to mix the honey and decoction.

9. At this point, you can add brandy (optional), approximately 6–8 tablespoonsful per pint of syrup.

Brandy is added for flavor and further preservative action. If this is to be a cough syrup, brandy adds some muscle relaxant and cough retardant properties. (There are some excellent-tasting fruit- and spice-flavored brandies on the market.)

You might also want to add a fruit concentrate for flavor and nutrients. This will dilute the syrup and make it more prone to fermentation unless you compensate by adding more sugar, glycerin, or brandy.

10. Once the syrup has cooled down, essential oils such as Peppermint, Anise, Cardamom, or Ginger can be added for flavor. Add 5 drops *total* of a single oil or a blend of oils per pint of syrup. Add these only 1 drop at a time, and test the flavor each time; these aromatic oils are extremely concentrated, and they can easily overpower your syrup.

11. Remove the syrup from the heat and bottle it in clean bottles for use.

A 5:1 (Syrup to Herb Ratio) Medicinal Syrup

This syrup will have a 1 to 2 teaspoons dose level.

1. Weigh 50 Gm of the cut herb or herb compound.

2. Measure 500 ml of distilled water.

3. Make a decoction that when completed is strained or expressed.

4. Prepare a concentrate by placing the decoction into a water bath, and at 140–160° F., reduce it to 125 ml.

5. Transfer this concentrate to a saucepan and add 200 Gm of white sugar.

6. Stir this mixture over a gentle heat until the sugar is completely dissolved.

7. Remove from the heat, cover, and when cool you will have 250 ml of medicated syrup.

8. Pour into small storage bottles.

Using this method, I recently made a syrup from a decoction of "Redwood Chai," a non-caffeine blend of herbs (Carob, Ginger, Cinnamon, Orange Peel, Clove, Chicory, Licorice, Cardamom, and Fennel) which was formulated by Julie Rothman, herbalist, and owner of *Flower Power Teas* in Santa Cruz, California. The consequent Chai syrup quickly attained a "nectar for the gods" status in my community; misty-eyed recurrent tasters revered it as El Dorado, liquid Elysium, Formicidae heaven…the Kingdom had definitely come by spoonfuls—I highly recommend it.

Garlic Syrup

This expectorant syrup is most useful for relieving spasmodic cough and lung congestion, and will be found especially appropriate for children.

Avoid using metallic containers or utensils when making this syrup.

1. Slice and bruise 3 oz. of fresh Garlic.

2. Measure 1/2 pint of vinegar.

3. Measure 1 pound of white sugar.

4. Macerate the Garlic in the vinegar for four days.

5. Strain and press.

6. Add the sugar.

7. Agitate vigorously, or gently warm the liquid until the sugar is fully dissolved.

8. Bottle in small clean bottles.

Compound Syrup of Blackberry Root

1. Weigh out 2 oz. of cut Blackberry root.

2. Combine with 3/4 oz. each of powdered Cinnamon, Cloves, Nutmeg.

3. Simmer the above mixture in 1 pint of distilled water for 1 hour.

4. Strain and press.

5. Add 1 pound white sugar and dissolve it completely.

6. To this syrup add 1 1/2 fl. oz. of brandy.

7. To this mixture add 1 drop each of Clove essential oil and Cinnamon essential oil.

This syrup supplies the well-known astringent virtues of Blackberry; it is also aromatic and a gentle stimulant.

Black Cohosh Syrup

1. Measure 4 fl. oz. of Black Cohosh tincture.

2. Add to 6 oz. of a prepared simple syrup.

3. Carefully evaporate to 8 oz. (1/2 pint).

4. Bottle in clean 2-oz. size bottles.

This makes a pleasant tasting syrup useful for coughs and other respiratory afflictions. The addition of 1/2 fl. oz. of Lobelia tincture to 1/2 pint of this syrup will give an exceptional relaxing expectorant and antispasmodic syrup useful for treating conditions of difficult breathing, alleviating dry coughs, and calming irritable contractions of the diaphragm.

Blackberry fruit	**Hawthorn**
Black Cohosh	**Marshmallow**
Burdock	**Mullein**
Cayenne	**Nettle**
Chamomile	**Peppermint**
Comfrey root	**Plantain**
Dandelion root and leaf	**St. John's Wort**
Echinacea	**Uva Ursi**
Elder berries	**Valerian**
Fennel	**Yellow Dock**
Ginger	

HERBAL HONEYS

Honey is deposited in honeycomb by the honeybee, *Apis mellifica*, our planet's premier herbalists and medicine-makers. Honey is a peculiar fluid, consistent with the other delightfully peculiar products that honeybees gather and create, such as royal jelly, propolis, pollen, and beeswax. In its freshly produced state honey is fluid, but upon aging it separates into two layers, a rather solid granular lower layer and a liquid upper layer. The granular layer is composed principally of dextrose or grape sugar, the upper layer being mostly levulose or fruit sugar. Honey, normally consisting of 70 or 80 percent sugar in an aqueous solution, has a sweet taste (although I have a quart of decidedly bitter-tasting Dandelion honey in my pantry) and a somewhat aromatic odor followed by a faint acidity. In addition to its sugar content, honey consists of wax, pollen, coloring, and aromatic constituents. It resembles sugar in its properties, but it is more laxative. Honey is emollient, demulcent, nutritive, and mildly laxative. Its emollient and demulcent properties are most beneficial for relieving dryness and pain in the throat and for treating cough and difficulty with swallowing. Combining honey with a strong infusion of Sage is a classic preparation for relieving hoarseness and respiratory congestion. The eminent German hydrotherapist, Father Kneipp, maintained that if a little honey were added to herbal remedies, it would greatly enhance their efficacy, as it acts as a medium to promote better assimilation of the nutritive components with the body's tissues.

The advantages of using honey

over syrups as a simple vehicle lie primarily in the user's belief system that honey is more nutritious and health-promoting than white sugar. I am one of those who believe this; however, I am also one who realizes how difficult it is for bees to supply enough honey for themselves as well as for all of us. In light of this, I think that syrups are excellent delivery vehicles that can be used more often, and the amount of sugar that is taken in these instances is of relatively little consequence. Focus on health and well-being; it deposes the tyranny of those little diet demons our minds love to create.

Thank you little furry ones for the sweet nectar of your lives.

Herbal Honeys

To Prepare Herbal (Medicated) Honeys

Herbal (medicated) honeys are thick liquid preparations closely allied to syrups, differing because honey is used as the base instead of sugar. They are simply a mixture of honey with certain medicinal agents (tinctures, glycerites, powders), and are normally prepared extemporarily.

Glycerin is sometimes added to medicinal honey preparations to prevent granulation and subsequent separation of the honey into layers. Some folks add glycerin for the purpose of better preservation (which is probably redundant since honey is an excellent preservative agent on its own). The glycerin is added in the proportion of 5 percent of the amount of honey.

To Prepare Aromatic Honeys

Aromatic honeys are prepared by adding aromatic essential oils to a honey-glycerin base. These aromatic honeys preserve forever, and with the addition of the glycerin, will not readily crystallize, so they need not be reliquefied by the use of heat (which readily evaporates volatile oils).

Aromatic honeys are excellent to use as vehicles to deliver essential oils for flavoring tea, coffee, salad dressing, hot breakfast cereals, toasted raisin-cinnamon bagels, etc., and they are well used as digestive aids taken after meals. Some essential oils that are good to experiment with are: Cinnamon, Ginger, Angelica, Peppermint, Bergamot, Rose, Lemon, Orange, Geranium, Dill, and Cardamom.

To each 1/4 cup of honey add 1 or 2 drops of essential oil and stir them in. As when flavoring a syrup, add the oil only one drop at a time, for these oils are very intense, and with some essential oils two drops can be too much (this is rectified by adding more honey).

OXYMELS

An oxymel is a specialized sweet and sour herbal honey, a sweet honey mixed with a little sour vinegar. This combination is used as a carrier for herbal infusions, decoctions, concentrates, tinctures, and so forth. Oxymels are used as a gargle or as a vehicle for intense herbal aids such as Garlic, Cayenne, and Lobelia.

OXYMELS

To Prepare an Oxymel Base

1. Mix 1 pound honey with 1/2 pint vinegar.

2. Place the mixture in a pot and simmer to a consistency of syrup.

3. To this carrier, one normally adds a medicinal agent (infusion, decoction, concentrate, tincture) to prepare it as a gargle or an expectorant medicine.

Garlic Oxymel by the Late Dr. John Christopher

Dilute a small portion; use this as a gargle and take 2 tablepoonsful internally.

1. Measure 8 oz. (250 ml) vinegar into a glass pot.

2. Add 1/4 oz. (7 Gm) crushed Caraway seeds and 1/4 oz. crushed Fennel seeds.

3. Bring this mixture to a boil and simmer for 15 minutes.

4. Remove from the heat and add 1 1/2 oz. (45 Gm) of fresh pressed Garlic.

5. Let this sit until cool.

6. Press and strain the liquid.

7. Add 10 oz. (300 Gm) of honey.

8. Place onto a low heat and simmer to a consistency of syrup.

Lobelia Oxymel by the Late Dr. William H. Cook

This is an effective preparation to use for relieving dry and irritable coughs, and congestion of the lungs.

1. Macerate Lobelia (preferably the fresh plant if available; dry plant works too) in enough apple cider vinegar to cover it completely.

2. Press it after 7 to 14 days.

3. Mix with honey at the proportion of 3 pounds honey to 1 quart of tincture [for a smaller amount use 340 Gm (3/4 lb.) of honey to 250 ml (8 oz.) of tincture].

4. Evaporate in a water bath to the consistency of thin molasses.

5. Bottle and refrigerate.

ELECTUARIES

An electuary (more commonly referred to these days as a *confection* or *conserve*) is a delivery vehicle that has been prepared by mixing an unpleasant tasting, finely powdered herb with honey (sometimes including a little sugar) or fruit pulp, creating a sweetened and flavored mass that can be molded into portions about the size of a marble (nib or an aggie-sized) suitable for oral administration. When made with honey or the addition of glycerin, electuaries retain their original soft condition for a long time; if made with fruit pulp, the moisture gradually evaporates and the mass becomes dry and hard. If essential oils are to be incorporated in an electuary, they should first be triturated thoroughly with some sugar to ensure their uniform distribution throughout the soft mass (see "*Trituration*," Chapter Twenty-Five).

If you're close, the attempted metric/avoirdupois conversions in this chapter might push you over the edge. Sorry.

ELECTUARIES

Rose Electuary

To make a Rose electuary from the petals of garden and/or wild Roses, which is useful as a mildly astringent, pleasant-tasting vehicle for deliver of other powders:

20 Gm	Rose petals in very fine #60 powder (2/3 oz.) (see "Powdering," Chapter Twenty-Five)
160 Gm	finely powdered sugar (5 oz.+)
30 Gm	honey (1 oz.)
40 ml	Rosewater (1 1/3 fl. oz.)

1. Heat the Rosewater to approximately 150° F. (65° C.); remove from the heat.

2. Pour in the Rose powder and rub it to reduce the Roses to a pulpy mash.

3. Gradually add the honey and sugar.

Orange Electuary

To make an Orange electuary for use to administer very bitter powders:

1. Grate 120 Gm (4 oz.) of fresh outer peel of Orange.

2. Slowly add 360 Gm (12 oz.) of sugar, mixing it in thoroughly.

Laxative Electuary

Standard dose is 15 to 30 Gm (1/2 to 1 oz.).

Sometimes honey and sugar are not necessary, as in the following laxative electuary:

40 Gm	Prune deprived of seed
40 Gm	Dates deprived of seed
40 Gm	dried Fig
40 Gm	seedless Raisins
10 Gm	Senna in fine powder or Cascara sagrada in fine powder

1. Pass all the ingredients through a small hand-cranked meat grinder (attainable at most antique/collectible stores) to produce a uniform paste.

2. Store in a tightly covered jar in refrigerator.

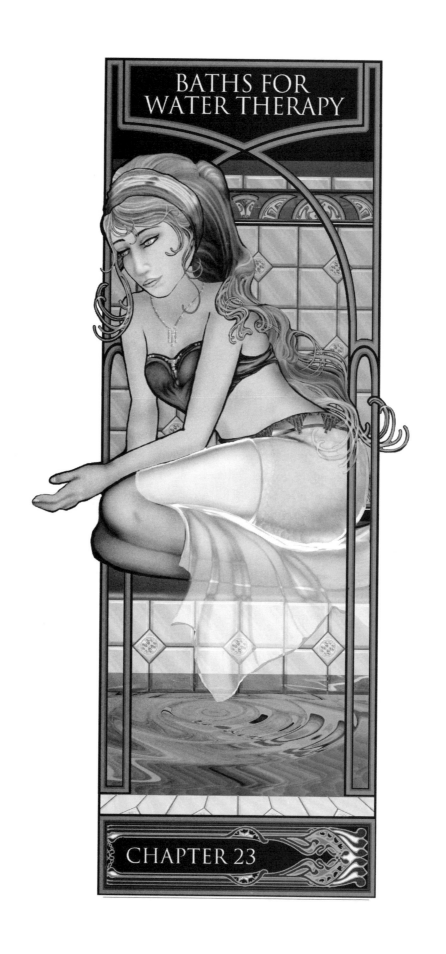

BATHS FOR
WATER THERAPY

CHAPTER 23

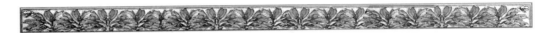

I considered giving this chapter a controversial title, possibly incorporating terms like passionate immersions, or wet bodies, or secrets of water erotica revealed, for, as it is titled, on first encounter many readers might pass over it (packaging is the gist of most products these days). For the most part in our culture, we have lost appreciation for and interest in the profound therapeutic effects of simple hot, warm, and cold water applications. We have forfeited most of our conscious knowledge of how to tap into the healing energetics of water by merely varying its temperature, getting in it for a short while and back out. This is unfortunate for, with its characteristic ability to affect human circulation by transferring heat to and from the body and from here to there in the body, water therapy lies at the very heart of health maintenance and natural medicine.

Water's solvency and fluidity have been major players in most of the medicinal preparations we have discussed so far, and in many of them water is one of their primary ingredients. I am compiling this chapter on baths and other forms of water application, because intuitively it feels important also to explore the nature of water as an externally applied tonic and medicine. My instincts make it clear to me that simple water therapy, or *hydrotherapy*, is an important compo-nent of any book that promotes home-crafted medicines and independent domestic health care. I've learned a great deal by undertaking this task, as I too had limited exposure to and experience in using water/bath therapy. I have relied on the publications in the early 1900s of professional practitioners of hydrotherapy, such as physicians J. H. Kellogg, A. Stillé, and G. B. Wood, along with the teachings of my now deceased friend, Wade Boyle, N.D., along with other specific information that I found here and there to guide me in my own understanding and experimentation. So I offer you the following basic principles of water therapy, and, after having applied much of it myself, I wholeheartedly encourage you to work with this information to further educate yourself about the phenomenal uses and pleasures of full body and partial immersion water/bath therapy. At the very least immerse yourself in the information about the strategy of the "whole body, cold water plunge," and then do it. I'm confident you will enjoy your experiences as you experiment with these techniques on your own wet body.

You'll need a good bath thermometer.

A chapter on hydrotherapy has to begin by first dipping its toe in the water. Water is an enchanting phenomenon, exhibiting remarkably diverse physical properties and modifications in its chameleon-like chemical antics. In its pure state, water is a transparent liquid, lacking color, taste, and smell. Pure water has been highly esteemed by science's assumption that its specific gravity is unity (1.0), and forms the term of comparison for the specific gravities of all other solids and liquids, earmarking water as the apple of gravity's eye.

Not to be totally unyielding, this provocative substance allows itself to be compressed, but only to the merest extent. When reduced to 32° F. (0° C.), water freezes and becomes solid, forming transparent crystals of ice, and when raised to 212° F. (100° C.), it boils and transforms into an elastic gas. Water's thermo-antics have also been honored by scientists by selecting it as their standard for specific heat, marking it as the official glint in the sun's resplendent eye.

As steam, water's bulk increases nearly 1700-fold, and its celebrated liquid specific gravity diminishes to merely half that of atmospheric air where it ascends sun bound, leaving gravity to court other elements for the time being. This impetuosity is understandable, for the essence of water's parental lineage, hydrogen and oxygen, is obviously a gaseous one, and it is only judicious for an offspring to commingle with family whenever possible. Then inevitably, while frolicking with its airy kin, gaseous water condenses into minute drops (which explains why steam appears opaque). And likewise, in a bigger picture, the over-saturation of air with water vapor causes a similar condensation in the atmosphere where water makes its appearance, this time with an expansive gesture as opaque clouds, preparing for its inevitable return as rain to the patient and willful arms of Earth's gravity.

At the temperature of 39° F. (4° C.), pure water attains its maximum density where one cubic centimeter weighs precisely one gram, and increases its bulk and decreases its specific gravity when either heated or cooled. Therefore, as steam, water expands and rises into the air, and as ice it expands and floats upon itself.

In the world of liquids, gases, and chemical compounds, water is definitely not known as abstinent, for it is a voracious entity with the power and appetite to dissolve many salts and more or less all gases, including common air, the constituents of which are always present in natural water. Therefore, natural water is rarely found in its purest state.

Globally, water is forever uniformly present in the atmosphere in the guise of an invisible vapor, even in the driest weather, and, as we all have experienced, exerts a vital influence on comfort, and on the animal and vegetable economy of our planet. Water unites with other bodies either in liquid or solid form, producing in the former case solutions, and in the latter case hydrates; therefore, when a vegetable or animal body is deficient in water it is considered dehydrated.

Water as the universal solvent has a profound influence in the operations of nature. Water by far constitutes the major portion of the mass of all living beings, and it is as essential to their organic physical nature as it is to the molecular actions and movements by which life is manifested. Water constitutes the basis of nearly all the secretions of the body, and nine-tenths of the weight of the blood. Consequently, water can be seen as an important article of food, which not only directly supplies one constituent of the body but also supplies a means of promoting the

This chapter is both an ode to the mind boggling restorative power of simple water baths and a therapeutic reference for treating acute physical discomforts and chronic maladies. But the heart of the chapter is its introduction to you of the quick cold-water plunge which is probably the most efficient, reliable, and free health tonic known to the human body. Enough said —see page 254.

solution of solid food in the gastrointestinal organs, facilitating its absorption. Water is also the solvent of all the body's secretions and excretions, and the vehicle by which the excretions are ushered out of the body.

But obviously not all natural water is suitable for food. The greater part of the water in the world is contained in the ocean; another large portion consists of spring and river waters, which (apart from the issue of pollution by civilized human beings) are commonly so mineralized as to be unfit for ordinary drinking; or of other water in certain sluggish rivers, stagnant ponds, and marshes, which contain too large a portion of animal and vegetable matter to be palatable or wholesome. (I would include chlorinated tap water somewhere on the "unsuitable for human consumption" list too, and I'd place artificially fluoridated water at the very top of that list.)

SOURCES OF WATER FOR HUMAN USE

Common fresh water can be divided according to its source. We are aware of rain, snow, spring, river, well, lake, and marsh water. These divisions are not so useful, however, as the source of water is not always indicative of its quality. From water's extensive solvent powers, it is obvious that in its natural state it must be more or less contaminated with foreign matter. Common water from different localities and sources possesses innumerable shades of differences. What is more useful for us as consumers and manipulators of water is to view water as soft and hard.

Soft water contains only a sparse amount of impurities, ordinarily tastes good, and when used with soap readily forms lather. *Hard water* is impregnated with mineral salts, most commonly sulfate of lime, which often doesn't taste so good, curdles soap, and is relatively unfit for most domestic purposes.

Rainwater and *snow water* are the purest kinds of natural water; in effect they are produced by natural distillation where ground water evaporates, leaving any dissolved materials behind, condenses in the atmosphere forming clouds, then returns to the earth as relatively pure rain or snow. Rainwater, however, as it lingers in its cloud form, ordinarily dissolves and thereby contains atmospheric air. It is carbonic acid that is dissolved and gives this water its lively fresh taste.

In its purest state, rainwater is best collected in large vessels away from buildings and at a time well after the rain has first begun to fall. Otherwise rainwater will be contaminated with the dust and various organic and inorganic matters that float in the atmosphere or have been dissolved in the air, and by impurities derived from rooftops, etc. Speaking of rooftops, rainwater can be collected in a relatively pure state even in cities by taking advantage of a heavy rain after it has descended for a considerable time and washed away every impurity, and is collected as it flows from roofs and spouts.

Snow water has a peculiar taste, because when water freezes the ice crystals formed are free of any and all compounds that may have been dissolved in the water. Therefore, when snow is newly melted it contains no air constituents (no dissolved carbonic acid) and this accounts for its rather stale, lifeless taste. Melting snow and exposing it to the air for some time allows it to take up the constituent gases of the atmosphere, and it will taste like other natural waters. Rain and snow water are both well used as food, and in the preparation of herbal medicines, fomentations, and baths. Water equal in purity to distilled water can be obtained by melting perfectly clear and transparent ice under conditions that protect it from dust and other impurities. Also sea water, with all its dissolved salts and minerals, can yield ice of as great a purity as river water (sea ice that is crystalline with a bluish cast has very little salt in it—gray or opaque sea ice is salty).

Spring water's purity and taste depend entirely on the strata through which it flows; it is usually found to be purest when it passes through sand or gravel. The refreshing taste of many spring waters is mainly due to the presence of the carbonic acid they have dissolved. This water usually contains a trace of common salt (sodium chloride), and generally other impurities, depending on the location of the spring. When these saline compounds (salts) are increased beyond a certain quantity, the spring is called a *mineral spring* where we collect various mineral waters, some of which we bottle for drinking, or sit in at spas for pleasant, healthful soaking.

River water is generally less impregnated with salt matter than spring water, due to its considerable proportion of rainwater and to the fact its volume of water is so proportionally large compared to the surface of its (mineral source) bed. However, even though river water is normally freer from saline matter, it is more apt to have certain insoluble matter of a vegetable and earthy nature mechanically suspended in it, which frequently impair its transparency.

Well water, like spring water, is liable to contain various impurities. The purity of well water is often proportional to the depth of the well and to the consistency with which the water is drawn and used.

Artesian or *overflowing wells* and springs, because of their great depth, generally bring forth deliciously pure water.

Lake water (aside from the issue of pollution by civilized human beings) offers the human community very pure and wholesome water.

Marsh water is generally stagnant and contains vegetable remains undergoing decomposition to the delight of innumerable fascinating plants as well as a myriad of mud and muck-seeking, jumping, scooting, moist, and warty creatures. However, this water is considered unwholesome for most human beings' domestic and medicinal purposes.

Water, therefore, is known as good (for Homo sapiens' use) if it is lively, clear, without smell, and does not curdle soap; and upon being evaporated to dryness, leaves an insignificant residue. This form of water answers well for the cooking of grains and vegetables, cleaning up, satisfying thirst, hydrating one's body, and for the preparation of herbal potions and healthful baths.

EFFECT OF WATER ON THE HUMAN BODY AS A TONIC AND RESTORATIVE AGENT

In general, water acts primarily as a direct means to modify the temperature of the body. Water at a temperature higher than the body is a direct stimulant of the circulation, and therefore stimulates all the body's functions. Cold water, on the other hand, diminishes a portion of the body's heat, and therefore is a direct tranquilizer or sedative to circulation and other functions. However, when applied correctly, cold can indirectly become a potent stimulant of bodily functions and a healthful tonic. This happens because a salient property of a living organism is to react against whatever tends to depress it. Ordinarily, the more vigorously and abruptly the depressing influence is exerted the more powerful the organism's reaction. (That can give wedlock a run for its money.) Therefore, cold applications to the body in a certain measure and for a given time produce a diminished activity of function, which is quickly followed by a degree of activity greater than that which originally existed. In this circumstance, the primary effect of heat and the secondary effect of cold resemble one another quite closely. However, cold and heat are relative terms; they do not designate any definite temperature. So we can use 98.6° F., the approximate temperature of the human body in health, as a standard and whatever is higher than this may be described as heat; whatever is lower as cold.

The term *bath* means the complete or partial immersion of the body in a fluid or in a vaporous medium such as steam. The effects of different baths on the system are very dissimilar according to their temperature, the area of the body being immersed, and the duration of time the individual is subjected to the bath's influence. For consistent remedial results, the original temperature of the bath (tepid, warm, or hot) is to be maintained during the whole time the individual remains in the water. At the end of a few minutes, the temperature should be tested with a thermometer and, if required, hot water added. The sensations of the bather are usually an inaccurate thermometer.

Heat and *cold*, as noted before, are relative terms. Objects are recognized as cold by the body when they have a temperature less than that of the skin—and the reverse. For convenience in this discussion of the physi-

ological effects of water, as well as for describing therapeutic application of various forms of baths, we can use the terms that have been commonly applied: very cold, cold, cool, tepid, warm, hot, very hot. It is not easy, however, to fix the limits of temperature to which each term should be applied, and this seems to have given rise to much discussion in the hydrotherapy world.

The following table of temperatures appears agreeable to most hydrotherapy texts and is convenient for our practical application:

Very cold	32° to 50° F.
Cold	50° to 65° F.
Cool	65° to 75° F.
Tepid	75° to 85° F.
Warm	85° to 98° F.
Hot	98° to 104° F.
Very hot	104° F. and above.

WHOLE BODY BATHS

THE COLD BATH (QUICK COLD PLUNGE)
(APPROXIMATELY 32° TO 65° F.)

The effects of cold water on the living body are complex. They include the direct abstraction of heat, and are followed by a multitude of fascinating reflex effects due to the mutually responsive relations between the skin and the body's internal organs. The interior of a healthy body maintains a certain average temperature or within two or three degrees of it, in spite of the temperature of the surrounding medium. The loss of heat by the contact of cold water with the skin is more or less completely balanced by the generation of heat through the organic changes which are steadily active in every tissue. This immediate and powerful reaction of the body to cold, along with its efforts to replace the heat that has been lost by restoring the equilibrium of the body temperature, is referred to, in hydrotherapy circles, as a *thermic reaction*.

The brief application of cold to the skin is so quickly followed by thermic reaction that the effects seem to be those of direct stimulation, mimicking the body's initial reactions to the application of heat. However, when the body undergoes a continual abstraction of heat by a prolonged immersion in cold water (or any cold medium), all the vital processes are depressed; there is a diminished production of heat, the skin grows pale and shriveled, the internal organs are overloaded with blood, the pulse beats slowly, the secretions are diminished, and the muscles grow lethargic.

When a person plunges into a cold bath, she or he is first sensible of a sudden sensation of cold upon the surface, accompanied by an oppression of breathing, causing this function to be performed in convulsive gasps. This is called *the shock*, and is caused by a rapid contraction of the cutaneous capillaries pushing a rush of blood back to the lungs and other internal organs. In a short time the difficulty of breathing disappears, the temperature becomes agreeable, and if the person now leaves the water, a warmth of the surface of the body comes on, termed *the glow* or *the reaction*. This is followed by a sense of invigoration of the entire system and an upliftment of the mind and emotions. (Try it, you'll love the glow, invigoration, and upliftment parts.)

However, should the person remain too long in the water, for whatever reason, another train of symptoms becomes apparent. The sensation of cold soon turns to an unpleasant degree of chilliness, followed by tremors. Soon, the surface of the body shows a bluish tint as the blood accumulates in the internal organs. Upon leaving the water there is no reaction, or at best a feeble one; the surface of the body remains cold; the extremities benumbed; and headache and difficult respiration ensue with a sense of depression and lassitude.

The goal in proposing a health enhancing quick-cold (plunge) bath is the tonic influence produced by a sudden, powerful impression on the nervous system, followed by due reaction. A tonic is an agent which, systematically applied, gives tone to the tissue, aiding in the restoration and maintenance of the functions of nutrition and assimilation and increases the body's vital resistance. The tonic effect of cold water is constant and regular whenever water is applied at a temperature below that of the body.

Cold water is a physiological tonic that awakens quintessential nervous activity without putting a burden on any vital organs and without hampering the activity of any bodily function. The tissue activity set up in the heat-producing tissues of the muscles (as the result of exposure of the skin to a cold medium for a short time) is participated in by every cell and tissue in the entire body.

By quickly touching the body's whole skin surface with waters having temperatures of 90° F. or below (the more below the better, short of bouncing on ice), the skin, with its vast network of sensory, motor, sympathetic, vasomotor, and thermic nerves, arouses every nerve center, every sympathetic ganglion, every sensory and motor filament in the entire body to heightened life and activity. Every blood vessel and cell in the entire body is awakened and quickened with vital impulse. The

In my opinion, the glow of exhilaration, and the invigoration and buoyancy of body and mind which accompany the reaction from a quick immersion in cold water, along with good food that you relish eating, pursuing enjoyable exercise and periods of repose, drinking lots of pure water, establishing and maintaining adequate intestinal flora, focusing on happy thoughts, and playing in the sunlight are the most valuable means of arousing to activity any and all flagging energies of the body. These are the most simple, inexpensive, and reliable means for individuals to prune chronic and acute disease off their limb of the family tree.

The cold plunge produces a reliable tonic effect by lifting the body's whole vital economy to a higher level and increasing vital resistance to all the causes of the pathological processes.

The reaction produced by tonic application fills the skin with blood, and if it is repeated daily the blood is finally fixed in the skin, rendering the skin vibrantly wholesome.

When there is any serious infirmity of the heart, lungs, or kidneys, or illness of any organ essential to life, the temperature of a bath should not be lower than 75° F. (a cool bath). If local applications of cold water cause any chilliness at all they should be discontinued.

reaction produced by tonic application fills the skin with blood, and if it is repeated daily the blood is finally fixed in the skin, rendering the skin vibrantly wholesome by permanently increasing its vascular activity, relieving internal congestion. Tissue building is accelerated, more blood is in circulation, more oxygen is absorbed, more CO_2 and urea are eliminated, and all the vital functions are quickened, thus causing the stream of life to flow at a more rapid rate.

Early morning baths or plunges in the sea, lake, or river, in a tub, or a naked roll in the snow are immensely invigorating; and in the summer months cold baths before bedtime are of great service by rendering sleep more sound and refreshing.

Any individual who has been wearied by laborious effort in a heated atmosphere will find her or his muscular strength immediately reinforced by a cold spray, shower, or bath. When fatigued, a quick application of cold water to the face and head has a delightfully refreshing effect. The relief, brightened expression, and increased vigor which follows this simple bathing of the head, face, and neck with cold are the results of the reflex stimulation of the nerve centers of the brain and spinal cord and the tonic reaction which follows such an application. When the whole surface of the body instead of merely a small area is acted upon, the effect is proportionally greater.

Water, by its accessibility, its convenience in use, its abundance, and its high specific heat, more readily lends itself to human beings in producing restorative and permanent tonic effects than any other agent.

However, it must be pointed out that it is essential to the efficacy and safety of a cold bath that a body's stock of vitality must be sufficient to create, immediately after its immersion in the water, those general sensations of warmth and invigoration pictured above. In other words, cold baths are always contraindicated when, from debility, the system is too weak to produce a reactive glow. In all seasons, baths at a lower temperature than 50° F. are considered unsafe for children and for old persons who are not in good health. Extremely feeble persons are in the greatest need of tonic treatment, and yet have the least tolerance for cold water. These folks must be attended to by an experienced hydrotherapist who knows how to employ the gentlest measures for administering tonic applications, such as cold wet-hand rubs, cold friction (rubbing the body with coarse material dipped in cool water), the salt glow (rubbing the skin with moist salt and sprayed with cool water which produces a circulatory reaction), and alternate hot and cold applications to the spine.

When there is any serious infirmity of the heart, lungs, or kidneys, or illness of any organ essential to life, the temperature of a bath should not be lower than 75° F. (a cool bath). If local applications of cold water cause any chilliness at all they should be discontinued.

It is important to mention the necessity of avoiding the use of the general cold bath in cases of extreme exhaustion from violent exercise, or when, with or without exhaustion, a sensation of chilliness exists. A cold application should never be used when the surface of the skin is covered with cold perspiration, or immediately after a meal.

Some techniques and physical conditions that aid the energies of the body so that it can develop a prompt and vigorous reaction, making the toning energy of a cold bath most efficient:

Before the bath

• Wear warm clothing or expose oneself to the air of a warm room.

• Take a short hot bath or shower of some sort. If preferred, begin with a shower at about the temperature of the skin, and gradually increase it. A very high temperature may be borne this way without pain. Raising the temperature of the skin has great value as a preparation for the application of cold. The skin is not only rendered more susceptible to the influence of cold, but is prepared to react after a cold application because of the increased nervous and vascular activity, and the large amount of heat stored up. When there is rheumatism with painful joints, or the skin is cold, fatigue, neuralgia, anemia, or lack of energy, this preliminary heating of the skin is of the greatest importance and value.

• Drink hot water or some other hot beverage.

• Exercise more or less vigorously according to one's strength, but not so much as to bring on perspiration or fatigue. Vigorous exercise or a hot bath taken just prior to a cold bath increases the initial rise of temperature because muscular activity increases heat production to such a marked degree that the cold application finds the heat-producing process already in full play. Hence, it is more able to produce a strong thermic reaction.

• Friction of the skin until warm and well reddened.

• Having warm, dry, or slightly moist skin.

• Being in a state of general health and vigor.

Pertaining to the bath itself

• The water should be a low temperature (the lower the temperature the more prompt the reaction).

• Wet the head before the rest of the body.

• Immersion should be short and sudden.

After the bath to encourage reaction

• Employ heat in the form of warm clothing, or hot, dry air, and/or by drinking a hot beverage (a steaming cup of green tea or hot Chai gives supreme pleasure at this time).

• Exercise vigorously.

• Brisk friction of the skin surface with the hand, rough towel, or skin brush.

• A high external temperature of whatever means available, favors reaction, both by lessening heat elimination and by increasing heat production.

Conditions to take into consideration which can prevent or delay the thermic reaction

• *Old age*, not necessarily referring to the number of years an individual has lived, but more specifically to the condition of his or her arteries. Individuals with progressed hardening of the arteries react with difficulty, and thus very cold baths must be avoided unless the area of the body immersed in the bath is very small.

• *Infancy*, very young children react poorly.

• *Exhaustion*, either of a temporary nature from excessive exercise, or from lack of sleep, or of extreme nervous exhaustion due to the weak condition of the nerve centers upon which prompt reaction depends.

A tepid bath can soothe and invigorate a tired laborer and uplift a weary traveler following a long or stressful journey.

• *Obesity*, due to relative anemia of the skin

• *Unhealthy* or *inactive skin*

• *Very low temperature of the skin*

• *Profuse perspiration*, but only when accompanied by great fatigue

• *Extreme nervous irritability* or *distress*

• *An immediately preceding or impending chill*

• *Extreme aversion to cold applications*

A simple method for testing a person's ability to react healthfully to a cold immersion is as follows:
• Dip the corner of a towel in ice-water.

• Hold the saturated towel against the bared forearm of the person for one minute, covering a surface of at least ten or twelve square inches.

• Do not rub the surface, simply maintain contact of the cold wet towel with the skin.

• On withdrawing the towel, dry the surface by light pressure with the dry end of the towel.

• Cover to prevent slow cooling by evaporation, and note the length of time required for the occurrence of reaction, as shown by the return of redness and natural heat.

• A good reaction should show distinct reddening of the surface within 1 or 2 minutes after the application of ice water. General chilliness produced by this application indicates an irritability of the nerve centers and of the vasomotor nerves which regulate the contraction and expansion of the blood vessels, along with an inept activity of the reflexes. A mottled blueness shows considerable cardiac weakness.

THE COOL BATH
(APPROXIMATELY 65° TO 75° F.)

The actions and uses of the cool bath are similar to the cold bath, but they are less powerful. They are, therefore, better used for children, for training those individuals who have a strong aversion to cold, and for those who are somewhat debilitated.

THE TEPID BATH
(APPROXIMATELY 75° TO 85° F.)

The temperature of this bath is closely approaching that of the body, therefore the shock and subsequent reaction are slight. This bath is not calculated to have much modifying influence on the heat of the body; rather, its peculiar effects are employed more to soften and cleanse the skin. However, in spite of the fact that the tepid bath is generally employed for comfort and cleanliness and not as a remedial agent, for frail persons and very young children, it might be better suited than lower temperature baths.

To help bolster the health and vigor of the more delicate individual, it is best to use this bath about noon, when the first process of digestion of breakfast is over; immediately after the bath take a brisk walk in the open air. In cases of fatigue and irritation from overexertion or a long journey, this tepid bath can be quite beneficial to soothe, invigorate, and uplift the worker and traveler.

THE WARM BATH
(APPROXIMATELY 85° TO 98° F.)

The temperature of the warm bath, though below that of normal body heat, nevertheless produces a sensation of warmth, as its temperature is above that of the skin's surface. The warm bath cannot be deemed, strictly speaking, a stimulant. The first effect of a warm bath is to produce a sensation of warmth upon the surface of the body which diminishes any tenseness of pulse. It also diminishes the frequency of the pulse (especially if previously accelerated), slows down the respiration, lessens the heat of the body, and relaxes the skin. The circulation in the skin is noticeably affected, and the bulk of the body is increased as evidenced by the increased pressure of any snug-fitting bracelets and of rings worn on the fingers or toes (it snugs up certain body piercings as well).

With regard to using a bath to help reduce fever, a cool or cold bath is not recommended. A bath of 88° to 95° F., which would produce little or no fall of temperature in a healthy person, seems to decrease temperature in one who is experiencing fever (for treating recurrent or intermittent-type fevers, see the section below, "*Partial Body Baths, Employing Cold Water*"). When a person's temperature is three or four degrees above normal body temperature, the difference in the temperature of the hot skin of his or her body and that of the bath water is much greater than ordinary, and consequently the temperature-reducing effect of the bath is proportionately greater. (A water temperature of 80° to 85° F. makes an impression on the hot skin of a nervous, feverish individual similar to that produced by water at a temperature five or even ten degrees lower on a normal person's skin.) Baths of 88° to 92° F. are highly effective in reducing temperature if sufficiently prolonged (30 to 45 minutes); a bath of this temperature has the advantage that it does not provoke a thermic reaction to any considerable degree and therefore does not increase heat production either during or after the bath. This bath is usually tolerated without difficulty by feeble individuals experi-encing fever who would do poorly with a more intense application, and will be effective in lowering their body temperature if needed.

The secondary effects of prolonged immersion in a warm bath are muscular relaxation, sometimes to a considerable degree. Even after leaving the bath, there is an inclination to lassitude with a tendency to perspiration which can continue for some time — a pleasant experience. This bath often acts as a soothing remedy, producing a proclivity to sleep, and helps relieve certain diseased actions and states accompanied by abnormal irritability. This makes a warm bath quite helpful in eruptive fever conditions (such as measles) in which the pulse is frequent, the skin exceptionally hot and dry, and the general condition characterized by restlessness. The restorative effects of a warm bath depend on its temperature and the time a person remains in it. Twenty to twenty-five minutes (making sure to maintain the temperature of the water at 85° to 98° F.) is commonly recommended, but this is best regulated by whatever effect is being produced.

Warm baths are beneficial in the onset of any inflammation of mucous membranes, especially those of the nose and throat, in some congestion of internal organs, chronic rheumatism, and in spasmodic afflictions, especially of children. These baths are remarkably beneficial for relieving convulsions in children (convulsions may be very serious and need medical diagnosis); they not only relax spasms, but they soothe nervous irritation. If the convulsions are severe, it is helpful to also apply cold water to the head.

When a child is given a warm bath, care must be taken not to expose him or her to the cold air for the purposes of drying the

A bath of 88° to 95° F., which would produce little or no fall of temperature in a healthy person, seems to decrease temperature in one who is experiencing fever.

The secondary effects of prolonged immersion in a warm bath are muscular relaxation, sometimes to a considerable degree.

body. The best technique is to envelop the child in a warm flannel sheet or warm blanket (including a huge wraparound hug with the gesture), and place him or her in bed at once. This way the child will not get chilled.

Warm baths are contraindicated in lung illness or when there is congestion or an engorgement of blood in the head.

THE HOT BATH
(APPROXIMATELY 98° TO 104+° F.)

Water is recognized as hot when its temperature is above the temperature of the surface of the body, or between 98° to 104° F. Above 104° F. it is termed as very hot. Aside from the healthy, stimulating reaction generated by the body from a quick cold bath immersion, the hot bath is far more stimulating than the preceding baths. This is evidenced by the excitement of the pulse, the quickening of respiration, the sensation of fullness in the head, the flushing of the face, the reddening of the skin, profuse perspiration, and the throbbing of cerebral vessels. At a temperature of 120° F. a full-water bath becomes unendurable and hazardous for most individuals, although small areas (as in the hand or foot bath, or in the application of a fomentation) can be gradually trained to endure a temperature of 130° to 135° F. Vapor (steam) baths, Turkish baths, and saunas can be tolerated and enjoyed at temperatures of 112° to 120° F., and up to 220° or even 250° F. for a short time by trained persons. I've actually met some of those puzzling individuals who enjoy that experience.

Heat is *primarily* an *excitant*. It is the most powerful of all vital excitants, as evidenced by the heat of the sun being the direct source of animal and vegetable life, stimulating all protoplasmic activity. In the human organism, heat can increase vital activity, elevate the temperature, and excite the brain and nerve centers.

The *secondary* effect of heat is depressant, manifested by the body's atonic reaction to it (the reverse of the tonic reaction is discussed in the section on cold baths). This atonic reaction shows itself as lowered temperature manifested through reflex action, which produces lessened heat production and increased heat elimination with general diminished tissue activity.

A general application of heat first slows, then quickens the pulse.

Short hot applications to the skin surface cause dilation of the small veins, which draws blood from the internal parts and increases the excitability and energy of voluntary skeletal muscles. These short hot applications also powerfully excite the nerves and nerve centers, and these excitant effects are soon followed by depressant effects or atonic reaction.

Prolonged hot applications increase heat production and can give rise to mixed effects of excitation and exhaustion, either of which may predominate. Excitation may involve circulation, respiration, and heat production. Exhaustion may involve nerve impulses and muscles.

Prolonged hot application lessens the energy and excitability of voluntary skeletal muscles. Very hot applications increase the excitability of the involuntary smooth muscles. Neutral temperatures have no influence upon the excitability of the voluntary muscles; the sedative effect produced by neutral temperatures depends rather upon the influence on the nerves of the skin.

Precautionary techniques

A hot bath should never be greatly prolonged, because baths at any temperature above that of the body cause a rapid accumulation of heat and rise of temperature. This can mimic the unpleasant symptoms and effects of sunstroke. The duration of the hot bath should be 5 to 20 minutes according to the temperature. If the intention of a hot bath is mainly to induce excitement, it should be of short duration. The bather is not to be exposed to its action long enough to cause exhaustion. When the sensation of heat is very great or one feels strong palpitations of the heart, it is time to leave the bath.

Before immersing oneself into a hot bath, the head should be rubbed with hot water. This relaxes the blood vessels of the head and lightheadedness (anemia of the brain) is avoided. While partaking in a full hot bath, care must then be taken to avoid cerebral congestion. To prevent this overengorgement of the blood vessels in the brain, apply a cold compress or ice-cap to the head when hot applications are being made to any large area of the skin. It is also important to avoid overexcitement of the heart. Therefore, in general, very hot applications are contraindicated in cases of weak heart, arteriosclerosis, advanced age if debilitated, and infancy (below seven years), and also with folks previously injured by sunstroke or heatstroke.

The hot immersion bath is probably most useful for producing powerful eliminative effects primarily through increased sweating. This bath is taken at 104° F. and above for 10 minutes. When followed by a dry pack, this bath is very efficient for promoting intense sweating. A dry pack consists of completely enveloping a person after a hot bath in a cotton sheet and warm dry blankets; the head only is excluded. A cool damp cloth should be placed on the person's forehead.

The hot bath is also a powerful derivative in that it can draw blood and other fluids from one part of the body to relieve congestion in another. I've read a number of reports where this has been used successfully in treating bronchitis and bronchial pneumonia in children; it relieves the overfilled vessels of the lungs by congesting the vessels of the skin and muscles. This effect is manifested very quickly as the child's coughing stops and the breathing becomes easier. The child is placed in a bath of 104° to 106° F. and removed as soon as there is a strong reddening of the skin. This can be done 2 to 4 times within a 24-hour span as necessary. The child may be placed in the bath up to the pit of the stomach while cool water is gently poured over the upper part of the body.

The hot immersion bath has proved itself valuable in relieving suppressed menstruation and amenorrhea (the absence of the menses). This bath is administered at the time menstruation is due at 101° to 105° F. for a half hour or more. This may be repeated twice a day for two or three days in succession. A hot bath taken at 102° to 112° F. for 15 minutes is also an effective measure for dysmenorrhea (difficult and painful menstruation) with scanty flow. And the hot bath may also be administered in painful menstruation when the flow is profuse, but when using it for this purpose it should be of a short duration of only 3 or 4 minutes at a temperature of 105° to 110° F.

The very hot bath above 104° F. for 5 to 7 minutes followed by rubbing the chest and body with a coarse towel or some other

The hot immersion bath is probably most useful for producing powerful eliminative effects primarily through increased sweating.

Heat is primarily an excitant. The secondary effect of heat is depressant, manifested by the body's atonic reaction to it. This is the reverse of the tonic reaction of cold water.

type of friction device relieves congestion of the mucous membrane when dealing with chronic bronchitis. If this condition is complicated with asthma, this technique generally affords prompt relief. Following this, the individual should be gently cooled and oil rubbed on the skin.

For relieving the discomforts of chronic rheumatism, the hot bath at 102 to 106° F. can be quite helpful. Rubbing the joints with a coarse cloth or with the hands and massaging the joints during the bath aids the circulatory reaction and increases the bath's beneficial effect. A prolonged tepid shower is recommended following this hot bath.

In muscular rheumatism, the hot bath relieves the pain by encouraging the elimination of the toxins that are the source of the condition and by relieving congestion with its derivative effects.

In gastric and intestinal colic, stomach and intestinal pain are quickly relieved by the very hot bath up to 110° F. for 10 to 15 minutes.

The hot bath is also valuable as a palliative measure in cases of gallstones and kidney stones.

The pain of cystitis or inflammation of the bladder is diminished by taking a very hot bath of 104° F. and above, but this condition is aggravated by cold, so the gradual cooling to a neutral temperature is imperative. Other measures (herbal nutrition and emotional upliftment) are well used concurrently to remove the causes of the inflammation.

Heat prepares the skin for cold applications, rendering them more acceptable to those individuals who feel resistance to cold applications. As discussed in the section on cold baths, an initial application of heat as- sists the tonic reaction one will experience from a quick cold application to the skin.

Hot baths are contraindicated in cases of organic diseases of the brain or spinal cord, such as sclerosis and inflammation of the spinal cord, and in cases of cardiac weakness and hypertrophy, and arteriosclerosis. In feverish disorders, as the body temperature is rapidly increased, hot baths are naturally contraindicated.

COMPARATIVE SUMMARY OF THE CHIEF EFFECTS OF COLD AND HEAT

From *Rational Hydrotherapy* by J.H. Kellogg

COLD

General

Primarily a depressant. *Short application* is an excitant by tonic reaction. *Prolonged application* is a depressant

Special

Skin: Action, diminished activity. *Reaction*, increased activity, diminished sensibility

Heart: First quickened, then slowed. Increased force

Vessels: Action, contraction. *Reaction*, dilation

Nerves: Benumbs and paralyzes Excites by tonic reaction

Muscles: Short application increases excitability and capacity Prolonged diminishes capacity and excitability

Lungs: Slows and deepens respiration. Increases amount of respired air. Increases CO_2

Stomach: Increased HCL and motor activity

Kidneys: Congests and excites

Body heat: Short application increased heat production. Prolonged, diminished heat production

Blood: Increased blood count, especially leukocytes

Metabolism: Increased CO_2. Increased urea and improved oxidation

HEAT

General

Primarily an excitant. *Short application* is a depressant by atonic reaction. *Prolonged application* is excitant and then depressant

Special

Skin: Action, increased activity. *Reaction*, diminished activity, diminished sensibility

Heart: First slowed, then quickened. Decreased force

Vessels: Action, contraction then dilation. *Reaction*, contraction

Nerves: Excites. Depresses by atonic reaction

Muscles: Short application lessens fatigue effects. Prolonged lessened excitability and capacity

Lungs: Quickens and facilitates respiration. Diminishes amount of respired air. Decreases CO_2

Stomach: Decreased HCL and motor activity

Kidneys: Renders anemic and lessens activity

Body heat: Short application diminished heat production. Prolonged, increased heat production

Blood: Decreased blood count, especially leukocytes

Metabolism: Decreased CO_2. Increased urea and general protein waste

COMPARATIVE SUMMARY OF THE CHIEF EFFECTS OF COLD AND HEAT
BY J.H. KELLOGG, continued

Reaction consists of a series of vital processes following the application of either a hot or cold medium to the skin or the mucous membrane. The reflex vital activities induced by cold applications are much more pronounced than those by heat, and they differ in their character, depending on a variety of circumstances as discussed above in the section titled *"The Cold Bath."* However, the vital reactions produced by applications of heat are clearly defined and quite constant in character, and these may be advantageously utilized.

Tonic *reaction* of body to cold	Atonic *reaction* of body to heat
1. Vasodilatation	1. Vasoconstriction
2. Skin red	2. Skin pale
3. Pulse slowed	3. Pulse rate increased
4. Arterial tension increased	4. Arterial tension diminished
5. Skin action increased	5. Skin action decreased
6. Temperature lowered	6. Temperature lowered
7. Feeling of invigoration	7. Languor
8. Muscular capacity increased	8. Muscular capacity decreased
9. Amount of respired air increased	9. Amount of respired air decreased
10. Heat production increased	10. Heat production decreased

From the above it is apparent that the general and usual reaction effects of heat are of an atonic or depressant character. For most purposes it is doubtless true that the tonic reaction effects resulting from quick cold application are to be preferred to those from hot applications; nevertheless (as discussed in the section—*"The Hot Bath"*), the peculiar effects obtainable from heat are sometimes better suited to the case in hand than those arising from cold. Often the dread of cold water on the part of an individual can be so intense it makes its use inadmissible without a course of gradual training. In this case the effects obtainable from heat are particularly serviceable, and its employment may prevent the development of an irreversible aversion to cold.

PARTIAL BODY BATHS

EMPLOYING COLD WATER

A single short application of cold water brought in contact with the general surface of the body is always restorative and invigorating in its influence. According to the circumstances under which it is experienced, the actions of cold water can be stimulant, astringent, tonic, refrigerant, sedative, or debilitating. Relying on these actions, cold water can be used to refresh and invigorate after hard labor, to check feverish and inflammatory processes, to stimulate a sluggish and overburdened nervous system, to arrest spasm, to relieve congestion and pain, or to diminish excessive secretions and bleeding. A cold water bath seems to energize whatever you decide to do following its application; if you choose to be mellow, it relaxes you, if you want to be activated, it stimulates you.

Cold water is one of the best applications for a variety of local inflammations, such as *burns, scalds, chafed skin*, and the *stings* of insects. Cold is one of the most immediate and potent means of arresting bleeding, whether from the lungs, stomach, bowels (bleeding from these organs can be serious problems and need medical diagnosis), nose, uterus, or from wounds. In such cases it should be applied as near as possible to the source of bleeding. A prolonged application to the upper portion of the back relieves congestion of the nasal mucous membrane, and is therefore useful in nosebleed. A friend of mine, Dr. Don, has been a practicing physician for more years than he probably cares to mention. He uses ice as his initial first aid treatment. He explains that the simple application of ice promotes the healing process of all forms of injury as it cleans the wound site, reduces the onset of inflamma-

tion, inhibits the action of opportunistic microorganisms, arrests bleeding, and hastens the repair of tissue. I suggest applying the ice (cold) treatment for 5 to 10 minutes. When it is removed, the body's natural thermic reaction will kick in (see discussion of thermic reaction in "*Whole Body Baths*"), raise the temperature of the area, and enhance vascular activity, quicken vital functions, and promote rapid delivery of the body's healing agents for efficient repair.

Cold water in the form of baths and wet wrappings is well employed in many cases of recurrent or intermittent fevers where there is a fall of temperature to normal at periodical intervals, as in malarial fevers. The use of cold water as a drink for tending to fevers is instinctual as well as reasonable.

It is possible to induce a warming reaction in cold body parts by rubbing them with snow or ice in a warm room, and you can warm cold feet by taking off shoes and stockings and rubbing your bare feet with snow, then immediately drying and dressing them again to promote a thermic reaction.

The application of cold fomentation around inflamed joints or soon after an acute injury to a joint is of great benefit as an astringent agent to help contain swelling, pain, and inflammation. To restrain local inflammatory processes, thereby relieving the pain and swelling of a sprained or strained joint, keep the sprained part raised high, and during the first 24 hours soak the joint in cold water or wrap it with a cold or iced fomentation (so as to suppress as much as possible the body's natural warming reaction to cold). Then, after the first day, use hot soaks.

The repressive power of cold water is reliable in the treatment of burns and scalds. One need apply the cold water immediately after the injury and continue this steadily. This will help remove the heat of the burn, lessen inflammation, and reduce damage to tissue.

Heatstroke or sunstroke is an emergency, and first aid measures need to be initiated as soon as possible. In this situation there is not only an excess of blood within the cranium, but the blood is excessively hot. A person who can't be taken to a hospital immediately should be wrapped in wet bedding or wet clothing and immersed in cool water or even cooled with ice friction and fanned while waiting for transportation (cool the individual until the heat of the skin and fever drops, but beware not to overcool them).

There is no better palliative for hemorrhoids than frequent cleansings (ablutions) with cold water, especially after a stool; this is most efficiently applied with a sponge.

EMPLOYING HOT WATER

A short hot application over the region of the stomach diminishes the secretion of HCL, at least in cases of hyperacidity. Prolonged application of heat over the region of the stomach after eating increases the amount of hydrochloric acid secreted by the organ.

Prolonged application of heat over the region of the liver and other viscera increases their activity.

Short hot application on the abdominal region relieves visceral congestion.

SITZ BATH

The sitz bath, also called the hip bath or the sitting bath, is one of the oldest and most useful of water therapy procedures. It has fallen into disuse in our professional health care system, as has hydrotherapy in general,

due most likely to its relatively labor-intensive nature. Yet, with just a little ingenuity, this process can be made a vital part of domestic health care and home therapy.

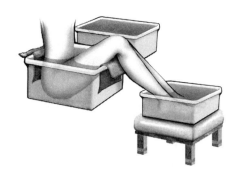

Sitz Bath

The hot and/or cold sitz bath acts simply to increase circulation to the organs of the lower abdomen and the pelvis. This in turn relieves congestion in other areas of the body such as the head and lungs. At the same time, this also tonifies the organs of digestion and the sexual organs. Hot baths relax while cold baths tonify the soft tissue structures; neutral baths have a calming effect on nervous system control of these areas. It is a valuable remedy in weaknesses and ailments of the womb, prostate region, genitals, and in irritations of the pelvic organs.

During a sitz, a hot foot bath is applied to minimize possible congestion to the pelvic region by pulling excess blood and lymphatic fluid to the lower extremities. The hot phase of a sitz bath is concluded with a cold immersion. This acts to prevent congestion of circulation and to reestablish the natural tone of (heat-generated) ultra-relaxed soft tissue.

The tub that is required for a sitting bath should be of such a form and size that the individual may be comfortably seated in it by leaving the feet outside and hanging the limbs to the floor, and the feet placed in a separate and smaller tub (foot bath) during the application. Large plastic wash tubs are just about all one can find these days to use for this. I set two of them in the bathtub, one for hot, one for cold, and extend a hose from the spigot to the tubs with which to fill them and maintain their temperatures. Obviously, the larger the bath tub, the better.

It is very important that the circulation in and to the legs not be interfered with by pressure from underneath the legs by the tub's edge. Placing a thickly folded towel on the tub's edge beneath the legs or elevating the foot bath tub sufficiently to raise up the legs avoids this problem. When using sitz tubs that have been placed in a bath tub, the bather can use the tub's sides to assist their movement. Otherwise, to make it easier for the bather to get up and down, it helps to elevate the sitz tub on blocks. For added comfort, place a folded towel on the bottom of tub along with one draped over the back and over the sides of the tub.

The physiological effects of a sitz, as in other baths, depends upon the temperature, the duration, and sometimes the mechanical effects (rubbing of the skin with hands or friction cloths) that are combined with the bath. The temperature of the sitz-bath may be cold, cool, tepid, warm, hot, or very hot depending on the purpose of the bath. The bath may be administered two or three times a day.

During a cold sitz or a prolonged tepid sitz, the bather's body should always be covered with a flannel sheet and/or blanket, or rubbed with an attendant's hands or a coarse towel to prevent chilling, and the feet are to be kept warm either by the hot foot bath (104° to 110° F.) or by hot towels wrung out and placed around the feet and legs.

The materials needed for a sitz bath

• A washtub (two tubs when doing an alternate hot and cold sitz)

• A foot tub or simple dishpan

• Towels and washcloths

• Flannel sheet and/or blanket to cover the bather

• Hot water and cold water

• A bath thermometer

The process

1. Assemble above materials.

2. Place towels on bottom, back, sides, and front of tub.

3. Fill sitz tub and foot tub with appropriate temperature and appropriate amount of water.

In general

• If it is to be a *hot sitz*, use 106° to 110° F. water with a 110° to 112° F. foot bath. Include enough water so level is about 1/2" above the navel.

• Bathe for a 3 to 8 minute duration.

• If it is to be a *cold sitz,* use 55° to 75° F. water with a 105° to 110° F. foot bath.

• Include enough water so level is about 1/2" below the navel.

• Bathe for a 3 to 8 minute duration.

• If it is to be a *neutral sitz,* use 92° to 97° F. water with a 105° to 110° F. foot bath.

• Include enough water so level is to the navel.

• Bathe from 1/4 to 2 hours duration.

• For an alternate hot and cold sitz, use the above temperatures.

• Bathe 2 to 5 minutes hot, 20 to 60 seconds cold. These can be repeated as desired.

• Always start with hot and end with cold.

• Assist disrobed bather in and out of tub, making sure she or he is comfortable.

• It is very important to prevent chilling of the bather. Cover her or him with a flannel sheet and/or a blanket if necessary.

• While the bather is in a hot bath, apply cold compresses or ice bag to head and back of neck to prevent cerebral congestion.

• Finish a hot sitz bath by pouring cold water over all the parts that were submerged in the hot water.

• Finish a hot foot bath by pouring cold water over the feet.

• Assist bather out of the sitz tub and dry with towels.

• Have bather lie down for at least a half hour.

INDICATIONS AND CONTRAINDICATIONS FOR SITZ BATHS

There are certain indications and contraindications for using this water tool. Basically, the indications for the cold sitz are the same as the contraindication for the hot sitz and vice versa. Contraindications for the alternate sitz are a combination of the contraindications for both the hot and cold sitz.

Hot sitz indications: painful spasm; acute abdominal pain; intestinal pain; or painful inflammation of kidneys (a serious condition, needs medical diagnosis); uterine pain; throbbing or stabbing nerve pain from the ovaries, testicles, or intestines; sciatica; lumbago; suppressed menses; painful hemorrhoids; congestive headache.

Hot sitz contraindications: hemorrhage; excessively profuse menstruation; pelvic congestion; atonic conditions or prolapsed organs.

Cold sitz indications: incontinence; constipation; benign prostatic hypertrophy (BPH) and any incontinence due to BPH; prolapsed uterus; herniated bladder; herniated rectum; excessively profuse menstruation.

Cold sitz contraindications: acute inflammation; any painful conditions; spasms; colic; acute lung condition; and heart problems.

Alternating hot and cold sitz indications: pelvic congestion; congestive headache; prostatitis; vaginal infection; pelvic inflammatory disease (PID, a serious condition, needs medical diagnosis); chronic urinary tract infections; improving nerve pain (neuralgias); insomnia; hemorrhoids; fissures; postpartum constipation.

Alternating hot and cold sitz contraindications: see contraindications under both hot and cold sitz.

Neutral sitz indications: acute urinary tract infection (never employ a hot or cold sitz for this acute condition); intense itching of anus or vulva; to calm mental or emotional overexcitement or sexual overexcitement (that sounds like an oxymoron to me).

QUICK COLD SITZ

A quick cold sitz (30 seconds to 2 minutes) produces active dilation of all vessels of the lower abdomen, increasing the movement of blood through these parts. The thermic reaction produced heightens the nutritive processes in the parts concerned. At the same time it excites contraction of the muscular structures of the viscera along with the musculo-ligamentous structures which support the abdominal and pelvic viscera. This has great influence on the bladder, all pelvic organs (male and female), and all structures that are involved in the acts of urination and defecation. It is good to note for those concerned that during the first moments of the cold sitz there is an increased activity of the heart and a temporary rise of the blood pressure.

COLD SITZ

The cold sitz (55° to 75° F., 5 to 8 minutes duration) produces a profound tonic effect on the body and must be frequently applied. The cold sitz is most frequently employed to bring about flowing effects upon the internal pelvic organs. This cold sitz is an excellent application for individuals who are at least moderately vigorous, and who suffer from congestion of the liver or spleen. It is very useful in atonic genito-urinary organs and in the nocturnal urinary incontinence of children (however, this needs to be introduced and employed in such manner that the child does not view it as punishment). It is equally valuable in chronic congestion of the prostate, in atonic weakness of seminal vessels, and in constipation, and in lack of tone of the bladder of both men and women. The cold sitz must not be used in cases of acute inflammation of the pelvic or abdominal organs, in painful conditions of the bladder or genital organs, in sciatica, or in cases of lung congestion.

COOL SITZ

A cool sitz-bath (65° to 80° F.) is derivative when continued for 15 to 20 minutes, or long enough to cause a decided reddening of the submerged skin which will attest to adequate dilation of the surface vessels. The special use of this bath for decongesting the internal organs lies in the persistence of a large quantity of blood that has flowed to and is fixed in the skin. This, accompanied by the contraction of the internal vessels which is produced at the same time by the irritation of the cold, aids in the decongestion of the internal parts.

PROLONGED COOL SITZ

The prolonged cool sitz-bath at 65° to 75° F. for 15 to 40 minutes causes prolonged contractions of the vessels of the pelvic and abdominal organs. This action makes this bath an excellent measure for relieving chronic congestion in this area. A hot foot bath must always be given simultaneously and the pelvic area should be rubbed so as to maintain strong surface circulation. This friction is important to assist the decongestion of the pelvic organs. The prolonged cool sitz also renders excellent results, when combined with other measures of treatment, and in relieving chronic excessively profuse menstruation (when not due to endometriosis). It is also useful in any bleeding from the bladder, the intestines, the uterus, urethra, and rectum, in hemorrhoids, and chronic inflammation of the prostate.

In many cases a temperature of 75° to 80° F. is preferable to a lower temperature, especially for individuals who have not been accustomed to cold water applications. In some cases it is desirable to begin the bath at a temperature of 85° to 90° F. and lower it after the first few minutes to 75° F. The duration of the bath should be 15 to 20 minutes. This should always be accompanied by a hot foot bath of 104° to 110° F., but no hotter than this.

The cool sitz-bath and the cold sitz-bath are to be avoided with individuals who have any kind of heart condition that would be adversely affected by a sudden increase in arterial pressure. It is also contraindicated in all acute inflammations and infections involving the organs of the abdomen or pelvis, painful conditions of the genito-urinary organs, any conditions of the pelvis accompanied by muscular spasms, spermatorrhea accompanied by frequent losses of fluid (see warm sitz), or sciatica. However, in many cases in which the cold bath is contraindicated, a sitz at 85° F., gradually cooled to 75° F., may be employed with benefit. The length of this bath should be 15 to 20 minutes.

QUICK COLD-HOT SITZ

The quick cold-hot sitz bath is also referred to as a revulsive sitz. It is a very short cold sitz, a simple dip in the cold water for a few seconds followed by a very hot sitz of 115° to 120° F. for 3 to 8 minutes duration. This extreme contrast of temperature is a powerful sedative measure in painful affections of the pelvic viscera. It has been used quite successfully in cases of ovarian or uterine pain that has a severe throbbing or stabbing characteristic, cramps, colic, severe pain in the intestine, often accompanied by spasmodic contraction of the muscles, and in painful conditions of the prostate, bladder, and rectum.

WARM (NEUTRAL) SITZ

The warm (neutral) sitz bath is 92° to 97° F., and the duration may be from 15 minutes to an hour or two if you have the time. There is no appreciable thermic or circulatory reaction produced, which is the beauty of this sitz. It exercises a pronounced calmative effect upon the viscera of the pelvis and lower abdomen, and the genitalia.

The neutral sitz is an exceedingly useful means of relieving nervous irritability and congestion of the pelvic viscera. It is of great service in the treatment of painful and inflammatory affections of the genito-urinary organs in both men and women, such as itching of the vulva and anus, hemorrhoids, frequent urination from irritability of the bladder, spermatorrhea arising from excessive irritability of the genito-urinary center, nervous irritability of the spermatic cord and testicles, and also chronic backache from rectal and uterine disorders.

The neutral sitz subdues inflammation and may be employed in subacute and even acute inflammatory conditions of the abdominal and pelvic regions, such as acute catarrh of the bladder and urethra, subacute inflammations of the uterus, ovaries, and tubes. It is especially helpful for relieving nervous pains of the fallopian tubes and the testicles. It is indicated as a sedative means in cases of spermatorrhea accompanied by excessive sensibility or painfulness to touch of the urethra and ejaculatory ducts.

This sitz bath is highly useful in all cases of pelvic disease in which cold applications feel inappropriate on account of pain or the inflammatory conditions that may be present.

VERY HOT SITZ

The very hot sitz bath is 106° to 120° F., and the duration is 3 to 8 minutes if the bather can handle it. It is suggested to begin with a temperature of 100° F., rapidly adding hot water until the maximum temperature is reached. A hot foot bath of 110° to 120° F. is taken with it. At all times, keep the head cool with cold compresses. Following this bath, cool the surface of the body gradually and be sure the bather does not experience any chilly sensations to the area being treated, for this will undo the benefits of the bath.

The general effects are essentially the same as those of the hot immersion bath. At temperatures above 110° F., especially if the bath is continued beyond 3 or 4 minutes, the effect is to excite the pelvic circulation, and to concentrate the blood in this portion of the body. This bath is an excellent means of restoring the menstrual function when it has been suspended as the result of general chill or from other causes.

The hot sitz bath is a powerful analgesic, an effective in-home, non-drug measure for the stilling of pain. For the best effects, it should be followed by a short cold application. Therefore, this bath is of great value in relieving the pain and discomfort of sciatica, and neuralgia or nerve pain of the ovaries, testicles, and the bladder. In general, this hot sitz is of great help for relieving pain in all affections of a non-inflammatory character involving the viscera of the pelvis and lower abdomen.

A shallow, very hot sitz is an excellent measure in relieving the pain of inflamed hemorrhoids.

FOOT AND LEG BATHS

HOT FOOT BATH

This bath requires a suitable receptacle for the feet, and a supply of very hot water, with cold water for tempering. (See also "*Herbal Baths*" below.)

The hot foot bath should be of as high a temperature as can be borne, so as to redden the skin of the immersed parts effectually.

Ideally the vessel used should be sufficiently deep to allow the legs to be immersed in the water nearly to the knees. The temperature required for most positive effects is 104° to 122° F. The foot bath should begin at a temperature of 100° to 104° F., and should be gradually increased until 115° to 122° F., reached in about three minutes. The duration of the bath may be from 5 minutes to half an hour. The feet should be completely immersed in the water, and the effect may be intensified by increasing the depth of the water up to the knees. To produce the true revulsive effect (drawing the blood from one part of the body to another), the feet should be dipped in cold water after the hot soak. This sudden cooling of the skin will encourage a tonic circulatory reaction. At a temperature of 103° to 110° F. the hot foot bath is very useful for balancing the circulation, by the dilation of the blood vessels of the legs, relieving congestion of the brain and other organs in the upper half of the body. The very hot foot and leg bath (as well as cold applications to the feet) stimulate the involuntary muscles of the uterus, intestines, bladder, and other pelvic and abdominal viscera. The hot foot and leg bath are well used in the treatment of insomnia, lung congestion, dysmenorrhea, suppressed menstruation, ovarian congestion, and pelvic pain from other causes. It is a simple and valuable remedy in the early stages of mucous membrane congestion and local congestion of the head, chest, or abdomen. It may be made more stimulating by the addition of common salt or mustard powder. In foot baths, mustard relieves headaches and cerebral and other internal congestion, especially uterine congestion that is accompanied with dysmenorrhea.

The very hot foot bath is exceedingly

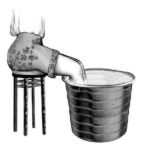

Foot and Leg Bath

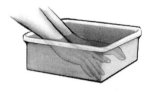

Hand Bath

useful in a case of sprained ankle joint—to be employed the day after a cold application is used first to subdue inflammation and swelling. (See below, "*Cold/Cool Foot Bath*"; also see above "*Partial Body Baths—Employing Cold Water.*")

A hot foot bath is contraindicated in any sensory loss to the feet or in cases of peripheral vascular disease.

COLD FOOT BATH (45° TO 55° F.)

The cold foot bath is of great service in producing reflex, revulsive, or counterirritant, and other effects. The sole of the foot is one of the most important areas in the body, having direct connection with the nerve centers that control the circulation of the pelvic and abdominal viscera. The reflex effects cause contraction of the vessels and muscles of the uterus and the organs connected with it. The blood vessels of the brain, the stomach, the liver, the bladder, and the intestines are made to contract at the same time. Intestinal peristalsis and contraction of the bladder are also excited.

The revulsive effects of the cold foot bath are very strong and continue for a long time—longer than those obtained from hot foot baths. The short cold foot bath (duration of 20 to 60 seconds only, for it is only the primary effect that is desirable) is useful in cerebral congestion and uterine hemorrhage.

COOL FOOT BATH (60° TO 70° F.)

The prolonged cool foot bath is well used as an anti-inflammatory measure in cases of injury to the feet and ankle, such as sprains, strains, and inflamed bunions. The feet must be well warmed by rubbing or by heat before the application is made.

THE ALTERNATE FOOT BATH

This foot bath is a more highly excitant measure than the cold foot bath.

In cases in which the feet are constantly cold and in cases of persistent sweating of the feet the alternate foot bath is most helpful. The feet are placed in hot water for 2 to 3 minutes, then in cold water for 20 seconds to 1 minute. They are then returned to the hot water for 2 minutes, then replaced in the cold water, this operation being repeated a number of times daily.

This alternate bath is also especially useful in treating chilblains and in eliminating any local stagnation of circulation that can lead to gangrene.

HAND BATHS

Immersing the hands in very cold water exercises a powerful influence upon the cerebral vessels and vessels of the lungs. The immersion of the hands in cold water for a sufficient length of time is capable of slowing the pulse and the respiration, and lessening the pressure in the cerebral arteries. Immersing them in a hot bath produces the opposite phenomena. The cold hand bath or simply holding cubes of ice in the hands is an excellent means of checking nosebleed, and has been used to check the bleeding in pulmonary hemorrhage very quickly.

HERBAL BATHS

Herbal preparations added to a bath enhance skin stimulation. At the same time the body absorbs through the skin a great number of the medicinal components of herbal formulations. The action of an herbal bath enhances the blood supply to the layers of tissue close to the skin, and the herbs' medicinal and tonic actions benefit the body organism in general. Western therapeutic science has substantiated these facts with their official experimentation and by authoritatively announcing its findings (mostly to itself) has finally caught up in this area of therapeutics with centuries-old folkloric herbal science. Further clinical data is still required, however, to convince the more resistant medical authorities and practitioners. In Europe, the work of two extraordinary herbalists, Herr Kneipp and Monsieur Messegue, made the use of medicinal herbs in baths a relatively common procedure. I suggest we lay practitioners move on with our empirical herbal research and let medical science catch up with us again later.

Possibly the best, and certainly one of the most sensually delicious ways of absorbing herbal remedies through the skin, is by bathing in a full-body herbal bath. Life in general is more fun when you're naked. A full-body herbal bath is certainly more exotic than a tincture, naughtier than an elixir, and a heck of a lot more pleasant than swallowing a capsule or a pill. Herbal bath therapy is economically administered in one's home and is practical when administered as a weekend course of treatment or as a regularly sustained system of self-pampering health care.

To prepare a herbal bath, one merely has to pour a quart of strong herbal infusion, herbal decoction, or concentrate into the bath water, swirl it around, take off the clothes, slip into the brew, lay back, and relax; high tea is served.

Often volatile oils are placed into the bath water for their aromatic and medicinal effects. Add a total of 10 to 15 drops to an already full bath. *Agitate the water to thoroughly disperse the oils before getting in.* It is important to bear in mind that when using essential oils, one drop goes a long way. These oils easily penetrate the skin and some may cause skin irritation or sensitivity if not properly diluted or if used in high concentrations. Some people have sensitivity reactions to essential oils; therefore, it is wise to test oneself first by applying the dilute oil to a small skin area before using on larger areas (dilute the volatile oil in a little vegetable oil).

Partial body herbal baths and herbal sitz baths are generally prepared in the same fashion. An **herbal foot bath** is prepared by pouring a quart of tea into a vessel that is large enough to contain the feet and to this preparation enough hot or cold water is added to cover the feet to the desired height and the desired temperature. This can range from a shallow foot bath where merely the soles of the feet are covered, to one that extends up to the knees.

Herbal hand baths are prepared by simply placing one's hands into a container of undiluted herbal infusion or decoction. When using essential oils in a foot or hand bath, put 5 to 7 drops into the container of water and disperse fully by agitating the water before getting into it.

Instead of preparing an infusion or decoction of the herbs beforehand, a couple handfuls of dried herb can be put into a cotton muslin bag and the opening of the bag held tightly around the hot water tap. Turn on the hot water and let it flow into the bag. This will make a fresh infusion as the hot water flows through the herbs into the bath. Once the tub is filled, tie off the bag and let it continue to soak in the bath water. This method is better used in partial baths and not normally in a full baths for, in the latter (except for small children's little baths) it becomes quite diluted.

Often a warm, sensually aromatic bath is prepared for a friend to savor and indulge. If aromatic volatile oils are used to provide the magic of the moment, it is imparative to agitate the surface of the water briskly before entering — particularly if it is a gentleman bather — for undiluted aromatic oils can burn tender, delicate skin which usually makes up one of the first parts of the male anatomy to plunge through the water's surface. This experience can radically alter the serenity of the moment for him if the oils are concentrated on the water's surface. Although probably to a lesser extent, this experience can also be disturbing to a lady bather's bottom.

Of course, one can simply harvest medicinal and aromatic plants, throw them into the hot bath water, and climb in with them. Normally, this preparation is only appreciated by individuals who also enjoy swimming in fresh water ponds, or in kelp beds, and don't mind the water flora (and attendant fauna) touching their skin. My first herb teacher, Norma Myers, used to soak herself in herb and seaweed baths routinely, but she was a wild woman; she thrived in that lifestyle.

Any herb that can be taken internally can also be used in a bath. The following are some suggestions for particularly good herbs to use for special occasions:

• Relaxing herbs that help relieve tension and promote restful sleep—Lavender (*Lavandula spp.*), Linden blossoms (*Tilia spp.*), Chamomile (*Matricaria recutita*), Peppermint (*Mentha piperita*), Lemon Balm (*Melissa officinalis*), or Valerian (*Valeriana officinalis*); for children use the more gentle Red Clover (*Trifilium pratense*), Chamomile, and/or Linden blossoms.

• For relief of itchy skin—Chickweed (*Stellaria media*), Black Walnut leaves or bark (*Juglans nigra*), Hyssop (*Hyssopus officinalis*), or Chamomile; for dry itchy skin fill a sock with oatmeal and tie it at the top, steep this in the bath water for a while, then rub the skin with the bag.

• For relief of muscular tension and pain—Mugwort (*Artemisia vulgaris*), Chamomile, Horsetail (*Equisetum arvense*).

• To help circulation use any of the following stimulating herbs—Rosemary (*Rosemarinus spp.*), Yarrow (*Achillea millefolium*), Marigold (*Calendula officinalis*), Cayenne (*Capsicum minimum*), Ginger (*Zingiber offici-*

nalis). Use small amounts of the Cayenne and Ginger.

These are only a few of the limitless possibilities one can come up with.

SUMMARY

I'm giving you the above suggestions and precise techniques as helpful guidance. If you are a water person and inclined to use the bath as a means of health care, you will need to use your intuition and good judgment as you implement these procedures in your home. And, of course, the bather will be the final judge as to how good and helpful it all feels. When the results you seek are manifested, please make notes on these successful experiences. If you make mistakes, learn from them and annotate your experiences. These notes will be invaluable to you and to others as we relearn how to employ the remarkable healing energy of hydrotherapy and simple herbal baths.

POULTICES AND FOMENTATIONS

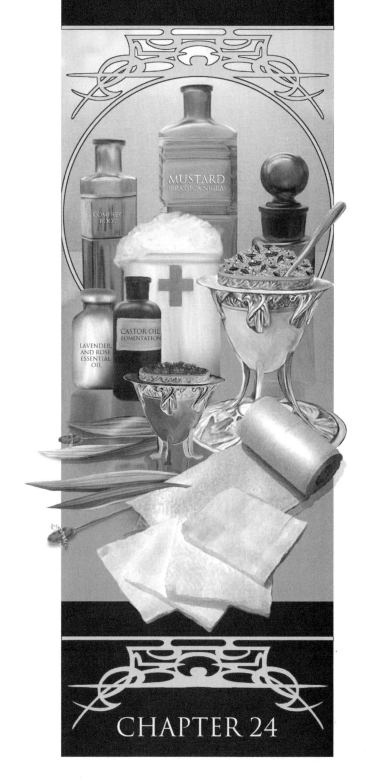

CHAPTER 24

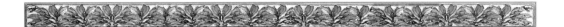

There has been an inspired reawakening of Western herb lore in the minds and hearts of the citizenry in North America. Individuals within nearly every society of our diverse culture are seeking knowledge about the utilization of self-medicating materials that were once commonly used in the homes and communities of our ancestors. One by one, we are rediscovering the simple vehicles that efficiently deliver the healing virtues residing in our garden's herbs and weeds. We are restocking our home pharmacies with herbal preparations and reviving the personal and family dignity of taking care of ourselves. This is the era of our reconnection with plant spirit; we are about to harvest the health-promoting independence of our greenselves.

Continuing the progress of this reconnection, we will review in this chapter the laying of simple herbal waters and succulent pulps upon our skin. This time-honored process is well used in concert with the vehicles discussed in the accompanying chapters.

At this point, I trust you are comfortable with the terms "self-medication" and "self-medicating." I realize we lay folk, over the last ninety years, have conditioned ourselves to believe and feel that "therapeutics," "medicine," and "medicating" are professional mysteries which are the sole domain of licensed medical doctors, and only a doctor by using medical pharmaceutical products can competently and safely medicate us. The medical/pharmaceutical licensing and marketing lobbies have successfully conjured this collective illusion. Yet I believe the current search for therapeutic "alternatives" and disease-preventive measures by ever-increasing numbers of individuals, along with the obvious swell of self-education in personal health care, illustrates our grassroots disenchantment with this tenet.

If you feel uncomfortable with the ideas of self-medicating, I respectfully suggest that it is time to root out and possibly reconsider the beliefs that underlie these feelings. Boundless numbers of us in this society are extremely intelligent human beings, fully capable of making excellent decisions about our lives, particularly when given access to valid information as a base on which to work. And in response to this collective calling there is an ever-increasing number of knowledgeably responsible books, seminars, hands-on workshops, and intensive school programs supplied by highly competent herbalists, teaching people how to use herbs safely, responsibly, and effectively for individual and family health care (see resource guide). We have every right to medicate our own persons, and the freedom to do so. (I believe the ninth amendment to the constitution focuses attention on this inalienable right.) And unless the state, in fact, does own our children, we have the same right and responsibility to find out what is best for them. The knowledgeable use of herbs administered in the home in place of pharmaceutical drugs is frequently a far more pragmatic, benign, and responsible choice for an ailing child's (and adult's) well-being. In the face of media blitz with its perennial promise of medical miracle cures waiting around every corner, we have allowed ourselves to lose sight of the true healing intelligence and wisdom each of us possess. We merely need to recall and revive this basic human function. Healing is inspired, not ordained.

In line with these thoughts, we will extend the previous chapter's focus on baths by looking at the uses of poultices and compresses, as these are some of the simplest and most pleasant feeling (bath-like) vehicles for the home delivery of herbal health care.

POULTICES

Classically, a poultice (a.k.a. cataplasm) is a soft, mushy preparation composed usually of some pulpy or mealy substance which is capable of absorbing a large amount of liquid and of such consistency that it can be applied to any flat or irregular surface. This herbal material is made into a paste, using hot liquids, and is spread thickly upon cloths and applied directly to the body while hot. Poultices owe their primary virtues to the moist heat which they contain and therefore must be renewed every few minutes, or somehow kept warm by other means. An exception to these mechanics is the Mustard (*Brassica nigra*) poultice, which supplies its warming action through a volatile component produced when its crushed seed is mixed with water. In herb land, however, the scope of the term *poultice* has broadened and now covers a wide range of preparations, some of which are applied hot, some cold.

Poultices and fomentations in their most simple form are merely local baths that utilize *warmth* and *moisture* to relax tissue and relieve pain. Beyond this, herbal preparations can be incorporated in these soothing hot waters to add further assistance with their unique therapeutic properties. Therefore, herbal poultices can be any of the following:

Emollient, which by supplying warmth and moisture are useful for reducing pain and inflammation and assisting the ripening and suppurative (pus-generating) process. Emollient poultices can be made of Flaxseed meal (powdered Flaxseed), Oat meal, bran, bread, and milk, Plantain, Marshmallow root, or mashed vegetable materials such as Cabbage, Turnip, Potato, or Carrot.

Medicated, which are intended to exercise a specific influence on a part of the body, independent of warmth and moisture. These are made of any or a combination of a wide variety of medicinal plants, such as astringents, styptics and vulneraries, anodynes, disinfectants, etc. They are used to penetrate and reduce enlarged or inflamed glands, eruptions, abscesses, lacerations, boils, etc.

Counter-irritant or *revulsive*, which, by inducing a local irritation or inflammation as they stimulate capillary dilation and action, cause skin redness. This counter-irritation draws stagnant blood and other materials

If you feel uncomfortable with the ideas of self-medicating, I respectfully suggest that it is time to root out and possibly reconsider the beliefs that underlie these feelings.

from deeper tissues and organs to the surface, thereby relieving deeper congestion and inflammation. These poultices also act as derivatives which draw pustular materials from the body through the skin. These poultices are made using stimulating herbs such as Mustard, Ginger, Cayenne, Garlic, Rosemary, etc.

Optimally, medicated herbal poultices are prepared from fresh herbs which have been chewed, chopped, mashed, bruised, or blended in an electric blender and mixed with hot water, apple cider vinegar, or some other hot liquid. A blender suits us well for these preparations, for it is important to break up the cell walls in order to gain access to the properties contained in the plant juices.

Dry (dehydrated) herb that has been rehydrated also can be used to make poultices. You can rehydrate a dehydrated herb by gently heating it in a little water, apple cider vinegar, milk, or other liquid that seems appropriate. Once the herb has absorbed the liquid and softened, it is ready to use for preparing a poultice in the same way that you would use a fresh plant.

A poultice can be used again and again during each session. However, it needs to be re-heated each time before reapplying.

A hot poultice should be applied as hot as can be borne. To test its temperature apply it to the back of your hand—it should feel hot, but comfortable. To prevent the rapid loss of heat, it is helpful to cover the poultice with a thick insulating cloth while it's on your body,

First clean the area of the body by using a solution of 1 part apple cider vinegar to 1 part warm water, or simply soap and water; then a thin layer of vegetable oil is rubbed on the skin to protect it, and to prevent the poultice from sticking to the skin.

The vinegar-water mixture is also an especially good solution to use for washing and conditioning the area after the poultice has been removed.

MAKING A POULTICE

A Very Simple Poultice

1. Put powdered or chopped fresh herbal materials into a clean white cotton sock. Use two socks and alternate them.

2. Tie it at the top (tie it in a knot, or use string, or elastic).

3. Place this into a shallow bowl.

4. Pour enough hot water over the prefilled sock to soak the dry herb or heat the fresh herb.

5. With your hands, knead the wet sock until it is quite hot, yet bearable.

6. Apply this to the affected area until the poultice is cool.

7. Repeat steps 3 to 6 to reheat and reapply the poultice.

Eye Poultice

A poultice for the eye can be quickly assembled by merely dropping a tea bag in hot water for an instant, long enough to wet the herb, then cooling it enough not to burn the eyelid, and laying the hot moist tea bag on the closed eyelid. Fennel, Red Raspberry, Chamomile, or disinfectant herbs are excellent for this purpose. You can purchase strips of empty tea bags and fill them with the herbs of your choice or use commercial brand prefilled tea bags.

Emollient Poultice

A Flaxseed (Linseed) poultice is a good representative of this type poultice.

1. Grind a good handful of Flaxseed into a meal using a mortar and pestle or an electric coffee bean grinder.

2. Add some boiling water [approximate proportions of 300 ml (10 fl. oz.) of water to 120 Gm (4 oz.) of Flaxmeal].

3. Quickly stir the Flaxseed and water together until you have made a thick paste.

4. Spread this hot paste (at least 1/2-inch thick) onto a clean white cloth, leaving the edges of the cloth free from the paste and avoiding the formation of lumps in the paste.

5. Apply the poultice to the body as hot as possible, making sure it completely covers and even extends a little beyond the area being soothed. It helps to spread a little vegetable oil on the skin before applying the poultice to protect the skin and to make it easier to remove the poultice. Otherwise, it can stick to the skin.

6. When the poultice is lukewarm, another poultice should be ready to take its place, and the treatment should be continued as long as necessary.

7. Of course, you can help retain the heat by insulating the poultice. First lay a plastic bag directly over the poultice, then wrap a towel around it, and if appropriate lay a hot water bottle or heating pad on top of all this to supply prolonged heat.

Another convenient method to prepare a Flaxseed or similar poultice is to make several bags of various sizes out of cheesecloth. Fill the bags half full with Flaxseed or whatever agent you select, then sew up the open end (store these in the refrigerator or freezer to prevent the Flaxseed from going rancid over time). When needed, the appropriate size bag is submerged in boiling water for a few minutes. When the bag is taken out of the water, you will see that the Flaxseed has swelled and filled the bag. Squeeze out any superfluous water, lay the bag on the body, and cover it with insulating and or heating materials.

As a poultice, Flaxseed can be used for treating carbuncles, shingles, and psoriasis, and it can be combined with Marshmallow root powder to use for reducing swellings and inflammations, and for drawing out the pus in boils.

Flaxseed poultices mixed with Onion are commonly used to provide relief in lung conditions, especially with pleurisy, which calls out for a warm poultice (pleurisy can be a symptom of serious disease—get it checked out). After removing a poultice from the chest area, a second one can then be placed onto the upper back, which will cover and treat the back regions of the lungs.

Other Herbal Materials Used to Medicate a Poultice

The herbs Calendula, Comfrey, and Plantain are the reigning matriarchs in the clan of herbal poultices, with Echinacea giving service as their cardinal aide when further wound healing and enhanced immune-stimulating action is needed.

Calendula (*Calendula officinalis*) promotes the healing and regeneration of bruised tissue, burns, eruptions, abrasions, and so forth. Overall, this herb is one of the most efficient of all herbs to use as a poultice or a fomentation (fomentations are discussed later in the chapter). A Calendula poultice reduces soreness and inflammation, while its anti-microbial properties assist in the cleansing of a wound, fostering rapid healing.

Comfrey (*Symphytum officinale*) is our most valuable plant ally for repairing wounds, while at the same time it soothes and softens tissue. It is probably the most healing mucilaginous remedy in our herbal materia medica, having been used for centuries to treat external ulceration and all types of lesions and injuries ranging from small cuts and abrasions to large wounds and broken bones. A Comfrey poultice quickens the repair of the normally slow healing process of torn cartilage, tendons, and ligaments. A common name "Knitbone" refers to Comfrey's historic use as a poultice for treating skeletal fractures in humans and animals. It heals bone tissue. Its mucilage and tannins produce an astringent and contracting effect. By drawing a wound together at the surface, it reduces the need for stitching; and its generous al-lantoin content stimulates the regeneration of skin tissue, making the formation of scar tissue less likely.

Of all the herbs, **Plantain** (*Plantago lanceolata, P. major*) is probably the most accessible and abundant. In league with Dandelion, it is one of an herbalist's two most loyal and reliable travel companions. They can be found growing nearly everywhere on our planet. Plantain is used by herbalists to remove the ouch! from wounds, especially the venomous ouch prompted by stinging and biting insects and other skin-penetrating animals. Plantain (both the narrow leaf and broad leaf types) helps stop bleeding, neutralizes venom and toxins, soothes inflammation, and heals wounds. This plant applied as a poultice is also helpful in withdrawing deeply lodged splinters.

Echinacea (*Echinacea spp.*) is a highly effective wound-healing plant, generously stimulating the immune system. It is especially useful in treating sluggardly, long-standing wounds that are slow to heal. The addition of this plant to any of the above plant poultices complements and amplifies their qualities.

Plantain and Dandelion are an herbalist's most loyal and reliable travel companions. They can be found growing nearly everywhere on our planet.

A Field Poultice

This poultice is useful if you are the recipient of an insect bite. It can be a fresh one or an old one that just doesn't seem to get better, or any kind of benign, welting, itching, insect bite including tick, wasp, yellow jacket, or a bee sting. In case of a bee sting, remove the stinger by sliding the edge of a credit card along the skin up to the stinger and gently nudging it sideways out of the skin. Don't squeeze the stinger by trying to pull it out with your fingers; you will inject more venom doing that. In case of a tick bite, pull the tick straight out first.

1. Pick a handful of Plantain.

2. Wad it up by rolling it firmly between your palms, bruising and crushing it well, or put it in your mouth and chew it (which is actually better—dogs aren't the only ones having therapeutic saliva).

3. If you chew it, don't swallow the juice. It's okay to swallow the juice, but the Plantain-infused saliva is what contacts the skin as a poultice and "makes you better."

4. Make the poultice thick and slap it on the skin.

5. Then hold the palm of your hand on top of the poultice to supply some warmth and some caring touch to the injury.

6. (*Optional*) When you can, brew a pot of Plantain tea and drink it freely.
Change the poultice a couple times a day and keep one on the wound overnight with some form of a bandage. Repeat this daily until all is well again; and it will be, soon.

Onion Poultice for Earaches

To make and apply an Onion poultice for relieving the pain of an earache:

1. Cut a medium-size Onion in half and bake it at a low temperature until it is soft.

2. Place the warm flat surface of the baked Onion directly on the ear.

3. Secure it with a cloth bandage wrapped around the head Van Gogh fashion. Unlike Vincent's technique, however, the application of a baked Onion will soothe the ear and relieve the pain and suffering.

Onion Poultice for the Body

While the aroma of Onion is in the air, I should explain how to make an Onion poultice for the rest of the body. (The notable refinement of detail and characteristic finesse in the preparation of the following poultice I obtained from a conversation with my friend "Herbal" Ed Smith, herbalist and president of Herb Pharm in Williams, Oregon. And although he is more than likely responsible for a lot of other things, he should not be held responsible for the wording used here.) This is what you can do at home to relieve the acute condition of cough, croup, bronchitis, strep throat, kidney infection, eye infection, and whatever else hurts:

1. Chop 3 or 4 Onions fine.

2. Sauté them in oil (it doesn't matter what kind of oil). Make it a little on the greasy side.

3. Cook the Onions until they become translucent, but don't cook them too much. You want them to be hot and flexible, not mushy.

4. Now, slowly pour on some apple cider vinegar (just enough to almost, but not quite, float the hot and flexible Onions).

5. Turn the flame down for the next steps to prevent the Onions from sticking to the pan.

6. Add Cornmeal or Flaxseed meal. Both of these are high in fat, so they absorb, and later, radiate the heat. You can use flour in place of the Corn or Flaxseed meals, but poultice gourmets tend to frown on this substitution.

7. Using a spatula, mix together and knead the Onions, the oil, and the meal into a wet plastic mass (not too wet, not too dry, but peanut butter-like).

8. When this is done to your satisfaction, put it on a piece of cheesecloth, or muslin, or flannel cloth, fold it over like a fat omelet, and stick the edges of the cloth together.

9. Apply the hot Onion poultice to the body.

This poultice is rich in sulfurated volatile oils and therapeutic mucilaginous substances. You will want to create a complete seal between the poultice and the skin by making sure there are no air pockets that will interfere with the "osmotic transfer" of energy between the poultice and the body.

When treating the lungs, following a chest poultice, turn the person over and apply another Onion poultice on the upper half of the back.

Honey Poultice

Honey is one of the best poultices to apply directly to a burn. First, cool the burned tissue with cold water,★ if possible, then merely spread honey on the burn or wound and leave it there for about a half hour. Reapply if necessary. Honey immediately seals off the damaged tissue from the air, reducing the pain while it works to rehydrate the wounded tissue; all the other magical bee-formulated components of honey proceed to do what they do to embellish the repair. Honey is antiseptic and helps to avoid infection.

★ RECIPE FOR A HOUSEHOLD BURN CENTER

Into a 2 oz. (60 ml) amber glass bottle, pour 1 fl. oz. (30 ml) of Aloe Vera juice. Add to this 30 ml of pure Lavender essential oil. Cap the bottle and keep it in the refrigerator where it will always remain cold and available. Shake well and pour this blend directly on any and all burns to immediately cool and soothe the skin tissue. Then when the skin is cold, apply the honey.

Mustard Poultice (*Brassica nigra, Sinapis nigra*)

A Mustard poultice, also known as a *sinapism*, differs from most other poultices in both its preparation and its action. Note that you shouldn't use pure, undiluted Mustard, for it is very likely to blister the skin. Mustard is ordinarily diluted with about an equal weight of Cornmeal, Flaxseed meal, or some other form of flour (sometimes these are called a *diluent*).

Prior to mixing the powdered Mustard seed with the diluent, it is moistened with tepid or lukewarm water (140ish° F.), never with boiling water. When water is added to the crushed seed, its ultimate warming action is aroused as an enzyme acts upon a glycoside. A volatile "isothiocyanate" is generated, which is called "volatile mustard oil" (not to be confused with an aromatic volatile "essential" oil). The formation of the warming volatile Mustard oil is greatly inhibited if too high heat is applied, so never use boiling water for this preparation. This tends to diminish the crucial enzymatic action. It is also recommended not to use vinegar as a wetting agent, for it too inhibits the formation of the heat-producing Mustard oil. To assemble and apply the Mustard poultice:

1. Mix the dry Mustard with the warm water.

2. Mix the diluent with hot water.

3. Stir these two mixtures together.

4. Place a thin cloth on the skin to protect it and to avoid adhesion to the skin.

5. Spread the poultice thickly onto the cloth.

6. The poultice is allowed to remain on the skin from 10 minutes to a half hour in order to gain its rubefacient activity.

The action is usually at its height in about 15 to 20 minutes, even though redness is usually produced in a shorter time. If an individual's skin is quite tender or there is a weakened system, a short action may be more effective overall than a prolonged one.

On delicate, sensitive skin, the Mustard poultice need not remain on the body for more than 6 to 8 minutes, for its effect continues some time after its removal. Please keep in mind that if a Mustard plaster is applied too hot and kept on too long, the skin can become inflamed, blister, and become otherwise injured.

The constituents of Mustard applied as a poultice or bath produce a lively stimulation and arouse the nervous system. This acts to disperse any pain that is due to congestion. Employ the wonderfully deep-penetrating, rubefacient, decongesting, and pain-relieving benefits of this herbal poultice, but be very attentive to the proper dilution of the Mustard with the diluent, and closely monitor the reaction of the individual's skin.

In addition to bentonite, other types and colors of clay make excellent poultices as well.

Cayenne Poultice

As a milder substitute for the deeper-penetrating Mustard poultice, the Cayenne red pepper or Capsicum poultice will serve well, and it will not cause blistering. Cayenne can be used as a poultice by mixing the powder with bread and moistened with a little hot milk, or mix the Cayenne powder with some form of powdered grain and moisten with hot milk or hot water.

White Cabbage Poultice

This (vegetable) herb is good as a poultice for drawing out pus and other gloomy body exudates. Merely take the inner leaves of a common White Cabbage, wash them well, and dry them (the large middle rib is best removed and discarded for easier processing of the leaves). Bruise the leaves using a rolling pin or some other like instrument to soften them and place them on the affected area. Hold the leaves in place by wrapping a loose bandage or small towel around them. Leave the Cabbage poultice on for 1/2 to 1 hour, then replace it with a fresh one. You can add some powdered Myrrh gum or powdered Echinacea to this if there is any infection.

Applying raw Cabbage leaves as a poultice affords a slightly stimulating poultice, which is best used in conditions where one is treating a sluggish, ill-conditioned, offensive skin ulcer.

Root Poultice

These emollient poultices can be prepared from any of the tender culinary roots (and tubers) like Carrot, Turnip, Potato, or Burdock. Simply boil the tender roots, remove the skin, and mash them into a soft pulp. These make a mild, nutritive, emollient poultice. Like the Cabbage poultice, when needed, a raw version of these root poultices renders increased stimulating action. Peel and shred the fresh raw roots, mash them into pulp, and apply them to the skin.

Clay Poultice

Clay poultices are made using bentonite clay, water, and appropriate herbal tinctures. Pharmaceutical grade bentonite can be purchased in health food stores and pharmacies.

1. Dilute an herbal tincture with about half as much water (2 parts tincture to 1 part water). Use this mixture to add to the clay.

2. Slowly add the liquid to the clay, stirring until you have made a paste. (Start out with the proportions of about a tablespoon of clay to each tablespoon of liquid.)

3. At this point you can add a few drops of Lavender or Tea Tree essential oil (5 to 10 drops) and stir them in.

4. Apply this herbal clay paste to the body.

5. Apply it thick (at least 1/4 inch). This helps keep the poultice warm and moist. Clay poultices that dry out too quickly are not as effectual. You want them to remain wet (when they are most active) as long as possible.

To prepare a **bentonite clay poultice** for the mouth, teeth, and gums for reducing the inflammation and agony of an abscessed tooth, or to help reach down and disperse the stagnating energy of swollen throat glands, you simply prepare a medicated clay roll as follows:

1. Add enough water to some pharmaceutical-grade bentonite clay to make it into a malleable peanut butter consistency.

2. Using an appropriate amount of sterile gauze, roll the clay into a joint (a controversial cigarette-like contrivance) about the size of the pain rider's small finger.

3. Rid the clay roll of any air bubbles and squeeze its ends closed to seal them.

4. Pack the cylindrical poultice between the gum and cheek and leave it there for 1/2 to 1 hour, 2 times a day.

5. Rest, holding the poultice in place.

6. The effect of the clay can be enhanced by mixing some finely powdered Echinacea root or Goldenseal root with the clay powder before adding the water.

When treating swollen glands, one can add a couple drops of Poke root (*Phytolacca americana*) tincture to this poultice. It is quite helpful to use hand baths also to help pump the nodes in the neck. Administer the baths by placing both hands in a hot bath for 3 minutes immediately followed by a cold hand bath for 1 minute. Repeat this several consecutive times.

FOMENTATIONS

A fomentation (a.k.a. compress) is a form of poultice that is composed of liquids or lotions, absorbed in woolen or cotton cloths and usually applied hot. (Cold compresses are prepared for treating some headaches and sprains, and to stop bleeding.) Basically, a fomentation is yet another species of a bath employed to convey heat, combined with moisture, to the part of the body being fomented. A fomentation, like all therapeutic and tonic baths, is administered with the intent to soothe, nurse, and/or excite one back to ebullient, healthy activity.

MATERIAL TO USE FOR MAKING A FOMENTATION

Flannel cloths wrung out of hot liquid form the best fomentation material. In every process of fomentation there should be two cloths, one flannel ready while the other is applied. After the water has been wrung from the flannel, it should be *shaken up* and *laid lightly* over the body part. This involves a considerable amount of air which, being a poor conductor for heat transfer, retains the heat in the flannel cloth for a substantial amount of time.

When selecting a material to use for applying a fomentation, the fineness or the coarseness of the flannel is important to note. The coarser the material, the less readily it conducts heat, but it retains its warmth longer. It is therefore more efficient for fomenting. White flannel appears to retain heat longer than colored flannel. Of course, any absorbent material can be employed to apply a fomentation. Depending on the body part requiring the assistance, you can use gauze patches, stocking caps, menstrual

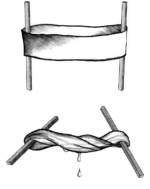

Sticks and Material Loop

pads, cotton gloves, jock straps, cotton bras, cotton socks, and so on.

For ease of wringing out boiling hot flannel cloths, one can employ the following technique:

Purchase two pieces of white flannel, each three yards long. (This is for use in large area fomenting; shorter pieces are appropriate for smaller jobs.) Sew the ends together making a very large headband-like device. This can now be wrung out of boiling liquid by means of two sticks inserted through the loop and turned in opposite directions. After the hot flannel has been wrung out, shake it up and lay the double-layered fomentation lightly on the body.

MAKING A FOMENTATION

To aid digestion in an individual whose stomach appears to be deficient in producing adequate hydrochloric acid, a simple hot water fomentation placed over the stomach for an hour or two after eating increases the amount of hydrochloric acid secreted by the peptic glands. A hot water bottle might be more convenient to employ for this purpose, but then where is the hot water bottle when you need it? And applications of heat over the abdomen can increase the activity of the digestive processes in the intestines and the functional activity of the pancreas and spleen. (In contrast, generally, whole body hot baths tend to diminish the secretion of HCL.) Hot applications placed over the liver region increase the flow of bile and stimulate all the other activities of the liver.

Simple hot water fomentations are remarkably soothing and revitalizing, but the use of herbal infusions and decoctions as the hot liquid further enhances their therapeutic action. Also, tinctures diluted with water can be used to medicate a fomentation.

Arnica Fomentation

A cold fomentation of Arnica (*Arnica spp.*) is well used to enhance peripheral circulation, helping to eliminate the pain of bruises, sprains, torn muscles, and tendons during the acute stage of an injury. A tablespoon of Arnica tincture to a half quart of cold water is used as the liquid in which a fomentation is soaked and laid on the injury. The injury is to be immobilized immediately and the fomentations are to be renewed frequently. Once the acute stage has run its course, one can apply warm poultices made of Comfrey root and Onion to give deeper action to assist the healing. Sprains can continue to trouble the individual long after the acute stages of the injury have passed. This is a good time to administer hot foot and leg baths or hot hand and arm bath, depending on the nature and location of the injury. These baths should be enjoyed for 20 to 30 minutes at a time.

Foxglove Fomentation

Foxglove (*Digitalis*) is a common garden plant that is toxic when taken internally, but is quite safe and useful when used externally as a moist compress. Dr. Rudolf Weiss, in his excellent book, *Herbal Medicine*, introduces this technique, which has been found to be of great value in promoting the healing of wounds that tend to persist for long periods of time. Foxglove leaves applied as a hot compress enhance the peripheral circulation of the skin and promote wound healing, especially those wounds that appear to be healing very slowly or not at all, such as chronic skin ulcers. I have found that a daily cup of herb tea made up of 1 part Comfrey root, 2 parts Burdock root, sweetened to taste, is a powerful adjunct for this task. *Never drink a tea of Foxglove, however!*

Poppy Fomentation

To help diminish pain, there is nothing as congenial than a hot fomentation made of dried Oriental Poppy (*Papaver somnifera*) heads. Drop 10 or 15 of them in water and heat the water. When it is quite warm, but not to hot to touch, pick out and tear the soggy Poppy heads in half and drop them back into the pot. When you finish doing this, bring the water to a boil, and simmer the Poppy heads for 10 to 15 minutes. The solution will turn a rich honey brown color. Dip your flannel into the hot decoction, wring it out, shake up the wet flannel, and lay it lightly on the painful area. When the flannel has cooled to warm, replace it immediately with a second fomentation. Repeat this 4 or 5 times. Leave the last fomentation on and cover it with plastic. Lay a towel over it, place a hot water bottle on this, and cover everything with a warm blanket. Let the individual lie quietly for about half an hour or so. While he or she is lying there fomenting, massage his or her feet and scalp.

Castor Oil Fomentation (Hot Pack)

It has been said and I must concur that the Castor oil hot pack (hot fomentation) is, without doubt, the high monarch of all herbal compresses; it is the Mohammed Ali, the Florence Nightingale, the '32 Ford Coup, the sensual Sultan of Swat of all poultices. I suggest that whenever you don't know what else to do for an ailing acquaintance, treat them to a Castor oil hot pack.

Mind you, a Castor oil fomentation can be a bit messy to administer. It's nothing a little attention to detail can't handle, though. It can take a while to produce noticeable, long-range results, but acute experiences of deep relaxation and central nervous system bliss are always noticed immediately. These are perfect experiences to initiate any healing journey.

A Castor oil fomentation can relieve muscular and skeletal pain, but more importantly, it can relieve the deep pain stemming from fibroids, internal scar tissue, congested lymph nodes, ovarian cysts, and infections. A series of Castor oil fomentations can restore health by invigorating scarred tissue and any deficient and sluggish glands or visceral organs.

Castor oil, which is derived from the Castor bean (*Ricinus communis*), is so similar to the natural oils of the human body it is easily received by human tissues and it is able to assist in their rejuvenation. Following is an abbreviated list of therapeutic chores expected by the judicious application of Castor oil fomentations: calming of nervous irritability and aiding sleep, detoxification of tissues including the liver when needed; reduction and healing of cysts, warts, and other unwanted growths; alleviation of uterine disorders and chronic infections; soothing the discomfort of bladder infection while promoting healing; and stimulation of the body's deep circulation, including lymphatic circulation. Castor oil fomentations promote general detoxification and deep relaxation which in turn rejuvenates all systems of the body.

To prepare and administer a hot Castor oil fomentation:

1. Cut several pieces of laundered white cotton flannel, cotton felt, or cheesecloth large enough to more than completely cover the area to be treated. (When fomenting the liver, it is best to use pieces of material large enough to extend from the navel, over the liver, and around to the spine, and from the right hip bone up to the breast/pecs.) I suggest you cut several pieces of material because it is best for this fomentation to be several layers thick.

2. Place the cotton material into a clean glass or stainless steel pan.

3. Pour 1 to 2 cups of Castor oil onto the pieces of material, soaking them through with the oil.

4. Place the pan of oiled cotton into an oven and heat it until the oiled material is very warm but still touchable. One can put a few drops of Lavender, Chamomile, Lemon, and/or Rose essential oil onto the pack at this point if this floral oil bouquet will be appreciated.

5. Wash the area of the body to be treated with a mixture of warm water and apple cider vinegar.

6. Take the fomentation from the pan and remove any excess oil so there is no dripping.

7. Place the hot fomentation over the area to be fomented. (If this is a liver pack, the person should be lying on his or her left side. Otherwise it will be a spleen pack, and that would be okay too.)

8. Cover the fomentation with a plastic wrap.

9. Over this lay a heating pad or a hot water bottle.

10. Wrap a large towel around all the above and tuck it comfortably under the body to hold everything in place.

11. Place a warm blanket over the individual and let him or her receive the fomentation for at least an hour up to several hours.

12. A gentle foot massage and head massage supplies a delicious touch to this healthful ritual.

13. When completed, remove the oil from the skin by using a gentle soap and then a wash of warm water and baking soda. (This mixture will soothe the area, especially if any minor skin irritation or rash has developed from the drawing action of the Castor oil.)

When all is finished, wrap the oiled material in a plastic bag and store it in the refrigerator. It can be reheated and reused several times, *but only on the same person.* Replace it with fresh material after six to eight applications.

Repeated fomentations over a period of time are often required to heal the above conditions. These can be given in a pattern of three days in a row, then four days off. Repeat this pattern for several weeks or until the ailing condition is history. Each time you receive the effects of this poultice you will feel like you've just taken a six-week vacation, one in which you never had to look for parking places or endure airport fiascoes.

Remember, the tricks for using poultices and fomentations successfully (although there are always some exceptions) are:

• Make poultices thick.

• Keep poultices and fomentations warm and moist.

• Allow them adequate time to do their work.

Incorporating time in any therapeutic formula is valuable; you asked for the help, so give yourself the space to receive it. Enjoy post-trauma time by relaxing and being patient. More than likely, stress and impatience had major roles in creating the wounds in the first place.

COMPLEMENTARY TECHNIQUES, TERMS, AND OTHER CONSIDERATIONS

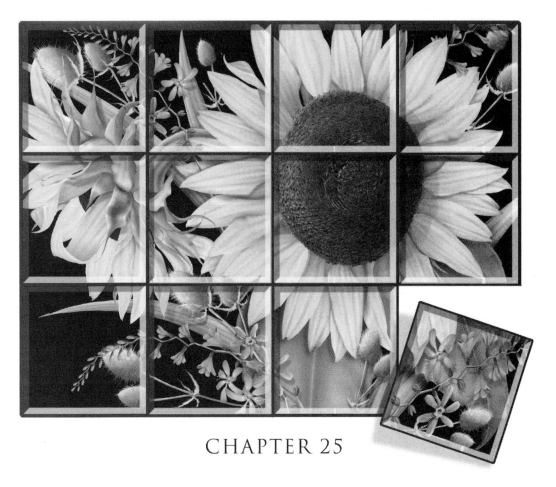

CHAPTER 25

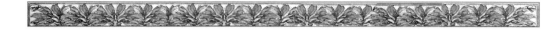

This chapter is the "grouting stuff" of the handbook, the informational mortar that should fill in any inadvertent cracks and crevices that might have occurred as we laid out the instructional tiles of the previous chapters. Arranged in an A to Z format, from *Absorbability of Herbal Medicines* and the *Art of Simpling* to *Making Liniments* and *Lozenges* to *Placebo Effect* and *Powdering* to *Weights and Measures* and the definition of *Wildcrafting*, this chapter is a cauldronful of definitions, techniques, concepts, and pertinent asides. The substance of the materials included supply sundry supportive, complementary details that should serve well to caulk the seams of our medicine-making vessel. Therefore, having said whatever it is that I just said…

ABSORBABILITY OF HERBAL MEDICINES

Medicines, in order to be systemically effective, must be soluble in some absorbable menstruum, or dissolvable in a body fluid. Medicines are commonly considered most readily absorbed when in solution.

Some folks believe that alcoholic solutions (tinctures) are generally more easily taken up by the body than water solutions (teas); as an herbal vehicle, tinctures are definitely more preservative. For these reasons, alcohol menstrua might be considered preferable to water except for the possible complications inherent with alcohol use. It can cause inebriation and can be habit-forming to some individuals. However, usual therapeutic dosage is well below a harmful level even in the long-term use (see "*Alcohol*," Chapter Six, for more details).

Water is harmless and readily absorbable, but has no preservative effect and can fail to dissolve and extract some desirable medicinal components (the latter is true for alcohol as well). When making an extract of dry plant material, a menstruum that combines alcohol and water is quite practical for tincturing. If a person is extremely alcohol-intolerant and doesn't want to chance taking any alcohol at all, it is advisable to use tinctures prepared with glycerin or vinegar menstrua or use herbal teas.

The administration of hard and difficult-to-digest medicines should be avoided because of their slow and uncertain rate of disintegration and absorption and their consequent unreliability. Certain compressed tablets, and, often, encapsulated, powdered whole herbs may pass completely through the intestinal tract without effect. It is very difficult to determine the quality or authenticity of commercially powdered and capped herbal ingredients, for the powdered herb which is encapsulated in a gelatin capsule is generally never touched, smelled, or tasted by the consumer.

Systemic medicines can act only when absorbed by the blood or lymphatics, so it follows that conditions must be right to obtain the most efficient results. Medicines administered by mouth act most readily when the stomach is empty, and slowly (sometimes not at all) when diluted by the contents of the stomach. A full stomach may greatly reduce absorption. However, if nausea or stomach upset occurs while taking herbal medicines on an empty stomach, a small amount of food can be eaten.

Syrups, mucilages, and resins are useful where a prolonged contact with the tissues is intended, provided they do not lessen the efficiency of the medicinal ingredients. Syrups are valued chiefly for their agreeable taste and the fact that the sugar content has a preservative action, provided the sugar is present in a 2:1 w/v proportion. However, a sick patient's stomach might rebel against a sweet or aromatized medicine.

Most medicines are best given at short intervals, and no matter what the stomach conditions the general American trend is in favor of administering herbal medicines in small and often-repeated doses (i.e., 10 to 30 drops of 1:5 w/v tincture, three to four times a day).

Medicines most likely act fastest when the circulation is active, and slowest when the circulation is depressed. When the stomach and/or the intestines are sluggish, medicines act more quickly when local stimulants such as Cayenne or Ginger are given with them. When diarrhea or vomiting occur during administration of medicines, certainly less is absorbed and a portion is lost through this heroic elimination.

ART OF SIMPLING

A *simple* is a common health-enhancing plant.

A *simpler* is one who knows how to use these plants…an herbalist.

The simpler:

• Uses local herbs, recently harvested.

• Uses only mild nutritional herbs with generous amounts of pure water.

• Uses these simples consistently over a long period of time.

• Cleanses the body, promotes healthy circulation, and creates a mild rise in temperature with baths and saunas to promote sweating.

• Uplifts, appreciates, and focuses on the individual's health.

One can always rely on this simpler's art to support health and heal ills.

CAPSULES

Capsules are used as a vehicle to deliver herbs in their dry form. They are useful for administering herbs in the following circumstances:

• When the herb is to be taken in small amounts, such as 1/2 to 3 Gm. An ounce is approximately 30 Gm.

• When the herb is intensely bitter or otherwise abominable tasting (like Saw Palmetto) or contains a lot of mucilage. The flavors of mild-tasting herbs don't need to be hidden in a capsule, and when possible they are better taken as a tea. These tonic plants (Red Clover, Nettle, Red Raspberry) usually require a larger dose to give a desired effect than is ordinarily provided by capsules.

• When an herb or herbal formula is to be taken regularly for a long period of time.

• When the whole herb can be taken including the woody material.

• As an excellent way to administer tinctures that have been infused in lactose powder (see "*Lactose Powder Infusion*," below).

• Capsulated herbs are very convenient to take, especially when traveling.

Drawbacks of using capsules

• You don't taste the herb, which, granted, can be quite merciful (like when taking Saw Palmetto. Did I mention that already?). However, this is a disadvantage when taking herbal bitters, as many herbalists believe their effectiveness depends on a neurological reflex triggered by actually tasting their bitter flavor. When put into a capsule this beneficial action may be lost or greatly diminished.

• You don't know what you are getting unless you fill the capsules yourself. (Of course this can be said about any type of commercial herbal product.)

• Short shelf life.

• Most capsules available on the market are made from gelatin. I have found that some of these capsules dissolve well and some don't. There are those that can travel the full length of your gastrointestinal tract from its oral commencement to its anal conclusion without dissolving, which with some pharmaceutical drugs probably does one a tremendous favor, but it's better that the capsules with your herbal preparations dissolve and release their contents while in the stomach. Check this out first before purchasing any quantity of empty capsules by first sucking on one for a while to see if it dissolves easily.

Some capsules on the market are made of plant starch or cellulose and tend to break down quite quickly. In my experience, these are less commonly used, more expensive, yet more efficient. In place of using capsules one can wrap powdered herb in edible rice paper cut to an appropriate size.

Capsule size

Small "0" capsules are best for children (if they'll swallow them), or for administering very strong herbs such as Goldenseal, Wormwood, Lobelia, or Cayenne. Larger "00" are more suitable for adults.

1 ounce of powdered herb will fill about 60 "0" caps or 30 "00" caps. One "00" cap holds about 1/4 teaspoon dried powdered herb.

Preparing the herb

Powder the herb finely so you can give a more concentrated dose, and so it is easier for the body to assimilate. If possible, powder the herbs as you use them rather than buying powdered herbs. Powdered herbs which have sat on store shelves deteriorate quickly and lose their effectiveness. Also, unless you know an herb quite well by smell or taste, it is nearly impossible to be sure that you are getting the herb you want when it is merely seen as a powder. Most green powders look similar; so do most brown powders, tan powders, yellowish powders, etc.

Procedure for filling capsules

1. Powder herb in coffee bean grinder.

2. Place powder in a small bowl. If using more than one herb, blend them together at this stage.

3. Separate the two halves of the capsule, and hold the empty capsule bottom between the thumb and the forefinger.

4. Punch or press the capsule bottom vertically into the powder until it is filled.

5. Push capsule ends together and place in another bowl.

6. Continue this until all caps are full or all the powder is gone.

Dosage

People ordinarily take 2 "00" caps full of herb 2–3 times a day with water (1 "0" cap, 2–3 times a day for children).

Storage

Store in tightly sealed bottles in a cool, dark place. Herbs begin to deteriorate fairly rapidly after they have been powdered. However, when put into air-free capsules, they keep for a longer time, approximately 1 year.

Circumstances that modify the effects of medicines

While the effects of herbal remedies are generally much the same on people, there are conditions or circumstances which tend to modify their action. These factors create the environment that makes healing and herbal therapeutics more an art than a science. The modifying conditions and circumstances are: 1) age of the patient, 2) the patient's sex, 3) weight, 4) temperament, 5) variations of temperature, 6) diseased tissue, 7) drug habit(s), 8) pregnancy, 9) menstruation, 10) idiosyncrasy, the peculiar susceptibility (or insusceptibility) of the tissues of certain persons to the influence of certain medicines, 11) placebo effect, the most profound, unpredictable, and potentially enlightening of all the modifying conditions.

CONCENTRATES

A simple method for increasing the potency of an infusion or decoction is to prepare a concentrate. (This process is not particularly suitable with sensitive or volatile plants.) In general, this is done best by using a large volume of tea, as it is easier to concentrate the brew without burning it. Concentrates are the common herbal base used to prepare syrups and fomentations. An easy method for preparing a concentrate is to place a strained and filtered infusion or decoction into a stainless steel or glass pot. Stick a chopstick straight down into the center of the liquid touching the bottom of the pot. Withdraw the stick and make a mark at the water line. Bring the liquid to a boil. Reduce the flame and gently simmer the liquid, slowly evaporating the water portion until the surface of the liquid marks a point half as high on the chopstick as the original watermark. At this point, one-half the volume of the original liquid remains, rendering the concentrate double the potency of the original tea; when it marks a point one-quarter as high as the original watermark the concentrate is considered to be four times the strength of the original extract, and so on until the concentrate is transformed into a tar and ultimately into a powder. Be sure to use low heat over a long period of time or the concentrate will "burn" and its therapeutic potency will be trashed. One can also concentrate a tea by placing it in flat trays inserted in a dehydrator.

DECANTING

The simple process of decanting is used to separate fluids from solids. It usually consists of allowing the solids to settle and deposit at the bottom of the vessel, and then carefully pouring off the liquid by inclining the vessel. You can also use a food baster for drawing off the desired liquids. This is a most valuable technique for separating water and marc from oil when making fresh-plant oil infusions.

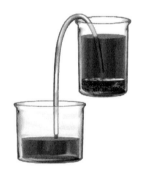

Siphoning Procedure

Siphoning. It is sometimes impossible to decant by pouring off the liquid, either because the holding vessel is too full or because of the light character of the precipitate (for example, with Usnea extract), the inclination of the vessel would cause a disturbance in the powder that would result in an admixture of the liquid and solid. A siphon can be helpful in a situation like this (see illustration). The best material to use for the siphon tube is flexible surgical tubing. Fill the tube with the liquid that is to be siphoned, and then insert the short end into the liquid that is to be drawn off. Place the long end in the receiving vessel. When a flow of liquid from the long end has been established, it need not be stopped until as much of the liquid as desired has been extracted.

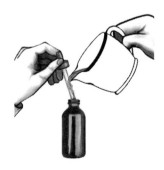

Pipette Guiding Rod

Guiding Rod. Some skill is necessary for decanting liquids without spillage from vessels of various shapes and when transferring liquids from a larger container into smaller dropper bottles. A guiding rod is most helpful in these processes, and it is good practice to develop the habit of using a guiding rod as illustrated. When dispensing liquid extracts into dropper bottles, use the bottle's pipette (dropper) as the guiding rod.

DIGESTION

Digestion, from the Latin *digerere*, meaning to separate or dissolve, is simply another maceration process in which the menstruum is heated, with the heat increasing the solvent power of the menstruum. Digestion differs from infusion and decoction in that the period of soaking is considerably longer (1 to 10 days), and the temperature at which the menstruum is held is much lower, usually between 100° and 140° F. This process is not used very often for the preparation of herbal extracts. I use it predominantly for the preparation of oil infusions (see Chapter Seventeen), and basically this is the process employed when making herb teas by *solar infusion* (placing the fresh and/or dried herbs in a clear jar with a water menstruum and letting the mixture set in direct sunlight for a day). A *lunar infusion* (Witch's elixir) is done in the same fashion, except that the subtle energy from the light of the moon is employed instead; a convivial chorus of cackles can expedite this process.

DISPENSATORY

The U.S. Dispensatory is primarily a commentary upon pharmacopoeias (U.S. as well as some foreign pharmacopoeias, particularly British), but it is broad enough in scope to include also every known medicinal or pharmaceutical article and its most important preparations. The dispensatory is the most comprehensive single work on medicines and their uses. In it you may find official, non-official, and common names of plants, descriptions, and botanical origins, and explanations of parts used. Notes on adulterants are included. It offers formulas for compounding preparations, and gives maximum and minimum doses. The actions of medicines (physiological, toxic, and medicinal) are fully but briefly discussed.

In reality, the dispensatory is an encyclopedia of drugs and their uses. It is not necessarily official, nor does it delineate the legal criterion used in this country. It includes a vast amount of material. Note that the information concerning the uses of botanicals is not written by herbalists and is often contrary to our experiences or what we might at times regard as standardized "b.s."

DOSAGE

It is better to err on the side of insufficient dosage and trust to nature than to overdose. This avoids harming the client. Giving no medication at all is always better than medicating aimlessly. Many medicines positively influence conditions of imbalance when given in minute doses, even though no explanation for the action can be given. The fractional dose of *Matricaria* (German Chamomile) or of Pulsatilla often effects a positive control over nervous phenomena that cannot be duplicated by more powerful agents or doses (for example, two Chamomile flowers in a cup of hot tea or 1 drop of Chamomile tincture in an ounce of water). Try it.

As a general rule, large and robust persons require fuller doses than small and frail individuals and the elderly require smaller doses than other adults. In general, beginning at age 65, dosage of most systemic remedies should run a gradually descending scale, while it may be necessary to increase that of eliminants such as gentle laxatives and diuretics. The weight of an individual also has to be taken into account. When giving medicine to children, certain rules must be followed. No absolutes can be determined in administering medicines to children, but one or the other of the following rules is often used:

Clark's Rule: Divide the weight in pounds by 150 to give the approximate fraction of the adult dose. (For example, for a 50-pound child, divide 50 by 150 = 1/3. Therefore, the dose is one-third that of the adult dose.)

Cowling's Rule: The age of the child at his/her next birthday is divided by 24. That is, for a child coming 3 years of age, 3 divided by 24 = 1/8. Therefore, the dose is one-eighth that of the dose for an adult.

Young's Rule: The dose is computed by dividing the child's age by 12 plus the age. So, for a child of 4 years, 4 divided by [12+4] = 4/16 = 1/4. Therefore, the dose is one-fourth that which would be given to an adult.

As I mentioned, no exact rule can be established, and these doses should be lowered in some instances, most notably when administering strong and intense medicines like Goldenseal, Cayenne, Poke, etc.

DOUBLE MACERATION

This is a process of macerating a plant in a menstruum for an appropriate amount of time, decanting it, pressing it, and then using that solution (tincture) as the menstruum for a second round, pouring it over an equal amount of herb as used in the initial maceration, thereby repeating the entire process. Supposedly, this technique renders the extract more potent. It is used by some commercial companies as a marketing gimmick in an attempt to position their products as superior. However, although this technique makes sense when extracting very mild herbs such as Cleavers, Mullein blossoms, Plantain, Nettle leaf, Red Clover blossoms, or even Ginkgo, with most plants, if one does the initial maceration properly and is using good-quality herb, double maceration is really unnecessary, and, in my opinion, needlessly squanders a lot of good herb.

DRUG

"Drug" comes from the Dutch word *droog*, meaning dried plant. Strictly speaking, a drug is a dried medicinal plant containing its entire ingredients. However, corporations cannot patent a natural plant for economic exploitation. Consequently, the Western pharmaceutical industry has emphasized and promoted chemical "drug therapy," giving themselves more economic control to manufacture and promote white powders and clear liquids. They also have fewer problems by not having to deal with organic materials that decompose and get buggy, and they generate immense profits from marketing patentable products. So today, by common cultural experience, a drug is thought of more as a modern chemical preparation than as a medicinal dried plant, unless of course that plant can get you high.

EXPRESSION (SEE PRESSING)

FILTRATION

Filtration is employed when the solid matter to be removed from a liquid solution is not present in large quantity. It is done by submitting the mixture to the separating action of certain materials which allow the fluids to pass through, but which block the passage of the solid particles. Sometimes filtration is called *straining* or *collation*. Actually, straining differs from filtration in that it affords less complete removal of suspended sedimentary matter from the fluid. It is useful when the solid particles are large enough to be easily retained by a coarser media than those generally employed for filtration.

The most common, easily attainable filtering material used in our work is a paper filter such as a coffee filter. It is advisable to use unbleached paper filters which have not been heat-sealed into preformed shapes, because it is suspected that the sealant is relatively toxic, especially when used to filter alcohol and vinegar-based extracts or any hot extract.

Collation is the preferred method of separation when the fluid is of a viscid (sticky or adhering) character, such as glycerites, oil infusions, and syrups. The filtering media employed here are cotton, muslin, flannel, or woolen cloth. These cloths can be used to line a wire sieve before the viscid fluid is poured through.

HERBS AND PHARMACEUTICAL MEDICATIONS

Herbs and pharmaceuticals are well-labeled as "complementary medicines." Regardless of rampant prejudice in favor of, and in opposition to either one or the other, they are of equal value; one primarily for heroic treatment of disease symptoms and crisis intervention, and the other perfectly suited for convalescent nourishment, nutritional toning/health sustenance, and disease prevention and treatment. Both are playing an important role in modern day health care and disease control. Both provide excellent service to humans and non-humans when used with a clear mind, compassionate heart, and a healer's intent.

• Normally, individuals having delicate constitutions are more prone to adverse or unpredictable effects.

• Herbal products that have been standardized (refined) to an arbitrary percent of any specific constituent in an attempt to exaggerate this component and elicit a faster (drug-like) action frequently demonstrate more (drug-like) side effects. This refinement process alters the natural synergistic energy of the herb and modifies the herb's natural ability to do many things and work on deeper fundamental levels.

• Alterative, adaptogen, and tonic actions are unique to herbal preparations. None of these actions are found in drugs.

• There are no drugs that can give the complex effects of an herbal bitter.

• The fast specific action of drugs dynamically support the surgical process in crises/disease management and cosmetic and corrective surgery.

• Relevant factors to include in the decision to use herbs or drugs:

• The individual's preference upon having been clearly advised and/or self-educated as to the risks and benefits of both types of medication.

• Effectiveness for desired results.

• Speed of action sought.

• Probability of dosage compliance, especially when prolonged treatment is necessary due to the use of a slower acting herbal preparation.

• Side effects (I regard this as more of a "wool over the eyes" or a "shmoozing" term. I don't see that any agent renders some quasi-predictable side effect that somehow proceeds beyond some intended or predicted effect; there are "the effects" an agent causes in "an individual"—the classic "different effects in different people" experience.)

HERBS COMPARED TO PHARMACEUTICAL DRUGS

	HERBS	DRUGS
ACTIONS	Often multiple	Usually just one (often using a single specific receptor site)
	Often enhances body's own healing ability	No drug does this
	Addresses causal factors of an illness	Mostly treats symptoms (can be life-saving in a crisis/emergency)
ACTIVE CONSTITUENTS	Many (synergistic)	Usually one
SIDE EFFECTS	Few and mild	Often many, can be severe
ONSET OF ACTION	May be slow (working on nutritional level)	Usually rapid and direct
COST	Variable (you can make your own)	Variable

HYDROLYSIS

Hydrolysis is a chemical reaction where a substance (plant constituent) reacts with water and is changed into one or more other substances, such as starch into glucose or natural fats into glycerin (glycerol) and fatty acids.

LACTOSE POWDER INFUSION

This is an excellent method for ultimately obtaining a dry preparation from a fresh plant or dry plant tincture without having to use heat. The process is suitable for administering tinctures and fluid extracts whose menstruum consist of water and/or vinegar and alcohol. It is not as suitable for those whose menstruum contain any portion of glycerin. Obviously, it is not a good idea to administer these preparations to lactose-intolerant individuals.

1. Mix a single tincture or a compound tincture with an equal weight of lactose powder [i.e., 30 ml (1 fl. oz.) tincture with 30 Gm (1 oz.) lactose powder].

2. Expose this mixture to normal room temperature in a shallow container. The menstruum will slowly evaporate, leaving the lactose saturated with the herbal constituents.

3. Triturate the dry powder to an even consistency. (See "*Trituration*" below.)

4. Fill the capsules with the dry powder or incorporate the powder in the making of lozenges, etc.

LINIMENT

This is more of a preparation thinner than salve, to be rubbed on the skin. Liniments are compounded and prepared exactly like tinctures, using vinegar, ethyl alcohol, or denatured rubbing alcohol as a menstruum. Liniments are prepared especially for external purposes, and it is a good idea to label them as such (i.e., "For External Use Only"). If rubbing alcohol is the menstruum, you might even draw a little skull and crossbones on the label in red ink.

Depending on the menstruum and the herbs, a liniment is employed for various purposes: to draw, to warm, and to dry an area of the skin; to disinfect cuts and wounds; to help heal wounds, bruises, sprains, burns, and sunburns; as an anodyne to soothe strained muscles and ligaments; or to work as a counterirritant (revulsive).

There is a classic herbal liniment formula whose praise is sung in the notebooks of every attentive herb student in America. This is *The Jethro Kloss Goldenseal & Myrrh Liniment*, the Florence Nightingale of compound rubs for injured athletes and sundry adventurers. This liniment will last forever and will always be there for you when you need it.

1. Mix together 1/2 oz. of powdered Goldenseal root, 1 oz. of powdered Myrrh, and 1/4 oz. of powdered Cayenne.

2. Add to this dry mixture, 1 pint of (rubbing) alcohol.

3. Let stand for seven days; shake well every day.

4. Decant and bottle.

According to Mr. Kloss in his classic herbal, *Back to Eden*, "If you don't have Goldenseal, make it without." I think a 1/16 to an 1/8 ounce of this endangered herb is more than adequate.

Of course, you can use ethyl alcohol as the menstruum in place of the rubbing alcohol, whereby this tincture can be used internally as well.

A lesser-known, quickly prepared liniment that is enthusiastically recommended by Mr. Kloss is a simple vinegar preparation:

1. Combine 1 tablespoonful of powdered Cayenne red pepper with 1 pint apple cider vinegar.

2. Simmer gently for 10 minutes.

3. Bottle it hot, unstrained.

This makes, "a powerfully stimulating external application for deep-seated internal congestion and inflammation, sprains, etc." The application of this Cayenne liniment arouses strong circulation upon the surface of the skin inducing smarting and redness, but does not injure the skin.

LOZENGES (ALSO CALLED TROCHES OR PASTILLES)

Lozenges are small, solid, flattened cakes of very finely powdered therapeutic herbal substance, prepared from a mass made with a base of sugar for its pleasant flavor and a mucilage prepared from Slippery Elm bark, or Comfrey root, or Marshmallow root, or from a mucilage prepared from gum Acacia (a.k.a. gum Arabic), or gum Tragacanth as an adhesive to give form and consistency. Water (plain or aromatic flower water) is used to supply the necessary moisture. Any suitable essential oil (Anise, Peppermint, Wintergreen, etc.) may be triturated (see "*Trituration*" below) with the sugar before this is mixed with the other powders.

Lozenges are placed on the tongue and allowed to dissolve slowly. They are especially useful when the herbal ingredients are intended to come into contact with the mucous surface of the mouth, throat, and upper respiratory tract. The remedial action of lozenges is generally designed to be local rather than systemic. (There may, however, be a place for a Damiana lozenge for enhancing staying power.) The action of a lozenge is normally expectorant, demulcent, sedative, or antiseptic.

The creation of the lozenge-mass is the critical step in making this vehicle. The dry herbal powders and sugar must be made into an adhesive mass that will be sufficiently plastic to enable it to be rolled into a flat cake without crumbling; at the same time it must dry quickly, and the lozenge must not become brittle due to insufficient adhesiveness. Mucilages are thick, viscid, adhesive liquids that are produced by dissolving gum in water, or by extracting by cold infusion the mucilaginous principles of Slippery Elm, Marshmallow, or Comfrey.

When making the lozenge-mass, using a (moist) mucilage is a preferred technique to mixing the dry gum powder with the other dry ingredients and then adding the water. In this method it is often difficult to avoid an excess of moisture.

Preparing a Mucilage

Using mucilaginous herb:

1. Macerate overnight 6 parts (6 Gm) dried herb in 100 parts (100 ml) of water.

2. Press it forcibly through cotton muslin.

Using gum Acacia (gum Arabic):

1. Combine 1 part gum Arabic to 2 parts water, let sit for several hours, and strain.

2. Or moisten 50 Gm Acacia with 75 ml cold water, set aside for several hours for the gum to dissolve completely, then add sufficient water to make up 125 ml.

Using gum Tragacanth:

1. Mix 18 ml glycerin with 76 ml water.

2. Heat to boiling.

3. Remove from fire and add 6 Gm gum Tragacanth.

4. Macerate for 24 hours, stirring now and then.

5. Strain forcibly through cotton muslin.

Preparing the Lozenge

1. Mix and sift the dry powders to be used (powdered herb and sugar, lactose infusions — see lactose powder infusion, above). If essential oils are to be incorporated, triturate them with the sugar at this time. The finer the powder, the better the quality of the lozenge.

2. Stir in sufficient powder to a prepared mucilage to make a mass of proper consistency. The quantity of mucilage to use always depends upon the character of the powder. If the powder is quite absorbent, more mucilage is required.

3. Once the final mass is prepared, it is ready to be formed into a flat cake by placing it upon a hard, level, dusted surface and rolling it with a cylindrical roller (which can be lightly oiled if necessary to prevent sticking). The thickness of the cake determines the weight of the lozenge, so it is more exact to have some means of adjusting the thickness. The herbs I use for making lozenges are not critically dose specific, so I usually avoid this rolling out (and cutting) process entirely by calculating an appropriate size portion for a dose, separating and rolling it between my palms into a little ball, laying it on a hard surface dusted with powdered sugar, and then flattening and shaping it with my fingers; then I do another one, then another....It is a mellow task that proceeds at about the same rate of speed and degree of excitement as filling capsules. You get into the rhythm of it, and in a brief, peculiar segment of your lifespan the job is completed.

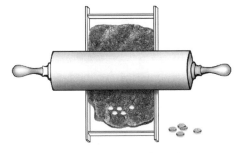

Lozenge Rolling Board

4. If you choose to employ the hard surface and roller technique, cut out each lozenge using a small, improvised, cookie cutter-type device.

5. Lay the formed lozenges out on a screen or on a large sieve to dry; a plate works in lieu of a screen; however, you have to turn the lozenges over with a tiny little spatula to dry them out underneath.

Making lozenges requires some trial and error to discern the right consistency for the lozenge-mass. Hold aside some of the powder and some of the mucilage. Be aware that mucilage deteriorates fairly quickly. Mix a mass, roll out a small portion of it (set the larger portion in a tightly covered jar to retain its moisture), and cut the disks, or form the cakes in whatever way you choose, lay them out to dry overnight, and see what you get. You can always go back to the main mass and adjust it for further experimentation by adding more mucilage or more powder. With sufficient stirring and kneading, the original mass will incorporate the modifying additions. Take accurate notes until you get it down. Make your first experimental lozenges tasty (1 part Wintergreen powder to 2 parts sugar makes a pleasant-tasting, aromatic treat); this way people won't mind testing these and giving you feedback as to the tenacity and basic "suckability" of your lozenges.

Remember, the finer the powder (#60 & #80, see "*Powdering*" below), the better the lozenge.

MARC

The term marc is from the old French word *marcher*, to trample (as on grapes). The marc is the insoluble residue remaining after extracting the soluble components of an herb with a menstruum (solvent), or the pulpy residue left after the juice has been pressed from grapes, apples, other fruits, vegetables, or herbs.

MATERIA MEDICA (THE MATERIALS OF MEDICINE)

Usually a materia medica is a treatise on the materials used in a particular school or system of medicine, discussing their history, source, physical characteristics, constituents, and actions. Preparations and doses are mentioned, and brief therapeutic and toxicological notes are usually given. A materia medica can be combined with therapeutics and these works are called *Materia Medica and Therapeutics*. These works include the same stuff which is found in a materia medica, plus extensive information on the physiological, chemical, and toxicological action, as well as the therapeutic usage of the medicines considered. A materia medica will reveal the individuality of its author. What the author includes is usually what she or he has personal knowledge of and interest in, or which meets with her or his approval. In this aspect it differs from a dispensatory, which is designed to be a book of general reference.

MEDICINE

Medicine is whatever you choose to help you focus on well-being, to help reduce any resistance to the flow of life force, and to revive your experience of health. Medicine is any agent that helps revive your physical, mental, and emotional vitality, and uplifts and promotes your natural state of wellness, joy, and prosperity. All medicines are equally creditable; different things resonate differently with different people.

MENISCUS

Due to the capillary attraction of a liquid to the wetted glass walls of a (graduated) cylinder or pipette, the surface of a liquid in these containers presents a cup shape called a meniscus. A line drawn through the bottom of the meniscus is normally selected as the point at which to read a measurement.

MENSTRUUM

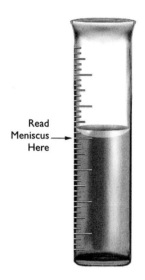

Read Meniscus Here

A menstruum is the solvent used to make extracts. The word menstruum comes somewhere out of the ancient language of lunar astrology. It is derived from the Latin word *menstruus*, monthly (from *mensis*, a month), which, according to Caspari's 1906 *Treatise on Pharmacy*, "was applied because of some influence which the changes of the moon, and consequently the time of the month, were supposed to exert upon the preparation of solvents."

Herbalists strive to prepare an extract that represents as much of the whole plant as is possible and practical. The best menstruum for extracting an herb will dissolve and bring into solution all the desired principles of the herb, will leave behind the principles which are not desired, and will retain the desired soluble constituents in a stable form that will not be injured by light, heat, or air during consequent use and storage.

The ideal menstruum for extracting a given herb's constituents is determined mainly by experimentation. The formula used to prepare a menstruum differs with each individual herb or type of herbal preparation. A menstruum may be pure water or pure ethyl alcohol; a mixture of alcohol and water; a mixture of alcohol, water, and glycerin; pure glycerin; glycerin and water; wine; vinegar (acetic acid); or whatever combination of solvents the medicine-maker determines to be the most efficient for making an extract of the particular herb at hand.

MAKING YOUR "MOJO"

In spite of the common notion a mojo is not an X-rated item. A mojo is four medicine power-roots that are housed in a small red pouch. One's mojo is carried in a pocket, hung on a belt, carried in a purse, or dwells in a frequently used drawer. This little red bag full of root allies is painstaking prepared and privately carried so the active spirit of the plants can assist an individual to remain in constant touch with her or his creative essence, freedom, wit, safety, and well-being. Preferably, the roots are wildcrafted; roots that the individual has personally taken from the soil with deep respect and full recognition of the powers embodied in the plant entities; roots that have been dug while the digger maintained clear, undisturbed focus on his or her requests for the plants' services; roots that have been anointed with specific herbal oil infusions that have been previously prepared for the making of a mojo. A mojo is personal, a mojo is private, a mojo is a man's and a woman's intimate herbal companion. It carries the visionary vibrations of their secret dreams, the passion of their desires, and the power of their intentions.

The taproot of the mojo tradition reaches back to the ancestral herbalists and ancient plant lore of the African continent. Transplants of this knowing appeared in this country in the West Indies and the deep South well over two hundred years ago. That is what I was told.

Once the appropriate wild plants have been approached and communed with, their roots are dug, carefully washed, dried, anointed with herbal oils, and placed in a small handmade red pouch, never to be seen again by anyone other than the carrier, the creator and possessor of that particular mojo.

With continual awareness and appreciation of their presence the visions of the roots' meaning and purpose are internalized by the carrier like the subtle vibrations of a powerful mantra consciously connecting him and her to Source energy. The carrier is self-empowered by the acquisition, preparation, and lifelong companionship of these wild medicine-roots. Magical occurrences are consummated by one's focus on a clear intention in a personal environment that includes absolute allowing with no resistance or doubt of any sort to detain the flow of the creative, manifesting energy; therefore the vibrations of a personally potentized mojo supports and sustains the ongoing magic and joy of one's life journey. The mojo assists its carrier to view life positively, to create deliberately, to attract delicious life experiences, to have what she or he truly wants.

The four roots traditionally used to activate a mojo (as this tradition was passed on to me) are:

1. Two (2) *Imomoea Purga* (Jalap) roots from the *Convolvulaceae* family. One of these roots having a more lengthy and slender form to energize "Him" (one's male energy, yang essence), and one shaped more round and circular to draw in "Her" (one's female energy, yin essence). Him and Her are the "power roots" known as *High John the Conqueror*. They draw in personal power protection, manifesting the impeccable warrior. This is star energy—the brilliance of the Sun. Both Him and Her are anointed with an oil infusion of Wormwood. Her is further anointed with oil of St. John's Wort (*Hypericum*), Him with a female ritual oil (one's own creation), then both roots are anointed with the carrier's own saliva (a personal intimate touch).

2. One (1) Bethroot (*Trillium erectum*) from the *Liliaceae* family. This root is known as *Southern John*. Southern John is the "wealth root." It assists one to develop a sense of personal worthiness bringing wealth of material benefits. One enjoys an endless abundance of friends, health, love, money, wisdom, humor, and joy. This root properly anointed is expansive with the vibrations of Jupiter. Southern John is anointed with oil (infusion) of Wormwood, oil of Mugwort, oil of Hypericum, and oil of Calendula.

3. One (1) *Alpinia officinarum* (Lesser Galangal or Small Galangal) root from the *Zingiberaceae* (Ginger) family. This root is called *Little John the Conqueror,* or sometimes *Chewing John*. It is the "wit root" which assists one to cut through fear and confusion, giving the power of clear thought, wit, and lucid expression. Properly anointed, it is the penetrating problem solver, active with the vibrations of Mercury. Chewing John is anointed with oil of Wormwood, oil of Hawthorn berry, oil of Mullein blossoms, and oil of Hypericum.

4. Focus clearly and pointedly on your request of the roots as you anoint them with the herbal oils. If any of the roots discussed above are not available to you, you will of course use roots that thrive where you live which you sense to be equally appropriate for preparing your personal mojo. Trust your intuition. Our plant allies live near us. Design and hand-sew the red bag yourself. Make pull strings to close the top, hang beads on them if so inclined, whatever; fashion the mojo to suit your style.

Gather your roots, prepare the herbal oils, select and sew some passionate red material. It takes time to do all this, time in which you are focusing on your strengths, acknowledging your personal beauty, tuning into your joy, your health, your power and worthiness, noting your absolute freedom to choose your thoughts and live your life as you wish, and to prepare in the present your ensuing journey into the future. Actualize your dreams, get your mojo working, enjoy your life, and thrive; it is your spiritual heritage. You are the healer and the dancer, joy is the music, the roots are your allies.

NATIONAL FORMULARY (NF)

A formulary is a collection of working formulas for the preparation of medicinal compounds. A formulary may or may not give the therapeutic properties of such compounds.

The National Formulary is a semi-official work that includes standard formulas and directions for pharmacists to make the preparations used widely across the country, but which are no longer included in the *United States Pharmacopoeia*. The NF is basically a treatise of oldies but goodies, medicines that were at one time official, but no longer are, and are still in popular use by the medical profession. National Formulary preparations are designated by the abbreviation NF. When a preparation is prepared exactly as directed in the National Formulary VI (for example), it can be identified as such by noting it on the label using the symbol, NF VI.

Herbal medicine-makers are advised to seek out the National Formularies which were published around 1926 and earlier, when the healing professions employed mostly botanicals for their medicines.

PHARMACEUTICS (PHARMACY)

Pharmaceutics is the science and art of preparing, compounding, using, and dispensing herbal or chemical medicines.

PHARMACODYNAMICS

Pharmacodynamics is a study of the way in which an isolated plant or chemical constituent affects the body, or a study of the power of plant and chemical constituents upon normal living organisms (otherwise known as the physiological action of drugs).

PHARMACOGNOSY

Pharmacognosy is from the Greek word *gnosis*, a knowing or recognition. It is the science of dried plants which deals primarily with information on the sources and constituents of plants. It embraces the knowledge of the history, distribution, cultivation, collection, selection, preparation, commerce, identification, evaluation, preservation, and use of plant and chemical medicines. Modern pharmacognosy texts focus on the microscopic and chemical qualities of plants. Older books talk more about quality of the visible (macroscopic) nature of herbs. If you can find one, an old copy of Youngken's *A Textbook of Pharmacognosy* is an invaluable aid for assessing herb quality.

PHARMACOKINETICS

Pharmacokinetics is the study of how the body affects an herb or drug (i.e., absorbs, distributes, metabolizes, and eliminates).

PHARMACOLOGY

Pharmacology is from the Greek words *pharmakon*, a medicine or drug, and *logos*, a study or science. It is the study of herbal or chemical drugs, their chemistry, their effects on the body, useful and dangerous actions, and dosage, and includes research into newly discovered plants and chemicals.

PHYSIOLOGICAL ACTION

Physiological action is the action of plant and chemical constituents upon what biomedical researchers call "healthy animals." It has been studied to a lesser extent in humans. Drug action in one species may be widely divergent from that in non-human or other human mammals. The maximum value that "scientism's" grim animal experimentation can have is to point out the direction and extent of activity a drug has upon certain types of tissue, and only in certain animals. This can be and frequently has been dangerously misleading. For example, thalidomide, a chemical tranquilizer drug once prescribed in Europe as a sedative to treat morning sickness, tested safe in the lab on mice, rats, dogs, cats, and monkeys. In humans, it rendered 10,000 children crippled and deformed at birth. Biomechanical differences between species are so great that it is impossible to study one species and expect to learn accurate and reliable information about another. This is amply illustrated by the fact that guinea pigs can eat strychnine alkaloid with no ill effects. Much of the information we have on the physiological action of drugs upon mankind has been acquired from accidental overdosing and cases of poisoning (as opposed to the deliberate overdosing and poisoning of other animal species), and to a lesser extent from drug proving. All significant medical breakthroughs benefiting humans have come from the clinical study of the disease process in human beings, *and primarily through improved nutrition and hygiene.*

PILLS

Pills are globular dosages designed for oral administration. They are prepared by incorporating an herb with other material in such a proportion that a cohesive mass is formed and this in turn is molded into a desired shape. For the past several hundred years pills occupied a place of major importance in pharmacy. The word "pill" was nearly synonymous with doctor and disease; and why not, with the very root of the word and the main mass of its spelling being the word "ill." But not all that long after the horse was replaced by the automobile and passion was replaced by TV, the pill started being replaced by the capsule. Most of what remains in popular use today to honor the tradition of this medical champion is The Pill, which of course continues to reign as an undisputed superstar in bedroom pharmacy. Making pills that have any aesthetic appeal whatsoever and won't quickly dry out and harden to the point where they will no longer disintegrate in the alimentary tract, requires considerable time, labor, and technical skill. Many of the advantages in administering herbal doses that the pill once possessed such as smallness of bulk with consequent ease of administration, concealment of taste, and relative permanence no longer exist, as these features are supplied today more economically and more efficiently for an herbalist by the easily acquired capsule. Therefore, I suggest that if you are determined to make a pill for delivering a dose of an unpleasant-tasting herbal powder, a very simple method is to roll the powder in a small piece of fresh bread. This works very effectively, unless, of course, you are on a grain-free diet.

PLACEBO EFFECT

The faith, hope, and beliefs an individual holds when she or he decides to re-experience his or her health, call forth the innate ability of the body to heal itself. These are probably the most dynamic aspects of any therapeutic results. The beliefs of both a client and a practitioner, their trust in each other, in the process, and in the form of medicines employed generate a significant (probably the major) portion of the therapeutic interaction. If a therapeutic process does not stimulate this profound energy, the chances of success are greatly diminished, no matter what medicines are used. The power of the client's belief in the potential for cure has been observed by all schools of health care throughout history. The use of placebos grafts research-based allopathic medicine back onto the common root stalk from which grew the methods of primitive medicine people as well as the science of the re-emerged shamans and herbal medicine folks of today. Modern placebo research forces the truly objective thinker to reassess all traditional therapies and view mainstream medicine's allopathic practice in a more accurate perspective as one of many diverse, equally effective health care modalities.

POSOLOGY

Posology is the study of dosage and its relation to different ages, sizes, weights, sex, idiosyncrasies, tolerance, time of administration, and conditions of disease in individuals (see "*Dosage*" above).

POWDERING

This is the subdividing of dried plant material. Dried herbs are powdered prior to dispensing or just prior to an extraction process in order that as much of the cell contents as possible can come in intimate contact with the digestive juices or a solvent. In pharmacy, the act of powdering is also referred to as *comminution* or *trituration*, which means literally to rub, crush, grind, pound, and pulverize into fine particles or into a powder.

The mortar and pestle is our classic device to use for this purpose. However, this can be quite laborious to use, which is why the electric coffee bean grinder (a mortar and blade) has become the second-generation mortar and pestle, the modern lay herbalist's pulverizing tool of choice. Metal hand-powered grain mills, small electric coffee bean mills, and older model (stainless steel type) Vita-Mix blenders are excellent tools for grinding all but the hardest of herbal material; however, nothing short of a rock crusher can pulverize dried Turmeric, dried Wild Yam, or dried Red Root. You have to shred dense plant materials like Turmeric and Wild Yam while they are still fresh (undried) by using a cheese grater or an electric food processor and then dry them. You need to use pruning shears or a heavy-duty lopper to process dense woody roots like Red Root and Oregon Grape root. Later you will be able to powder the thin dried shreds and woody slices for extraction.

The device used to measure the fineness of a powder is the *sieve*. If a sieve has 20 meshes (holes) to a linear inch the powder that passes through it is called a No. 20 powder, which is referred to in pharmacy as a "coarse powder"; a 40 mesh sieve renders a No. 40 "moderately coarse powder"; a 50 mesh gives a "moderately fine powder"; a 60 mesh count supplies us a "fine powder"; and an 80 mesh lays out a "very fine powder" indeed. Numbers 20, 40, and 50 are intended for herbs that are to be macerated and percolated, while 60 and 80 are used more for pills, lozenges, dispensed or capsulated powders, and suspensions.

From my kitchen drawers, I dug out four well-stained sieves I've had around my house for years. Measuring their screens, I found that one of the sieves has a 16-mesh count per inch (I guess that gives me a No. 16 "uncouth powder"); one has 30-mesh count; one has 28, and the fourth one is a bamboo sieve that refuses to conform in any way to a linear evaluation (an East meets West thing). Therefore, for our lay purposes a common household sieve or sifter will gives us a "coarse" to a "moderately coarse powder" (mcp) which is most often all we need for our work (except when making lozenges). "High tech" European sieves sold in department store kitchen supply centers will give you a finer powder.

Water softens and easily penetrates powdered herb, causing the powder to expand; however, alcohol has a hardening effect as it thoroughly dehydrates plant material, leaving behind only hardened cellulose and other plant solids. A menstruum containing 60 percent or more absolute alcohol tends to harden plant tissue, so a finer powder is more efficient for those plants requiring a strongly alcoholic menstruum (Cayenne, Myrrh, Gumweed, Milk Thistle, etc.).

Powdering should be done only just prior to your actual need for it. Once powdered, many of the plant's constituents dissipate rapidly with the passage of time; store your herbs in as whole a state as practical in order to inhibit oxidation and loss of volatile oils.

Prior to rendering resinous or gummy plants into powder, place them in the freezer for a couple of hours. The frozen, (temporarily) brittle plant material will grind up quickly and is far less likely to coat the inside surfaces of your machine with tenacious substance. If you choose not to do this, denatured rubbing alcohol is a good, inexpensive cleaning solvent (never to be used as a menstruum for internal use, however) which then can be removed from the machine with water and soap.

Powders. Herbal powders can be administered in capsules or orally as is by being placed on the tongue and chased by a drink of water or other liquid. If the dosage to be taken is large, you can first mix the powder with a liquid. Mixing powders with honey, syrup, or jam will assist in masking any unpleasant taste (see Chapter Twenty-Two, "Syrups, Honeys, Oxymels, and Electuaries"), and bitterness can be partially overcome by dissolving the powder in sweet fruit juice. Some herbalist practitioners believe that due to the fact the digestive process must extract the properties of the herb(s), this process provides a slower and more even absorption; therefore, lower doses of the powders are required to produce the results obtainable with extracts; however, many other herbalists believe powders are not as easily digested as teas, tinctures, etc., so powders require higher doses…Hmmm.

PRECIPITATION

Precipitation is the formation of solid particles in a previously clear solution. At times in pharmacy this is promoted intentionally, usually to "purify" a product. However in our humble work, precipitation and its formation of precipitates is ordinarily unintentional, unsightly, and not welcome; so we attempt to avoid it. For the purpose of appearance, it is usually easier to prevent disagreeable precipitates or other offensive appearances than it is to remedy them.

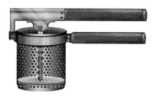

Hand Wringing

Therefore, if a resinous tincture is to be mixed with water, it is best that the water be cold and the tincture slowly added to it in a fine stream while stirring; never do the reverse by pouring the water into the resinous tincture. By following this procedure, the resinous particulates are still precipitated, but they are formed in such fine condition that they are easily diffused by shaking the mixture.

When you attempt to mix a strong (high percent alcohol that is high in alcohol-soluble components) with a weaker alcoholic extract (and maybe then water), the strongly alcoholic liquid should be gradually diluted with the weaker (and the water added last). Less precipitation occurs using this procedure.

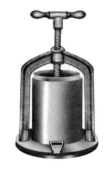

Potato Masher

PRESSING (ALSO REFERRED TO AS EXPRESSION)

Pressing is a process for separating liquids from solids which involves the use of some force. This is because pressing is employed in those cases where the amount of liquid is small compared to the quantity of solid matter that is to be removed. Pressing is employed to extract juices and oils from various fruits, nuts, and vegetables, from some fresh herbs and grasses (see "*Succus*" below), and the expression of herbal solutions from their marc.

Single-Screw Press

There are many devices appearing on the market today that have been designed for the herbalist to press his or her marc. Some of these devices work reasonably well; some don't. The renewed demand for tincture presses has in the past ten years been significant, and those engineers and machinists who are attempting to service this request have marketed their first prototypes. I deeply appreciate their efforts and have used a variety of these presses for a number of years. However it is obvious to me that significant modifications need to be incorporated in future product designs, the most salient starting place being the steel container which holds the material to be pressed; make it cylindrical rather than rectangular, please! And let me know when you have one for sale (see illustration of an old single-screw tincture press).

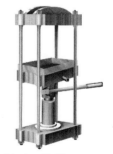

Hydraulic Press

When using a device like the hydraulic press or the screw-press, the substance to be pressed is first put into a canvas bag, or a cotton muslin cloth that has been wrapped tightly around the wet marc much like a burrito. As pressure is exerted on the herbal burrito, the pressure forces the liquid between the meshes of the cloth, and the marc is detained within. Unless, of course, the cloth bursts. This all too commonly occurring perplexity can be kept under some measure of control by applying the pressure slowly, giving the liquid time to exit gracefully through the cloth housing, and by using press cloths that are relatively fresh. If you insist on using one that is obviously battle worn, you're asking for the often ornery combination of marc and menstruum to extemporarily express itself as extended cleanup time.

The potato masher (purchasable in antiques and collectibles stores) is useful for expressing small parcels of marc; use it as you do a garlic press, and the hand-wrung process is performed as illustrated.

RULES (PROPOSED) OF MEDICINE-MAKING

As a teacher who values the creative potential of students more than the content of my teaching, I seldom express any rules of the art and science in discussion. I feel it is wise and important for a student to learn basic theory and skills from an experienced other, but then to pursue these ideas and skills in his or her own creatively evolving fashion. Therefore, I extend principles I feel give sound direction, but are certainly not gilded as sacrosanct. My eight prime principles of herbal medicine-making are discussed in Appendix C. However, there are 5 concepts that are rules in my work. I think these ideas can be accepted as such by almost everyone who works with plants and makes plant medicines. See if you agree.

Rule #1—First and foremost, harvest only plant communities that are healthy and are growing in great abundance.

Rule #2—The use of high-quality herb is essential for making good herbal medicine. Regardless of how practiced you are or how refined your technology of preparation, you can never make a preparation's quality better than the quality of the plant with which you begin.

Rule #3—Pay attention to detail.

Rule #4—Take detailed notes on all your work.

Rule #5—Have fun! If you're not enjoying yourself, something's out of harmony with you. Do something else you enjoy for the time being.

SOLUTION

A solution is the separation of the molecules of a substance (the solute, herb) and their diffusion through a liquid (the solvent, menstruum). The cohesion of the molecules of the herb are broken and uniformly diffused throughout the solvent. A substance that is not acted on by the solvent is said to be insoluble and ultimately becomes the marc. Mechanical division (powdering the dried herb) divides the solute into small particles, and these finer particles present a greater surface area to the solvent. Heat further favors solution because it drives the molecules of the solute farther apart, breaking up cohesion. *Heat is not safely used with alcohol solvents.* Frequent agitation is necessary to ensure complete extraction of soluble matter by maceration. If the mixture is not agitated at least once every 24 hours, a concentrated solution will envelop the material and prevent effective solvent action; consequently, only a small proportion of the soluble constituents will be taken up. So always remember to:

Shake Your Tinctures.

(Maybe there are six rules.)

When a liquid dissolves in another liquid it is usually said that the liquids are miscible. For example, glycerin and water are miscible, as are alcohol and water. Oil and water are obviously not miscible. A gas (vapor) dissolving in a liquid is called *absorption*.

SOLVENT EXCHANGE

Some herbs appear to be most efficiently extracted by using pure 190-proof ethyl alcohol for a menstruum. Examples of this are Milk Thistle seed (*Silybum marianum*), a popular liver regenerative and liver protective tonic; Chaparral (*Larrea tridentata*), useful for relieving arthritis and auto-immune conditions; Myrrh (*Commiphora mol-mol*), useful for treating infections and inflammation of the mouth and throat; and Calendula (*Calendula officinalis*), a mild and effective anti-inflammatory and lymphatic well used for children's health care.

If one wishes to use these extracts, but does not want to ingest any amount of alcohol (i.e., an alcohol-intolerant individual wanting to heal and nourish the liver with Milk Thistle), the following simple technique can be used to remove the alcohol and replace it with glycerin as a preservative after having first used the alcohol to extract the plant constituents.

1. Make an extract of the desired plant using 100 percent 190-proof alcohol as the menstruum (no added water).

2. Make note of the exact amount of alcohol used in the menstruum.

3. Decant and press the finished extract.

4. Measure the total amount of this extract after pressing.

5. Measure an equivalent amount of glycerin to the amount of alcohol used in the menstruum (as noted in step #2).

6. Pour the glycerin into the extract and place this entire mixture into a stainless steel or glass pot.

7. Over a low heat, gently warm the liquid extract/glycerin mixture until its volume is equivalent to the original amount of the extract in step #4. Keep the heat low, for glycerin will vaporize at 212° F. *The alcohol has boiled off and you are left with an alcohol-free glycerated extract.*

8. Cool, bottle, cap tightly, and store in amber-colored bottles.

A similar method of solvent exchange good for modifying small quantities of alcohol extract and a little more economical using less glycerin was shown to me by Karen Aguiar, herbalist and co-owner of The Herbal Apothecary, Sonoma County, California. She suggests: "Take 120 ml (4 oz.) of tincture, place in an enameled pot, add 60 ml (2 oz.) of 50 percent glycerin (which is a mixture of 50 percent absolute glycerin, 50 percent distilled water). Simmer gently on a very low heat until all the alcohol has evaporated. The finished amount should measure about 120 ml. You may need to add more of the 50 percent glycerin to bring up to 120 ml."

SUCCUS

A succus is simply a juice. The device I use for making an herbal succus is a Chop-Rite Health Fountain (Wheatgrass) juicer.

It's the only device I have found that performs this job, and it does it admirably, though laboriously. A succus is an elegant extract that will deteriorate readily. Unless it is to be used immediately, it must be either mixed with absolute alcohol to protect and preserve it: 3 parts succus to 1 part alcohol, or poured into ice cube trays and frozen. These succus cubes can then be taken one by one and dropped into a glass of water, or a cup of juice, or merely put in a cup and melted as needed. This preservative method of freezing an extract into individual dosage cubes also works well with herbal infusions, decoctions, and concentrates.

Freshly picked Cleavers is the only herb I prepare annually as a succus. Dandelion root and Plantain are two herbs, however, that I have juiced a number of times, and I highly recommend that an herbalist experience them in this form. The juice of the Dandelion root provides a vitally calming liver tonic and the Plantain juice blesses one with a magical (I mean this literally) vulnerary, anti-inflammatory, anti-venom/toxin, anti-microbial, astringent agent that is extremely useful in home and travel first-aid kits. It "fixes" spider/insect bites (most notably the Brown Recluse spider bite), poisoning, toothache, earache, inflammation of the skin, and makes a soothing dressing for fresh cuts, wounds, bruises, hemorrhoids, etc.; this résumé goes on and on. Wheatgrass is another fine tonic obtained as a succus. The juices of other medicinal grasses of the *Poaceae* family (formerly the *Gramineae* family) is an herbal materia medica that has yet to be studied in any depth. From a botanical family that includes many other power plants such as Wild Oat, Couchgrass, Rice, Wheat, cane sugar, Bamboo, etc., I think we will discover a wealth of other excellent medicines.

THERAPEUTICS

Therapeutics is the art of applying medicinal agents and other measures for the alleviation or healing of disease. This word comes from the Greek *therapeutikos*, inclined to serve or to take care of. In early Greek times the term *therapeutes* was applied to the slave who acted as a nurse or orderly.

Empirical therapeutics is that therapy for which no scientific support can be given other than that it has been repeatedly used with success. It does not take into consideration physiological or pathological mechanisms, but is based upon observations in past experiences of the effects of plant remedies and other remedial measures. This is the accumulated knowledge of our approximately 2,000,000-year heritage of human beings experimenting on human beings (provings). This profound, rich body of truly scientific knowledge is the accumulated wisdom and knowledge of healing and of healing agents repeatedly used with success and passed down to each of us by our ancestral healers. It is the bulk of this universal human heritage and wisdom that the novice community of Western medical technology feels compelled to refer to as quackery.★

In *Rational therapeutics* the method of action of a remedy can be "accounted for." It is based upon the use of medicines according to their known physiological, chemical, or biological action upon definitely known pathological conditions and body malfunctions.

Chop-rite Health Fountain (Wheatgrass Juicer)

★ The medical profession's favorite word, "quack," wantonly used to demean the perspectives and practitioners of (most) other health care modalities, is derived from the term quacksalver. Quacksalver is the archaic name for quicksilver (mercury), which is the highly toxic allopathic medicine used historically by university-trained medical doctors (M.D.s) to treat syphilis and other infections. Therefore, to be etymologically precise, today's practicing allopathic physician (the M.D.) is, by his and her professional heritage, the original and authentic quack, but the proponents of other modalities do not feel required to refer to them as such.

However, it must be noted that to this day the mechanism of many drugs in the *Physician's Desk Reference* (PDR) is "unknown."

The rational starting point of the medical discoveries of the Western medical world is basically the empiricism of folk medicine and Herbalism.

TRITURATION

Trituration is the process of reducing the size of particles by rubbing them in a mortar with a pestle. This renders a *crushing* and or a *mixing* effect as the pestle is plied under pressure in a circular motion. The most effective method of using the pestle is to begin in the center of the mortar and describe a circle of small diameter with the pestle on the substance, and gradually increase the size of the circle with each revolution until the side of the mortar is touched. Then reverse the motion, describing circles that are continually smaller in diameter until the center is again reached. This is repeated until pulverization or thorough mixing of all ingredients (powders with sugar, essential oils with sugar, etc.) is effected. Mortars with pestles having somewhat flattened ends are the best for this process.

Mortar and Pestle

UNITED STATES PHARMACOPOEIA (USP)

The U.S. Pharmacopoeia is an official manual of standards for the identification of drugs known as "official" in this country. The components and processes identified and outlined in this manual are the "top 40" of the day, so to speak, as compared to the NF's "oldies but goodies"; and like the National Formulary, those USPs published around 1926 and before will be the most valuable resource books for herbal medicine-makers. The abbreviation "USP" stamps a medicine or preparation as official, and as such any preparation bearing this official title must conform in all respects to the provisions of a U.S. pharmacopoeia (as designated by its number, i.e., USP IX).

Many countries compile and publish their own official pharmacopoeia. Originally, the U.S. Pharmacopoeia was revised every ten years by a committee of delegates from the American Pharmaceutical Association, medical and pharmaceutical colleges and associations, and the army, navy, and marine hospital services sitting in convention. Today, due to the continual swamping of the drug market with new patented drugs and drug recalls by pharmaceutical conglomerates, it is revised much more frequently. It is accepted as the standard concerning the quality, uniformity, purity, and integrity of the drugs and chemicals embraced by modern medicine. It describes them, gives tests, notes the usual adulterants and sophisticants, sets limits for impurities, gives instructions on preservation, and, most useful to herbal medicine-makers—it gives appropriate (official) menstrua and practical weight/volume ratios for each botanical tincture discussed (as does the National Formulary). Except for USP II published in 1830, neither the USP nor the NF gives therapeutic uses in any form except as may be inferred from the titles of some of their preparations.

VETERINARY DOSES

Herbalists are asked to advise in regard to giving herbs to animals in appropriate dosages. In general, sensible dosage corresponds to the weight of the animal, but there seems to be some exceptions. Cows, for instance, appear to be less responsive to medicines than horses when they are about the same weight. Cows are just more laid back than horses.

The following doses will work as a good starting place to develop experience.

Cats—1/8 to 1/4 the dose for an adult human

Dogs—Correspond to adult human dose according to weight (obviously a 12 pound Shih-tzu/Maltese cross—even though every bit as brave and tough—cannot take a dose appropriate for a 140 pound Rottweiler.

Horse—8 to 16 times the dose for an adult human

Cow—12 to 24 times the dose for an adult human

Goats and sheep—1 1/2 to 2 1/2 times the dose for an adult human

Swine—1 to 3 times the dose for an adult human

Llamas and ostriches—If you have them, your guess beats mine

VIVISECTION

Vivisection is the cutting, puncturing, or otherwise operating on, a living animal, usually without the use of anesthesia, for scientism's medical, physiological, or pathological "rational" investigation. This method of research renders confinement and usually extreme suffering for 70,000,000 of our companion animals each year. Ninety percent of these animals are referred to as "expendable mice and other rodents"; the "other rodents" being rabbits, squirrels, ferrets, guinea pigs, and hamsters. The remaining 10 percent of the animals used are apes, chimpanzees, monkeys, dogs, and cats (both strays and illegally seized pets), sheep, horses, goats, pigs, and exotic animals. This 10 percent in real numbers amounts to 7,000,000 non-rodent animals "rationally" violated yearly.

A growing portion of modern medical herbal research, which is eagerly referenced in most of today's trendy new herbals, is derived directly from biomedical vivisection. This helps sustain the market for animal testing. If this concerns you, please examine your sources as you pursue your herbal studies, considering the role you might be playing in perpetuating the demand and commercial market for this sort of rational "medical herbal research."

Vivisection is a technique that reductionist science instigated to bestow so called "rational credibility" upon itself. Currently, vivisection is employed by many other commercial industries as well to appease the insurance industry. Reviving the art, science, and language of Herbalism for enhancing human health simply does not require the pain and suffering of other species to generate credibility, nor is this required in any way for lay herbalists to continue developing insight into the use of plants for nourishment and well-being. I don't see how the carnage and abuse of non-human species will somehow render human beings more healthy and happy. It is my deeply felt opinion that the continued support of vivisection and animal testing for gathering herbal knowledge is not in the least bit what green Herbalism is about. Accessing research based on vivisection is more about individuals attempting to establish some form of "medical credibility" and recognition as "advanced herbalists." I suggest growing a garden instead, or adopting a puppy. Focus on life, nourishment, and health; deep insight and appropriate knowledge will follow.

WEIGHTS AND MEASURES

In the herb lab (as well as throughout the rest of the world), it is most useful to weigh herbs and measure liquids using the metric system. This system was developed by the French during their Revolution, supposedly to replace the many varied systems used at the time throughout the country. Most likely, however, the metric system was devised to defy the previous government's standard measurement system which was based on measurements of (royal) human anatomy. The avoirdupois system of measurement is one of those archaic systems the French snubbed ages ago, but we continue to embrace as the U.S. Conventional System. Our inch and ounce are possibly based on the length and mass of some late French king's nose or other item of his anatomy, whereas the prime unit of measure for the metric system is the meter. This unit is based on the circumference of the Earth as measured on a line through Paris and the north and south poles. The length of this line was divided by 40,000,000, and each division was called a meter (from the Greek word *metron*, "measure"). Other standards of length (centimeter, millimeter, kilometer) were further defined by dividing or multiplying the meter by various factors of 10.

The standards of weight (mass) and volume are also derived from the meter. The gram (Gm) and its divisions are used for weighing, while the milliliter (ml), also known as a fluid-gram, is used to measure liquids.

The gram is a unit of weight set by the mass of a cubic centimeter (cc) of water under standard conditions. A gram and a cubic centimeter of distilled water are essentially identical. In other words, a measure of 1 cc of distilled water weighs 1 Gm (at sea level, at 4° C.).

A milliliter is identical in volume to 1 cubic centimeter of distilled water; therefore, 1 Gm = 1 cc = 1 ml of distilled water (and for our practical purposes this holds for all other liquids we refer to in this manual).

This approximate 1:1 equality between the weight (the mass) of a solid substance and the volume of a liquid substance is very useful for determining weight to volume (w/v) proportions when calculating and formulating the strengths of liquid extracts. (See Chapter Twelve on making tinctures.)

APPROXIMATE (USER-FRIENDLY) EQUIVALENT MEASUREMENTS

Liquid measures

1 drop★ = 1 minim
15 minims = 1 ml = 1 cc
30 ml = 1 fluid ounce = 8 fluid drachms
1000 ml = 1 liter (approximately 1 quart)
500 ml = approximately 1 pint (480 ml = 1 pint)
1 teaspoonful = 5 ml = 5 cc
2 teaspoonsful = 10 ml = 10 cc
1 tablespoonful = 15 ml = 15 cc = 3 teaspoonsful

---

1 wineglassful = 60 ml (2 fluid ounces)

1 teacupful = 120 ml (4 fluid ounces)

1 glassful or cupful = 240 ml (8 fluid ounces)

1 gallon U.S. = 128 fluid ounces = 3.8 liters

1 British Imperial gallon = 154 fluid ounces = 4.6 liters

1 liter = 1.8 pints

Weights

30 Gm = 1 ounce (avoirdupois)

454 Gm = 1 pound (avoirdupois)

(*This is based on the new 1959 international agreement of English speaking nations.*)

1 kilogram = 2.2 pounds

Length

1 inch = 2.54 centimeters

1 meter = 39.37 inches

★ A "*drop.*" A rose by any other name is still a rose, but is a drop always a drop? This is questionable. A drop of water is supposed to be equivalent to a minim and in pharmacy-speak is often referred to as a "minim." But this is only true when applied to water, and then, only when the water is expelled from an "international standard dropper." The shape and quality of the surface from which a drop descends influences its size. However, even when using a standard dropper these presumptions are seldom true when applied to liquids other than pure water. Thick, viscous liquids such as syrups produce a drop five times larger than a drop of a heavy, mobile liquid like chloroform and three times that of alcohol. If we use a fluid drachm as a liquid measure, we will find that it holds 250 drops of chloroform; or 146 drops of alcohol, or 130 to 150 drops of an aqueous-alcohol tincture or fluid extract. It will hold 105 to 140 drops of oil, but only 45 to 110 drops of syrup. So, since there are 8 fluid drachm in a fluid ounce, for all practical posological purposes we can assume that 1 U.S. fluid ounce of most commonly used tinctures holds approximately 960 to 1200 drops. But none of this is any big deal, unless of course one is administering highly intense or toxic extracts or when administering medicines to infants. In these situations, measuring doses by the milliliter (ml) or the cubic centimeter (cc) instead of by drops would be more reliable.

A "*part*" of an herbal formula. When putting together a formula, herbalists design the formula and communicate its composition by referring to the number of "parts." Example: for treating and toning an irritated prostate gland, mix 2 parts Saw Palmetto, 1 part Echinacea, 1 part Damiana, 1 part Yarrow, 1/8 part Ginger. The question often arises, what is a part…? Is it a gram, an ounce, a cupful, a shovelful, a truckload, or a drop? Of course, the answer is it can be any of these measures. You retain the proper proportions as long as each measure used to make up a part is the same measure as each of the other measured parts in the mixture. It all comes down to how much mixture you ultimately want to make. If you chose shovelsful as a measure for each part in the sample formula, you'll end up with enough mixture for all the prostates in the NFL. So a more reasonable measure to use is the oz. (avoirdupois = 16 oz. to the pound) when compounding bulk herbs or the fluid oz. for blending liquid extracts. Referring back to the sample formula, you would blend 2 oz. Saw Palmetto, 1 oz. Echinacea, 1 oz. Damiana, 1 oz. Yarrow, and 1/8 oz. Ginger, ending up with 5 1/8 oz. of the formula. If you want only half that amount, make each part 1/2 oz. It doesn't matter what measure you use. A household coffee scoop (filled and leveled) works fine as a part measure as long as you use the same scoop throughout. (Taken from *The Male Herbal*)

Thermometer correspondence

In Fahrenheit's (F.) thermometer, the freezing point of water is placed at 32°, and the boiling point at 212°. The number of intervening degrees is 180. In the Centigrade (C.) or Celsius's thermometer the freezing point of water is marked zero and the boiling point 100°. From this information, it can be seen that 212° Fahrenheit is equivalent to 100° Centigrade.

To convert degrees Fahrenheit to degrees Centigrade—C = (°F − 32) multiplied by 5 and divided by 9.

To convert degrees Centigrade to degrees Fahrenheit—F = (°C multiplied by 9 and divided by 5) + 32.

Or find a good conversion table somewhere. *The New York Public Library Science Desk Reference*, edited by Patricia Barnes-Svarney, is the best science reference book I've found, published by The Stonesong Press Inc., MacMillan, 1995.

Solid weight—Liquid weight

1 gram is equal in mass to 1 cc of water at sea level at 4° C (39° F); a cubic centimeter (cc) is the approximate equivalent of a milliliter (ml). Therefore, for our purposes: 1 cc = 1 ml = 1 Gm.

WILDCRAFTED HERB AND ORGANICALLY CULTIVATED HERB

The term *wildcrafted* signifies that the plant has grown wild in nature without human intervention and ideally has been consciously harvested from unpolluted areas with full regard for the plant communities and care for ecological balance. These plants should never be fumigated or irradiated.

Please note, that as the medicinal herbs are becoming more and more popular, some wildcrafting practices are placing a great burden on a growing number of wild plant populations; therefore it is important to begin organically cultivating many of our herbal medicines rather than over-harvesting and wiping out wild medicinal plant communities. A good example of the destruction caused by mindless wildcrafting is the notable loss of fields of wild *Echinacea angustifolia* and *Echinacea purpurea* due to commercial over-harvesting. Organically cultivated *Echinacea purpurea* is every bit as effective. Wild Goldenseal is also currently under stress due to over-harvesting, as are Osha, Lady's Slipper, American Ginseng, Blue Cohosh and Black Cohosh, and a growing number of other native medicinals.

But let us not make a reactionary mistake of construing wildcrafting as something negative. It is not in the least; it is an herbal art and a craft that commands respect when

Wildcrafting is an ancient, honorable art and craft of harvesting Earth's gifts. It is a communion with the wild green as organic gardening is a communion with the domestic green. What we must take care of is to attract to herbalism more teachers of sustainable wild harvesting to guide and inspire young herbalists.

performed by a skilled artist and craftsman. Pursued with intelligence and understanding, wildcrafting is a process of harvest pruning, which when practiced knowledgeably never exploits or diminishes wild plant communities, but instead supports and enhances them. What is needed is not condemnation of this ancient, honorable craft, but more well-trained teachers and fervent, plant-loving students.

The term *organically cultivated* means that the plant has been cultivated by natural means on unpolluted land without the use of chemical fertilizers, sewer sludge, pesticides, or herbicides. Hopefully these plants are never fumigated, irradiated, or genetically altered (these lists of corporate foolishness keep getting longer and longer).

CHAPTER
26

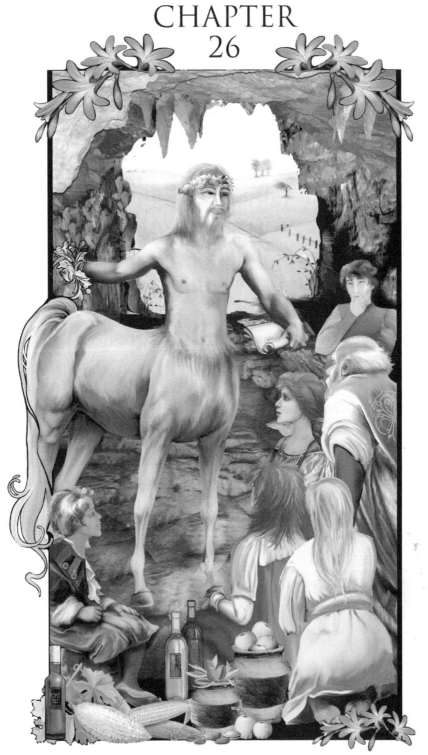

A PERSPECTIVE
ON MEDICINE

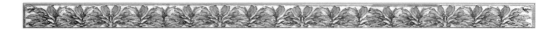

T'was a balmy summer afternoon. Chiron sat waiting in the cool shade of his summer cave on the northern slope of Mount Pelion.

The Centaur observed with deep affection the students who were entering the cave and sitting in a circle with him, his grand heart touched by their individual beauty and eager vitality.

Chiron was a renowned health seer, archer, musician, and visionary. It is said that he was the wisest and kindest of all Centaurs. He was learned and skilled in the use of herbs, potions, gentle words, and healing song. Over the years of his life, innumerable youths had been entrusted to his charge, amongst them some of the finest healers and warriors of Western story.

Chiron had summoned the students and their friends to speak with them about the function of medicine and about the art of health. Upon the students' request, he had agreed to share with them his knowledge of medicine: its value and role in the human journey.

The wise Centaur knew well that words don't teach, that it is only life experiences that teach, but he knew that words stimulate ideas in the minds of others, and therein he was aware of the great influence words possess. As always, he agreed to speak with those who asked him to. Chiron was happy to share any knowledge he had gained from his centuries of life experience on Earth, especially his knowledge of the uses of herbs and other medicinal substances for human beings in their quest for health, joy, and prosperity.

In a short while, all who were to participate in the discussion had arrived. The final person to join the circle was a woman called Artemis, who, upon entering the cave, walked over and hugged one of the students, her young nephew, Asclepius, and sat down beside him. She then looked with loving eyes at Chiron, her long-time friend, and nodded her head in warm greeting; the Centaur returned the salutation, with a gesture of delight and mutual appreciation.

Chiron then closed his eyes for a moment of thought. A tranquil silence filled the air. Thereupon he opened his eyes and looking to each of the individuals in the circle, he spoke,

"Thank you for the honor of this gathering, I am most pleased that you are here with me, and I trust that we will inspire and lift each other to realms of thought and vision that no gathering before has experienced in quite the same way. This meeting of spirits in this physical time and place is unique in all of creation, and I am delighted to be here with you.

"As health seers and self-healers we focus our attention on the nature of joy, health, and well-being; and frequently in our discussions with one another the question arises, 'What is the nature of medicine?' What is its action in the process of individuals experiencing their intrinsic health or re-establishing wellness from an experience of illness? If I may share my experience and insights, I'll offer you a perspective to consider, and as we have brought ourselves to this communion for mutual upliftment and stimulation of thought, please be free to contribute what you will during the time we are here together."

Transcribed from the herbal Akashic Records.

Chiron fell silent once again. Sensing permission and a concerted desire from the gathering for him to continue, he drew a deep breath, "Each of us is an absolutely free spirit, currently choosing to walk the physical spheres of creation, eagerly participating in this realm with a physical body, mind, and feelings. We are creators; this is our essence. Desire is the will of our spirit to create. With our mind we freely create thoughts, the vibrations of which are propelled into the universe, bolstered by the passion of our desire and attendant feelings. From this point of offering, we attract to us the experiences born of the content of our vision.

"Each individual is complete and independent in his and her ability to create. If, however, due to circumstances in one's life, an individual holds inner resistance to the manifestation of a desire and feels the need for assistance to allow the experience of that which he or she strongly desires, 'medicine' is a catalyst that can be empowered to help. With the power invested by the individual's belief in it, medicine in turn, bolsters the individual's belief that he or she can have what is wanted, reducing inner resistance, allowing and accelerating the materialization of this desire.

"It is important to note that the use of medicine is appropriate not only to help alleviate or prevent disease, but also when one feels it necessary to use an ally to assist in creating whatever is desired. Therefore, plants, prayer, foods, chants, minerals, the company or touch of another being, potions, ritual, music, incantations, charms, amulets, icons, fetishes, and all other manifestations a person strongly believes in can be utilized as good and powerful medicine." Chiron paused for a moment, then added, "I define the term 'good' as 'that which one wants.'

"Yet ever bear in mind that 'medicine' is simply a tool, a means to facilitate the clearing of a pathway in a person's life journey to whatever experience he or she wants. Medicine is not the creator of one's life experience; it is not the walker on the path, nor is it the healer. The human being is the walker; the human being is the creator, the self-healer."

Chiron paused, allowing for comments that might come forth; he looked to the individuals in the circle, and as no one spoke, he continued,

"I have found it most important to understand that during those times in one's life when illness is experienced, medicine does not 'fix' a person, simply because he or she is not broken. Human beings do not weaken, nor are they fragmented by their life experiences. One is never less than a perfectly whole being, regardless of the extent of his or her experience of dis-ease. As a human being travels in his life's infinitely varied experiences, his true nature flows forever undivided. Freedom, joy, radiant health, youthful vitality, passionate enthusiasm, abundant prosperity, creativity, and growth are—ever accessible—core components of each individual's whole self. These components, even when resisted, are never forfeited by one's temporary experience of the lack of any of them. They are perpetual qualities of one's ever-perfect spirit, one's true self." Chiron smiled joyfully to his friends, "Babies, young children, and playful adults demonstrate this reality each moment of their day…for they do not resist it. They are profound teachers."

A young woman motioned to Chiron that she had a question. Chiron was pleased and nodded to her. "Chiron, if feeling good, perfect health, and vitality are indeed our true and natural state of being, what then is the experience of disease and physical deterioration? If freedom is a basic component of human nature, why would one choose to feel bad; why do human beings ever diminish themselves by choosing illness and physical degeneration?"

Chiron listened closely to his student's words. "These are excellent questions, young Ceres, questions that reach to the very heart of each person's journey within this grand physical domain. Thank you, I will clarify my perspective on this. As I said a moment ago, humans are creators. This is the dynamic essence of our beings; and within this vast physical realm, everything is possible. There are no limits to what an incarnated spirit can manifest within any of his or her physical life experiences.

"On this planet, Earth, we live in an abundant arena of contrasts and differences from which we can compare one thing to another, one experience to another, and, from this infinite array of choices, decide precisely what we want.

"As you can see, this dense physical realm is a magnificent, inspiring environment for us creators to direct the creative energy that is summoned by our desires, and therein relish the exuberant feelings of this life force flowing through our being.

"As each of us create and manifest our ongoing series of ideas, beliefs, attitudes, and experiences—thereby ever creating one's self—we expand our knowing and grow in wisdom. We unfold the singular attributes of our spirit and offer a wholly unique perspective of consciousness to All that Is. Within this grand universal dance, each of is contributing entirely new dimensions to the lead edge of thought of which we are integral participants in this ever-evolving, ever-expanding universe. And it is because we are entirely free spirits pioneering on this cutting edge that we can make choices that might at times manifest experiences of bondage, frustration, and boredom, or symptoms of disease and physical deterioration. However, in the ever-changing nature of the physical universe, each and every experience is always temporary and changing, while our nonphysical spirit, our inner being, the creator, is eternal and forever ongoing.

"In light of this, one must keep in mind that venturing into choices that manifest an experience of dis-ease is not a process of breaking or diminishing or devaluation. It is quite the contrary. Illness, like any and all other experiences, is just one of our current life's transient manifestations. It is merely a signpost, an illustration, an intimate teacher, a passing experience indicating to us precisely how, from our current beliefs and mental attitude, our choices are flowing our creative energy relative to the broader intention of our inner being's true nature. We are in process of gaining knowledge and wisdom about ourselves, about who we are, and thereby, which choices harmonize with the individual nature of our unique spirit. We are steering ourselves on our particular paths of joy.

"Experiencing disease is merely another venture of our innumerable, ongoing human processes for pressing forward, feeling, probing, and extending our individual creative boundaries. Therefore, plunging oneself into life—which I strongly recommend all beings do with full passion—rummaging through this world's vast field of contrast, leaving no experience unconsidered—even though, sometimes, maybe even frequently, we get ourselves into trouble—is how each of us expands and evolves our valuable and indispensable being. Dear companions, our spirits have not projected themselves into this physical realm to be guarded and safe; we have come for adventure, to feel the delicious surge of passion, to flow life force as we create ever more glorious visions and experiences. Each of us is an ardent explorer, a seer, a warrior, and a monarch on a grand creative quest.

"Health and disease are the consolidation of one's current mental attitude. Illness—not feeling good—is a powerful indicator that we are holding inner resistance to following our inherent path of joy. We are diverting our vision from focusing on our bliss, there in disallowing the vital free flow of our Source energy throughout our being. We are holding to thoughts, beliefs, and actions that are contrary to our individual true nature—and they do not feel good to us, but we fail to acknowledge the truth of there inner signals and so, for the time being, manifest like experiences of discontent and dis-ease. Experiencing the contrasting information that illness can afford us concerning who we are and what we want is one way that we can grow. It is a segment of our ongoing adventure, a succeeding step in the unending sequence of movements in our life's dance; it is merely a motion forward in an unending series of forward motions that make up an individual's unique evolution.

"The experience of health teaches us in the same way. Each and every one of our life experiences is of paramount significance to the creative unfolding of our spirit's abiding journey and, therein, an integral part of the concerted evolution of all life, of All that Is. Blessed be diversity my dear friends. Each individual's path is unique, and where one stands at any moment is a mark of perfection in that being's creation. We are Spiritwalkers; each of us, in every moment, is a creator with a unique perspective to offer, powerful, adventurous, and forever whole. We do not break, and we are never diminished or devalued by *any* of our experiences.

"Once we determine that a manifestation we've attracted does not or no longer feels good, we can use this life experience as a platform on which to stand, providing us with a fresh perspective to determine and envision what we now want instead, and thereby focus the magnetic vibrations of our creative thought on that fresh vision and intent. Through this process, we progress our experiences, we grow, we expand, and we move forth in the rapture of our spirit's eternal journey.

"In like manner, once an individual who is experiencing illness makes a clear impassioned decision that she wants to feel good again, she has set the revival of her experience of health in motion. If she does not resist this experience, but rather focuses on those things and ideas that feel good to her spirit, envisioning her health, feeling her health, easing inner resistance, allowing the flow of ideas that ignite feelings of joy in her life, and letting these feelings become the seeds of fresh experiences, the return of her innate health is hers; it is inevitable. If she feels she needs an ally to help her find the state of mind that allows this transformation, whatever or whoever she believes will do this is good medicine for her.

"This is the nature of medicine; it is an ally. It matters not which medicine-path one chooses. All medicines are powerful when empowered by an individual's belief in them, coupled with one's focused desire to be well, or to have whatever else it is that is wanted. With the empowerment of one's creative thought and passionate will, medicine becomes a potent companion. It becomes wholly empowered to uplift, soothe, nourish, and assist.

"From this point of view, I observe one's true nature, that perpetual non-physical inner essence, remaining consummate and unaltered by any physical experiences that have been amassed. Our intrinsic health and wholeness are integral parts of our human nature, always and forever accessible; and each individual remains whole even in the midst of experiencing disharmony and illness, no matter how grave his or her immediate condition has been labeled. Recurrent stories of dramatic personal transformations and 'miraculous healing' demonstrate this most vividly. Health remains innate to our being, and it is always within reach when we desire it resolutely, focus our attention on it passionately, release inner resistance to our innate joy, and follow all intuitively inspired actions. The contrasting experience of the lack of ease in one's life merely leads us to an intense desire to experience ease, to put our life in harmony with the knowing of our inner being. And if one feels the need of a medicine to help realize this desire, then it is wise to embrace it, whatever nature of medicine it might be."

Chiron concluded and smiled at his companions. At that moment Artemis indicated that she would like to speak. Chiron knew Artemis to be a bright and wise teacher, and he welcomed the contribution of his knowledgeable peer. "Yes Artemis, please speak."

"Thank you, Chiron" Artemis said, and looking into the eyes of the young woman who had asked the question of Chiron, she spoke,

"I know you, young Ceres. You and your companion, Bacchus, seated beside you, have strong, distinct paths that you both follow with clarity and joyous passion. You offer little resistance to the flow of life force through you. You seldom react to what others do or say, but instead you set your own tone in life, which allows nothing to lead you astray from your chosen path. Your spirit grows passionately in its own individual way.

"And I observe you honoring with equal spontaneity the individual paths of others, allowing them, without judgment, disapproval, or rancor, their way of being, appreciating their singularity, enjoying their idiosyncrasies. You flow gracefully with the humor and beauty of life. From your strength of inner knowing and accordant action, you radiate your undiminished health, youth, and vitality. Your presence is uplifting to all whose lives you touch."

Ceres and Bacchus smiled at Artemis gracefully receiving her acclaim.

"You embody a path of passionate health," Artemis continued, "which we can look to as a model of harmonious nonresistance to one's own innate qualities of well-being."

Then looking to the others sitting in the circle, Artemis said, " So often I have discussed with Chiron and other health seers what we feel are the very foundations of health, the understanding of which can render any illness of mind and body both preventable and curable. I have found two simple principles that inevitably emerge. The first is to follow the guidance of your inner spirit always. This guidance which attends to each and every thought, comes forth to you through your feelings. Focus your attention on those thoughts that feel good to you, for these are the ideas and visions that are in harmony with the truth of your inner nature.

"Hold to the thoughts and actions that follow the instincts which come forth from within. It is only through one's intuitive inspiration that a person takes right action and gains true self-knowledge. It is not the idealism, morals, whims, and dictates of the outer world, or the observation of and reaction to other persons' experiences that give joyful, healthful guidance. I have seen consistently that when one's spirit and one's mindful personality are in harmony with each other, life force flows with ease, and life experiences consist primarily of joy, prosperity, and health.

"Invariably, our inner being holds clear awareness of the original intent of our incarnation, that unique cardinal path we originally chose for this life. In accordance with this we have a profound inner guidance system ever at work; in every thought, one's mind and personality are guided from within through a continual communication with one's spirit, using the intimate inner language of feelings. Those thoughts and experiences that vibrate in harmony with the vast knowing of one's inner being feel good, and those that vibrate in discord feel bad; it is that simple. This is why love, appreciation, enthusiasm, and so forth feel good to us, and why anger, frustration, guilt, jealousy, and blame feel bad.

"Chronic pain and disease are merely extensions of bad or painful feelings that one has endured or attempted to ignore and disregard over a period of time. Disease is initiated by any prolonged resistance or conflict between the specific choices of one's mind and the comprehensive knowing of one's inner spirit.

"The second principle is to hold sacrosanct in one's heart and mind the freedom and importance of all others to follow their chosen paths. Venerate, as you do your own, the wisdom and true guidance of another's inner being; honor their path, be they connected and in harmony with their inner self or not. They are learning and growing too. Judge them not; do them no harm; they are co-creating with you. They do not have to agree with you. Allow them their way and truly appreciate their individuality. The vibrations of appreciation are profound, akin to those of unconditional love.

"Each of us appears to be separate from one another, but nonetheless each is an integral part of the whole of life, and each being has her or his own path to follow. The questions of right or wrong, of good or evil are relative; what is right for one is possibly wrong for another. And, likewise all standards of morality and idealism are purely relative. Spirit has no rules. The unique individuality of every path is hallowed and is wholly essential to the evolution of All. Appreciating and allowing all others to be as they are, attracts full freedom to be oneself, and it is this vast field of diversity we access on this physical plane that allows each of us to find everything we need to support the realization of our desires.

"We have come into this realm eager to engage in physical life, to celebrate our individuality, to feel the joy of life force flowing through our being as we exercise our innate ability and freedom to deliberately create whatever experiences we desire. Through each of our life journeys spirit accesses the wonderful contrasts that compose the physical realm, indulging in the infinite choices this realm bestows that feed our creative nature; therein we grow in wisdom and knowledge and expand our being within the grand evolution of All that Is.

"Life only asks of us that we travel our individual journey with joy in our heart while allowing all others to do the same, appreciating their individuality, therein blessing all those around us. This is the art of health."

As Artemis finished speaking, Asclepius, sitting beside her, looked at her, respect and affection lighting his face. She was a renowned patron of the healing arts and a bright influence in his life, having taught him the artful way of animal and plant medicine. In the succeeding moment, however, an expression of puzzlement cast a fleeting shadow over his face. He gestured to his two teachers that he wished to speak.

"Dear Artemis and Chiron, I understand your ideas about the nature of health and illness and I appreciate the depth and practical significance of your perception. But, what about the symptoms of disease, shouldn't we clearly identify these and work to understand their cause? Wouldn't an in-depth diagnosis help someone attend to the discomfort of the symptoms and relieve a person's irritation?"

Chiron reflected on the young physician's question for a moment and then responded; "When one fully recognizes the power of the mind to create, Asclepius, he will use it only to focus attention on what he wants. If what is, is not that what you want, then do not energize the experience further by dwelling on it.

"Physical manifestation is a by-product of your vibrational offering. I am referring to the vibrations of the mental signals you project. Those signals you set forth are the vibration of what you are giving your attention to, by either your perceiving, your daydreaming, your imagining, your remembering, and so forth, in whatever way you are focusing in the moment. In other words, the signals you send out to the universe, those which in turn attract things to you, are all about what you are giving your attention to. The physical reflections of these signals are those manifestations you experience.

"It is best to walk lightly with understanding and enjoy these personal manifestations. Appreciate the enormous amount of information they supply, for they do you a great service by accurately illustrating to you where you are currently holding your predominant focus. You are continually molding your experience, this is ongoing, and the manifestations that occur are there specifically to give you the information that helps you to identify more clearly what you want.

"I repeat, Asclepius, we are creators. This is what we have come to this physical realm to do; it is our life. We are intimate extensions of the very same Source energy that has created and sustains this universe. We have come forth in these bodies intending to evaluate the lush contrast of this physical time space reality, letting that contrast evoke within us clarity of decision, because it is through the decisions that we forge, that we direct and flow the very same creative energy that creates all things. And it is the flowing of this energy that is life.

"The process of creating one's life experiences is all about attraction. It is about what comes to you as a result of your vibrational offering. When the manifestations you are experiencing feel joyful and fulfilling, you are creating in harmony with your inner nature; and these manifestations offer you new perspectives from which to envision and create even greater and more delightful experiences. Your creating never ends; manifestations come and go, informing you of what you are currently attracting; experiences flow one to another; the journey is forever ongoing.

"If the manifestations you are presently experiencing are not exactly what you want, let this insight stimulate you to examine more closely what you have been thinking, discussing, believing, remembering, assuming, or expecting that is attracting these phenomena into your experience.

"The laws that support the functioning of the universe reflect its vast transcendent intelligence. The simple universal law of attraction is a cardinal law. There is no law of projection. There is nothing that can project itself into your experience unless you allow this by concurrently attracting it to yourself. *You* are the sole creator of your life; you experience only that which matches your creative output, that which you somehow include in your vibrational offering. So, it is wise to focus your mental energy consciously on what you want, rather than including in your mental signal that which you do not want. Note those thoughts and experiences that feel good to you, those that are, therefore, in harmony with your inner being—your true nature—and focus your predominant attention on them. Attract them and others of like vibrational quality into your life experience, thereby intentionally creating the experiences you want.

"Therefore, prolonged diagnosis of disease—*dwelling* on the etiology of what you do not want—and attempting to discern the cause of these symptoms merely includes them strongly in your signal, and this is the vibration you will continue to energize. Hence this and other vibrations like it are what you will continue to attract unto you. Instead, I strongly suggest you use the opportunity to focus on your health; focus predominantly on what feels good to you. See your health; envision what you want. Feel these feelings; dwell on them instead and project these signals to the universe. Focus your passion on what you want to manifest in your life. Ask yourself why you want it. This further clarifies your desire as it magnifies the passion of your wanting and attracts more and more supportive, harmonious thoughts that further enrich and intensify your vision. Devote time to this task; this is your work as a creator. Create in your mind a vivid picture of what it is you want; and feel this desire. Feel it strongly. Feeling is the first step in the manifestation of your wishes, a powerful component of consciously creating your experiences.

"And by all means, avoid inner resistance to your wishes. Weed out any contrary, habitual thoughts and beliefs you hold. Do not contradict the manifestation of what feels good to you by dwelling for any extended period on imagined obstacles to its manifestation. Weed out any negativity that vibrates resistance. Seek the company of those who uplift you and see your health and beauty. Fully allow your desires to come to you in their perfect time; they will come to pass; enjoy the process of the returning experience of wellness; follow your inspired actions, for they will be in harmony with your creation; relish the journey."

As Chiron finished speaking, a man whom he had not previously met, spoke,

"Members of this circle, it is delightful to be here with you." he said,

"My name is Sachs, I am here with my young son, Tages, one of your students, Chiron."

"I have been an herbalist throughout my life. I help others learn to communicate with plants and to make herbal medicines." Looking to Chiron he continued, "In light of this creative process that you explain so clearly, Chiron, how is medicine best used by an individual? What is the wisest counsel to give one who is seeking a medicine for healing?"

Chiron smiled warmly, pleased to meet this new acquaintance. He welcomed the elder Sachs and greeted the young man sitting next to him. He then said, "When you use a 'medicine' to assist you in a creation, your perspective while using it is of paramount importance; for it is the perspective with which you take a medicine that formulates your vibrational offering. Decide clearly what you want to attract. Let the medicine assist you in allowing yourself to have that which you desire. One's belief in a medicine increases the expectation for receiving what is wanted. Enthusiastic expectation is a perfect state of mind for allowing the manifestation of one's desire, because, therein, any resistance to this manifestation is significantly diminished.

"Hold your primary intent for using a medicine clearly in mind. Employ the help of your medicine to accent your intention to experience health and well-being. Use it with the conscious intent to feel good, to manifest vitality, to attract prosperity or whatever else you seek. This clear intent, bolstered by your belief that the medicine will assist you strongly directs your signal to attract the experience of whatever it is that you want. This fertilizes the seeds of self-healing and intentional creating.

"Do not mis-create by using medicine with the idea of 'getting rid of' what you don't want, or to 'fix' something that is 'broken,' or to attack disease and so forth; for these vibrational offerings, in the attempt to exclude, will merely attract those very things you do not want by focusing attention on them. By focusing attention on symptoms or on past 'causes,' one is not moving away from the unwanted experience, but instead is lingering in the thoughts, statistics, visual images, and the feelings of their 'dis-ease,' prolonging the experience of that which is not wanted. Avoid reacting to what is. Rather, create the tone of that which you want.

"Symptoms of dis-ease are the manifestations brought about by an individual's past thoughts, beliefs, and mental attitude. It is important to realize that one has no power to change what has passed. One's full power, the power to change what is, lies solely in the present, wherein one can envision, feel, and consciously create the nature of future experiences.

"Once disease symptoms—reflections of inner disharmony—have ignited the realization that they are not what one wants, these manifestations have done their job. It is important to appreciate the powerful teaching they afford, but there is no longer any value in focusing further attention on them. Acknowledge that they stem from past attitude, and that it is this attitude, and its attendant thoughts, that must be revised in order to change one's experiences. Identify those thoughts and beliefs that illicit a sense of uneasiness within you, thoughts that do not feel good to you, but for whatever reasons you have continued to hold on to and prolong. These are the thoughts that resist the flow of your true nature. What is appropriate now is to decide what is wanted and to focus creative thought totally and passionately on the visions ignited by that decision.

"Regardless of present circumstances and despite the etiology of an illness's manifestation, one's full power as a creator of future experiences, as a self-healer, lies entirely here in the present. Use medicine as a mantra that magnifies the vibrations of your intent; let your medicines echo the vibrations of your impassioned desire to regain the experience of your innate health, vitality, and well-being."

Asclepius, who, at his young age, had already shown himself to be a remarkable physician, was clearly fascinated by the significance of Chiron's counsel on the use of medicine. He immediately asked him to elaborate on how, then, the knowledge and compassion of the herbalist and the physician can help heal another being.

"Physicians and herbalists, like medicine, can be distinct allies for a person who regards and trusts them. They are influential companions for anyone who believes they can help them and have requested this help. An attending herbalist or physician can skillfully soothe and mend another person's physical malaise and make them more comfortable, but herbalists and physicians do not 'heal' others, no one heals another." Chiron emphasized, "One can only heal oneself.

"When I use the term heal, I mean reconnecting to one's Source energy by one's removal of inner resistance to the flow of life force, so that inner ease returns, harmony between one's mind and spirit is reestablished, and the experience of one's intrinsic well-being is revived.

"A wise practitioner views illness not as an affliction, but instead as an explicit teacher in one's life. The experienced practitioner also knows that, if disease symptoms are merely palliated, and the teachings these symptoms offer are ignored, the individual will soon re-experience the effects of illness in the same or in yet another form. An external remedy offers no cure if a person has not established mental ease. If one's spirit is not heard, the rhythm of mind is broken, and the mark of a person's illness remains there.

"To assist another's healing, herbalists and physicians should consider using their thoughts more to visualize, less to analyze, seeing their client's innate health and well-being, not using the time so much to scrutinize a person's symptoms of dis-ease. Guide the person to reveal how he can restore his experience of health. *Ask him what he wants in his life* and once he identifies this, ask him *why* he wants it. Further indulgence in this liberated flow of desire will increase the passion of his vision and animate his determination. Enter into the joy and passion of the realizations that come forth, and accompany him in his vision wherever he wants to take it. Accompany him in the creative power of his daydreams, for these are the exhilarating passageways his spirit has opened to his heart and mind. Assure him of his ability to manifest his dreams and his worthiness to have, and to be, and to do whatever he wants. Encourage him to explore his bliss, uplift him and assure him of his well-being. Inspire him to find the desires of his true self and feel the deeply nourishing feelings of connecting in a positive way with them. This is a trusted ally's power and purpose, a gift of medicine, a practitioner's joy.

"A compassionate herbalist's or physician's finest service is to focus on their client's innate health, radiate an uplifting attitude, and assist the client to make heartfelt sense of their experience of illness. This juncture initiates a highly creative momentum. Referencing the client's experience of illness as a provocative manifestation of what the individual no longer wants to create, relating to dis-ease merely as a powerfully motivating experience from which to decide and envision what feels good and what is now clearly preferred, the practitioner assures the client, without a shadow of doubt, that this illness by nature is a temporary condition. The herbalist embraces the client's impassioned preferences as the birth of a resplendent idea upon which the client can build an ever more enlightened vision, generating greater and greater enthusiasm and vitality for attracting what is now clearly desired, releasing resistance to what is wanted."

At this point Chiron wished to elaborate on the topic of compassion, for he knew the confusion many individuals experience around this emotion and concurrent feelings of empathy. He was very aware how the focus of one's feeling of empathy can impinge on one's power to assist another's healing. Chiron took a few moments to choose his words precisely, then he said, "The truest essence of compassion is a very high, pure vibration—it stems from a deep understanding of well-being.

"The greatest compassion a health seer and counselor—a health ally—can offer another is, 'I know without a shadow of doubt that well-being is your true experience—that very high passionate vibration of well-being, having no resistance within it.'

"However, when most individuals use the word 'compassion,' they are looking at some suffering individual who is in a desperate situation and feeling empathy for where they are—and that is of no benefit at all.

"When a health counselor holds someone as their object of attention from a place of knowing their innate wellness—they may be temporarily not well—but as a health seer knows their true well-being, *they set the tone* of the consultation. The counselor floods the energy field with a pure, positive, resistance-free vibration; and the client's vibration readily acclimates to this higher vibration. They are attracted to it like a shivering man is attracted to a warm stove; and well-being becomes their experience. This is true compassion!

"But so many individuals get lost in the struggle. Many counselors search for something or someone who seeks their help, but then upon finding this, they get focused on the needy part. They acclimate to the needy part and feel the despair of it—and call this compassion. This only lowers an individual's vibration separating the counselor from his or her power to uplift and inspire.

"If a counselor is empathizing with the client's *struggle*—now, instead of maintaining the higher, faster vibration and bringing the other person to it, their experience is empathy with the client's lower, slower vibration and their feelings of discomfort.

"At this point it depends on how the counselor is feeling. True compassion feels very good, and when feeling this, whomever a health counselor holds as their object of attention will feel good also. This is true upliftment!

"*Set the tone of the consultation to a vibration of upliftment.*" Chiron stated with impassioned emphasis, "This is the health counselor's power of true compassion.

"What good can we do another unless we see them in their perfect health and hold this in our thought as we counsel? If we see them any less than this, what good are we doing them? We must inspire them to be their wholeness which includes perfect health. If we see them in their disease where can either of us go, except to merely palliate their symptoms?

"By holding this state of inspired vision and upliftment, you radiate it. As you think, you feel; as you feel, you radiate, and all is affected by your offering. This is the power of your influence as a health seer, herbalist, physician, and health ally.

"When a client experiencing temporary disconnection from their inner source of joy comes to you for assistance, your intent, as you are interacting with this person, is to bring them closer to remembering and appreciating who they are. This means appreciation and reassurance coming from you is in order. Focus your attention on them wholly. Listen to the words they offer, acknowledge their experience of illness, suffering, and discomfort, but behind it all hear the singing of their spirit. Therein abides their wellness. See their beauty and perfection, and offer soothing words like, "I assure you, it will be all right,' and 'It too will pass, things will get better.' When you offer your words of reassurance *from your place of knowing* that all is well, they will begin to *feel* it. This fresh feeling within them will be the first step in the manifestation of their re-experience of health. Encourage them to flow their energy to concordant feelings, to the ideas that inspire them and feel good to them, to the feelings that stem from deciding more clearly what they truly want.

"Use gentle humor. It is the unbounded expression of appreciation. Laughter is life force reflected through a physical being who is willing to be light enough to let it flow. Keep the session buoyant; relax, spend more time looking for things to appreciate, to laugh about, and to play with. Let cheerfulness deflect all oppressive doubt and depression. It is most efficient to view all that is right with the individual, focusing upon those areas in their life that feel good to them—and there are so very many when one looks from a perspective of appreciation and laughter—As these positive aspects are identified and felt, others, one after another after another, those aspects that are in harmony with their spirit make themselves known, and the appreciation for that which feels good in their own life grows. The temporary disconnection from inner joy dissolves." Chiron fell quiet for a moment, looked deep into Asclepius's eyes and continued, "and once a person finds himself, it no longer matters where he was when he was lost.

"See another's suffering only long enough to feel your desire erupting within you to help them, *but do not let their suffering take you to it.* See your client's health, don't use the time to dissect his or her dis-ease. Consider using your thoughts more to visualize, less to analyze. Instead, find within yourself the ability to imagine a better life for them. You have to imagine their wellness even in the reality of their experience of (temporary) illness and pain, and exercise the creative beingness you came here to live. Wish wellness for them, imagine wellness in them. Know they are well, regardless of what they say. *This is your power.* If you go to their way of believing in the moment, you give up your power.

"But, remember, my companions, you don't do this for them because they need it; you do it because it is *your* true nature, and because doing it also makes you feel good, and because joining them in a slower vibration takes you from the very Source that is you. Your greatest value to others is when you are joyful, when you are connected to who you are. Your greatest value to others is when you are radiantly healthy, when you are happy, to have, and to be, and to do all the things that are very important to *you.* When you are doing these things that make you feel good, that bring you joy and vitality, you are a catalyst inspiring others to an awareness of that. You have healed yourself, you are immersed in your natural wellness. Radiate health and well-being and all will be influenced by this. *You are a natural healer*, a health seer, a perfect health ally."

Chiron fell silent. The others remained silent as well, each traveling their own pathway amongst Chiron's ideas. A few moments passed, and Chiron added,

"Then while harmony between the spirit and the mind is being brought about, the very cause of the experience of illness being eradicated, one can apply the herbal oils and salves, administer the simples, the potions, and the tonics that usher good feelings and a strong sense of well-being to the body, therein most efficiently using such physical means as may be appropriate to soothe, tone, and complete the healing of the body.

"Show your companions how to make herbal brews and potions that sustain the body's vitality. Make with them those herbal preparations that help nourish their bodies and minds and soothe their afflictions, further assisting them to focus attention on all that feels good in their life. Remember, health is simply feeling good.

"And, as herbalists, whenever possible show these wonderful people to the gardens, to the fields and other places where plants live, for *the companionship of living plants* is truly the highest level, the premier expression of herbal medicine. Let folks' minds and hearts be uplifted by the silent language of the flower kingdom, words expressed through the pure positive energy radiating from the beauty and vitality of each living plant. Let the rhythm of human pulse be influenced by plants' enchanted connection with the cycles of absolute well-being and the jubilant abundance of Earth. Entreat yourself and your clients to meditate within these surroundings, this uplifting environment that assists one's mind to become calm and widen its outlook, allowing an individual to feel the visions of what he or she truly wants, rediscovering and confirming pathways to their bliss.

"And, finally, esteemed students and peers, communicate clearly to your clients that healing is a human function; it was not the counselor or the medicines or a supernatural power that healed them; it was they who healed themselves, for the final responsibility and the most compassionate act of health seers, herbalists, and physicians are to ultimately empower their client companions with the full realization that health and healing come forth solely from within."

Upon this final word, young Bacchus, who, although he loved listening to the teachings of his mentor, could contain himself no longer. He jumped up onto his feet saying, "Chiron, is it not time now to play; is it not time to honor this delicious flow of life by enhancing its surge with dancing and the taste of fine wines, ripe fruits, and spiced vegetables?"

"Yes," added Ceres, "and I have here loaves of fresh bread, sweet cakes, and rice puddings on which to feast." She laid out a spread of food that boggled the minds and aroused the palates of all present. Artemis had also brought sweet milk, and honey, and wheels of cheese to share.

Suddenly, in a rush of Nature's sweet magic, lush green vines could be seen growing from out of nothingness, lining the walls of Chiron's cave whereon clusters of berries, fat bunches of grapes and fruits, and the kindly buds of the hop family flourished in abundant display, all ripe for the picking. Dragonflies and damselflies, hummingbirds, and honey bees touched here and touched there, finding nectar-full flowers everywhere.

"And we have made potions, cordials, and herbal brews to share." said the elder Sachs, as he and Tages drug forth straw baskets and leather satchels brimming with colorful bottles and fat little jars full with aromatic liquids, twinkling powders, herbal blends for smoke, and other enchanting lore.

Chiron, delighted to his core, took out his lyre and began to play while others passed around flutes, cymbals, rattles and drums, and together they harmonized their rhythm and melody to the enchanting music of the spheres.

Outside Chiron's dwelling, hearing the festive merriment, Hermes as quickly as thought spread word of the magnificent affair throughout the land. Soon nymphs and satyrs wearing garlands of oak leaf and ivy, Psyche and Cupid, faeries and gnomes, Mother Nature, the Greenman, lovely Venus, and the great Pan himself arrived at Chiron's cave and were seen laughing and frolicking therein.

And as the music plays on, this joyous flow of life sings the songs of each individual's freedom, while the boundless creation of All that Is dances on and on into the wee hours of eternity.

So, side by side my friends, let's row our boats
gently down the stream…
creating everything we want,
making life full with all that we can dream…
we live in a child's garden, you know…
where it is always good to have fun
romping joyfully with the weeds…
pursuing the passion of our dance…
helping care for the garden's beings…
appreciating the grand diversity of us all…
And remember always,
Earth companions and co-creators,
be very, very good to yourselves…
and life will flow delightfully
with no resistance at all…
Our joy will illuminate the heavens…our youthful giggles tickling the moon
and the brightness of our spirits
will twinkle back to the shimmering stars…
The gifts of life are joy…that we are each beautiful and forever free…
have fun growing with all this herbal stuff…affectionately…

—JG, herbalist

> "Imagine for the pleasure of imagining, and your dreams will all come true."
> —T. ELDER SACHS

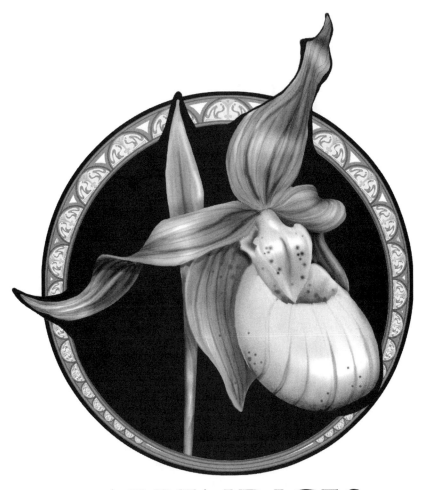

APPENDICES

APPENDIX A

THE UNITED PLANT SAVERS LIST OF "AT-RISK MEDICINAL PLANTS"

We have been seeking a clear vision as to which Native American medicinal plants are the primary focus of attention for our plant-protection efforts. This has taken the form of the "UpS At-Risk List," which has been defined and reviewed quite exhaustively over the last year, and has been agreed upon by the UpS Board of Directors. It consists of herbs broadly used in commerce, which due to over-harvest or loss of habitat, or by nature of their innate rareness or sensitivity, are at risk or of a significant decline in numbers within their current range.

STATEMENT OF PURPOSE

For the benefit of the plant communities, wild animals, harvesters, farmers, consumers, manufacturers, retailers, and practitioners, we offer this list of wild medicinal plants we feel are currently most sensitive to the impact of human activities. Our intent is to assure the increasing abundance of the medicinal plants presently in decline due to expanding popularity and shrinking habitat and range. UpS is not asking for a moratorium on the use of these herbs; rather we are initiating programs designed to preserve these important wild medicinal plants.

AT-RISK LIST

The wild medicinal plants on the following list have been proposed for inclusion on the "At-Risk List," but they are in need of further research. In some cases, the plants are abundant in one bio-region and quite rare in another. Some of these herbs are widely used in commerce, others are not widely used. United Plant Savers is watching these herbs and collecting information on levels of commercial usage while monitoring the viability of these plants within their current range. We invite your participation in this project. Please feel free to report on the health of populations of these plants in your local area. Also, feel free to propose other medicinal plants that you feel are presently in decline due to expanding popularity and shrinking habitat and range.

American Ginseng (*Panax quinquefolius*)

Black Cohosh (*Cimicifuga racemosa*)

Bloodroot (*Sanguinaria canadensis*)

Blue Cohosh (*Caulophyllum thalictroides*)

Echinacea (*Echinacea spp.*)

Goldenseal (*Hydrastis canadensis*)

Helonias Root (*Chamaelirium luteum*)

Kava Kava (*Piper methysticum*) Hawaii only

Lady's Slipper Orchid (*Cypripedium spp.*)

Lomatium (*Lomatium dissectum*)

Osha (*Ligusticum porteri, L. spp.*)

Partridge Berry, Squawvine (*Mitchella repens*)

Peyote (*Lophophora williamsii*)

Slippery Elm (*Ulmus rubra*)

Sundew (*Drosera spp.*)

Trillium, Beth Root (*Trillium spp.*)

True Unicorn (*Aletris farinosa*)

Venus' Fly Trap (*Dionaea muscipula*)

Wild Yam (*Dioscorea villosa, D. spp.*)

TO-WATCH LIST

Arnica (*Arnica spp.*)

Butterfly Weed (*Asclepias tuberosa*)

Calamus (*Acorus calamus*)

Chaparro (*Casatela emoryi*)

Elephant Tree (*Bursera microphylla*)

Eyebright (*Euphrasia spp.*)

Gentian (*Gentiana spp.*)

Goldthread (*Coptis spp.*)

Lobelia (*Lobelia spp.*)

Maidenhair Fern (*Adiaantum pendatum*)

Mayapple (*Podophyllum peltatum*)

Oregon Grape (*Mahonia spp.*)

Pink Root (*Spigelia marilaandica*)

Pipsissewa (*Chimaphila umbellata*)

Spikenard (*Aralia racemosa, A. californica*)

Stone Root (*Collinsonia canadensis*)

Stream Orchid (*Epipactis gigantea*)

Turkey Corn (*Dicentra canadensis*)

Virginia Snakeroot (*Aristolochia serpentaria*)

White Sage (*Salvia apiana*)

Yerba Mansa (*Anemopsis californica*)

Yerba Santa (*Eriodictyon californica*)

The term "spp" in the context of this list means "all North American species in this genus." We are using this category when there is reason to believe that through misidentification or intentional collection various species within the genus besides the officially recognized species are being utilized. We see this situation clearly when various species of Trillium are harvested to sell as "Beth Root," or when various species of Echinacea are harvested as "Echinacea angustifolia." We ask wildcrafters to consider the ecological impact of taking these herbs from the wild. Replanting in the wild, as well as careful stewarding of your collection areas, is of tantamount importance if the trade of wildcrafting is to continue. Although the herb may be abundant in your locality, it has probably already disappeared from other areas. You are the folks who have the best understanding of wild medicinal plants, and you can contribute greatly by providing seed and advising others on how to plant and grow these herbs. We ask manufacturers and consumers to assist in the conversion of these plants from wildcrafted sources to organically grown. If there is a demand for the wild herbs, then we will continue to lose them. If there is demand for cultivated herbs, then we create environmentally friendly jobs while saving the wild plants. Although it is an expensive proposition, the time is ripe to assure sustainability of the herbs we love. I would like to express my thanks to the hundreds of good folks who reviewed this list and gave their constructive comments: academics, herbalists, government workers, botanists, and lay enthusiasts. Your views were taken seriously, and by comparing the feedback of what is considered rare from your various bio-regions, we have been able to compile much information on which herbs need our help most urgently.

—Richo Cech, Horizon Herbs, UpS Board Member

United Plant Savers
P.O. Box 98
East Barre ,VT 05649
Tel (802) 479-9825
Fax (802) 476-3722
Email: info@www.plantsavers.org
Web site: <www.plantsavers.org>

APPENDIX B

Welcome to the Garden

I've been waiting for you.

I'd like to take the opportunity, while we are here together in the garden pages of this manual, to restate that in my opinion the supreme form of all herbal medicine is the direct association with a living plant. In my experience, the most powerful nourishment given us by herbal tonics is delivered by simply commingling with living plants growing in a garden, particularly when it is your own garden. This is why in my herb school, we start all our intensive "Roots of Herbalism" and "Foundations of Health" course curricula and our herbal medicine-making classes and so forth in the garden. We ground all our teaching in the garden where Herbalism is rooted and flourishes. This way, we never forget just whom we are talking about. This way, when we delve into other facets of our herbal studies, those that often and quite quickly become highly intellectual and theoretical, we don't misalign our perspective. We don't lose sight of the reality of our most knowledgeable herbal teachers, the plants. The garden is established as "Home." At any point we can step back into this reality from the abstract symbolism of our mental journeys and be immersed in the organic vibrations of herbal truth. The garden, from its Earth connection and its aesthetic nectar, is the only classroom qualified to satisfy the hunger and thirst of passionate student herbalists, and it is the only teacher who can answer all their questions…without speaking a word.

Growing your own garden is very simple. How does one do it? "Just put your hands and some seeds or roots into the earth and grow something." Placing a plant or a seed in the soil, watering it, and caring for it, makes a "mother" out of you, a nurturer, and if you don't think that is important, you will. Whether you are a man or a woman, a young girl or a young boy, the experience of taking a plant into your life, providing it a place to dwell, paying attention to it, checking on it every day or so, talking with it (and you do talk to it with every thought and feeling, because plants don't require ears or mouths to communicate), checking to see that it is happy where you put it, moving it if necessary (it'll let you know where it likes to be), talking with it some more, all puts sparkle in your life. And sometimes that's all we are looking for…a little sparkle to help polish the nervous system and clear the heart valves. You'll be thrilled, and if your thumb's not green at first, just keep on gardening, it'll turn green. Actually, green is the natural color of all human thumbs. They just get coated with ink, and grease, and makeup, and all that kind of day-to-day stuff of civilization. Gardening—

bending, kneeling, stretching, reaching, digging, smiling, spreading, picking up, setting down, pruning, watering, pushing, pulling, carrying, scratching, and so forth—are also very gentle, yet excellent forms of physical exercise, akin to that which wild animals get while roaming the fields, the seashore, and the countryside gathering their food.

Also, purchase a chime for your garden. Spend some time selecting it; find the one (or two or three) that resonates perfectly with the appetite of your aesthetic ear. You'll recognize it when you feel your inner being humming along with its tone. Buy or build some bird houses, a bird bath, and a couple of bat houses. (If you disapprove of bats, consider reconsidering this attitude; unless you fly at night *and* you are a whole lot smaller than they are, bats won't bother you; and they garble from the garden sky a myriad of flying insects that take great delight in bothering you.)

Arrange all the above things in your garden near your plants. The birds you attract eat bugs that eat plants, and most important, the songs of birds are the perfect serenade for plants. It has been discovered that no other form of music makes plants happier and more garden-active. Bats patrol the garden airways for you at night. The music of the chime announces the arrival of garden breezes; this uplifting euphony is for you the gardener. It makes your mind pause a moment while your insides beam. This is herbal medicine at its best.

One final suggestion—avoid combat maneuvers in your garden. Children of every plant, animal, and mineral species do poorly when raised in or near a battlefield. Gophers, snails, deer, and aphid are part of the garden phenomenon. Granted they can be a giant pain, we all can be at times, but poisoning, stabbing-traps, and gunshots destroy the serenity of a garden, and they are not enjoyable strategies. Plant-munching critters can be outwitted and outmaneuvered. Take the challenge. If some of the other local fauna outmaneuver you, a point for them. Exercise your sense of humor. Let your frustration stimulate your creative wit. Companions (of all species) teach; you learn, and the next step in the garden boogie is yours. We live in the Garden of Earth as members of a sacred *circle of giving*. All beings need food, and the earth provides it for us. At some point in the ongoing dynamics of this organic cycle, each of us becomes a morsel of food for another. Eating a succulent garden plant, no matter where it might be growing (or what species you are), is instinctive, wholesome participation in the circle dynamics; don't take it personally. We garden to grow, to feel good, to be uplifted, and to enjoy our life; warfare heads us in a different direction. And, if you happen to have a bad back or some other injury, don't be deterred by this. Gardening is well done slowly and easily; it is a timeless adventure that will adapt gracefully to your rhythm and movements.

A Note on the Puttering Reflex

Gardening is a human being's most efficient means for reviving the ability to co-communicate with plants. This ability is systematically developed by the reawakening and refining of one's innate "puttering reflex."

The puttering reflex is triggered automatically the instant you step into your garden. Since the event of your last appearance in the garden, the resident plants have been growing and anticipating your return, and they will have a variety of organic details they would appreciate that you attend to.

Upon reentering the garden, you sense this intuitively, and, in classic reflexive fashion—which seems almost involuntarily performed—you start tending immediately to the salient project nearest at hand. The perpetuation of the reflex loop is automatic as you hear the plants' requests and respond, hear and respond, hear and respond throughout the garden community. In short time, this "puttering" process shifts gears into enchantment, graceful movements, shameless humming, deliberate creativity, full on joy, and non-resistance to total participation in the well-being of your innate health. Time ceases to exist along with the sidecar full of pressures that habitually ride with time in your life. Garden puttering is a mild form of trance that you enter, and when you come out of this green space, both you and the garden are emotionally and physically transformed. It is an ambrosial adventure that enhances your immune system and tones your nervous system. Concurrently, the circulatory system is caressed by your complete disconnection with all time-related stress; the five senses are acutely activated; and like your muscles when enjoyably exercised, the more you use them, in turn, the more pleasure they give you. So, be well, putter forth, and play with the faeries.

Further note: The impulsive tendency to hug trees is an opportunistic ancillary response to the puttering reflex.

Green Thumb Technology of Independence— A Recommended Home Medicine Garden

Western States

The size of your garden site will suggest the plants to choose.

Plants that yield a good harvest, yet do not require too much room
(suggestions for an approximately 10' x 20' plot)

• Calendula (*Calendula officinalis*)

• California Poppy (*Eschscholzia californica*)

• Catnip (*Nepeta cataria*)

• Comfrey (*Symphytum officinalis*) (Plant it where you want it to remain!)

• Feverfew (*Tanacetum parthenium*)

• Garlic (*Allium sativum*)

• Hyssop (*Hyssopus officinalis*)

• Lady's Mantle (*Alchemilla vulgaris*) (Likes shade!)

• Lavender (*Lavandula vera*)

• Lemon Balm (*Melissa officinalis*)

• Motherwort (*Leonurus cardiaca*)

- Mugwort (*Artemisia vulgaris*)

- Mullein (*Verbascum spp.*)

- Pennyroyal (*Mentha pulegium*) (Loves wet areas)

- Peppermint (*Mentha piperita*) (It spreads in all directions!)

- Sage (*Salvia officinalis*)

- Wood Betony (*Stachys officinalis*)

- Yarrow (*Achillea millefolium*)

Plants that require a relatively large area to yield an adequate harvest

- Angelica (*Angelica archangelica*)

- Burdock (*Arctium lappa*)

- Chamomile (*Matricaria chamomilla*)

- Fennel (*Foeniculum vulgare*)

- Globe Artichoke (*Cynara scolymus*)

- Milk Thistle (*Silybum marianum*)

- Red Clover (*Trifolium pratense*)

- Scullcap (*Scutellaria spp.*)

- St. John's Wort (*Hypericum perforatum*)

- Vitex (*Vitex agnus-castus*)

- Wild Oat (*Avena fatua, A. sativa*)

Plants that do well in pots and boxes

- Basil (*Ocimum basilicum*) (requires hot sun!)

- Calendula (*Calendula officinalis*)

- Feverfew (*Tanacetum parthenium*)

- Lavender (*Lavandula spp.*)

- Mints (*Mentha spp.*)

- Parsley (*Petroselinum spp.*)

- Rosemary (*Rosmarinus officinalis*)

- Sage (*Salvia spp.*)

- Thyme (*Thymus vulgaris*)

Wild plants to encourage in your garden and around the house

- Blackberry (*Rubus fructicosus*) (Keep an eye on this one and maintain control!)

- Burdock (*Arctium lappa*)

- California poppy (*Eschscholzia californica*)
- Chickweed (*Stellaria media*)
- Cleaver (*Galium aperine*)
- Dandelion (*Taraxacum officinale*)
- Gumweed (*Grindelia spp.*)
- Horsetail (*Equisetum arvense*)
- Oregon Grape (*Mahonia spp.*)
- Milk Thistle (*Silybum marianum*)
- Miner's Lettuce (*Claytonia spp.*)
- Plantain (*Plantago lanceolata, P. major*)
- Self-heal (*Prunella vulgaris*)
- Shepherd's Purse (*Capsella bursa-pastoris*)
- Sorrel (*Rumex spp.*)
- Stinging Nettle (*Urtica spp.*)
- Teasel (*Dipsacus spp.*)
- Violet (*Viola spp.*)
- Wild Oat (*Avena spp.*)
- Yarrow (*Achillea millefolium*)
- Yellow Dock (*Rumex crispus*)
- Yerba Mansa (*Anemopsis californica*)
- Yerba Santa (*Eriodictyon californicum*)

Plants that require digging roots (although other parts of the plant are often used as well)

Divide the roots' crowns and replant whenever possible.

- Angelica (*Angelica spp.*)
- Burdock (*Arctium lappa*)
- Dandelion (*Taraxacum officinale*)
- Echinacea (*Echinacea purpurea*)
- Elecampane (*Inula helenium*)
- Goldenseal (*Hydrastis canadensis*) (an eastern woodland plant that requires shade and damp soil—can be grown in West Coast shade gardens)
- Horseradish (*Cochlearia armoracia*)
- Poke (*Phytolacca decandra*)
- Stinging Nettle root (*Urtica spp.*) (rhizomes are excellent reproductive organ tonics)

- Yellow Dock (*Rumex crispus*)
- Valerian (*Valeriana officinalis*) (Likes it wet!)

Medicinal trees
- Crampbark (*Viburnum opulus*) (actually a large bush)
- Elder (*Sambucus spp.*)
- Eucalyptus (*Eucalyptus globulus*)
- Fremontia "California Slippery Elm" (*Fremontodendron californicum*)
- Ginkgo (*Ginkgo biloba*)
- Hawthorn (*Crataegus spp.*)
- Vitex (*Vitex agnus-castus*)
- Willow (*Salix alba*) (Likes a wet area!)

Plants for the medicine of their beauty
- California Poppy (*Eschscholzia californica*)
- Clary Sage (*Salvia sclarea*)
- Foxglove (*Digitalis purpurea*) (all parts are toxic taken *internally*—see Chapter Twenty-Four, "*Poultices*")
- Mullein (*Verbascum spp.*)
- Nasturtium (*Nasturtium officinale*)
- Poke (*Phytolacca decandra*) (toxic)
- Oriental Poppy (*Papaver spp.*)
- Sunflower (*Helianthus annuus*)

Note: Herbs love good soil and water. In the most part, it is an erroneous myth that they do better without.

Fertilizer
- Aged animal manure
- Kitchen and garden compost
- Urine (diluted with water 1:5); do not put on leaves.

Pest control
- Healthy plants
- Safer soap
- Garlic-Cayenne spray
- Beneficial insects (i.e., ladybug, praying mantis)

• Picking snails and slugs off plants every morning throughout the season. This will drastically reduce their population the following years.

• Gophers are highly territorial, so remove one and your garden is free until another moves in.

• Moles don't hurt anything; they merely plow the soil and eat creepy-crawlers, not plants.

• To discourage deer (glorified cows), hang from your plants nylon stocking bags full of smelly little motel soap bars.

Herbs love good soil and water. In the most part, it is an erroneous myth that they do better without.

Equipment

• Dehydrator

• Pruning shears (Good quality)

• Root-digging tool (Strong trowel or Japanese hori-hori)

• High-quality garden tools

• Gloves

Eastern States

(Suggested by James Green and Leslie Gardner)
The size of your garden site will suggest the plants to choose.

Plants that yield a good harvest, yet do not require too much room
(suggestions for an approximately 10' x 20' plot)

• Calendula (*Calendula officinalis*)

• Catnip (*Nepeta cataria*)

• Coltsfoot (*Tussilago farfara*)

• Comfrey (*Symphytum officinalis*) (Plant it where you want it to stay!)

• Feverfew (*Tanacetum parthenium*)

• Garlic (*Allium sativum*)

• Hyssop (*Hyssopus officinalis*)

• Lady's Mantle (*Alchemilla vulgaris*) (Likes shade!)

• Lavender (*Lavandula vera*)

• Lemon Balm (*Melissa officinalis*)

• Lobelia (*Lobelia inflata*)

• Motherwort (*Leonurus cardiaca*)

• Mugwort (*Artemisia vulgaris*)

• Mullein (*Verbascum spp.*)

• Pennyroyal (*Mentha pulegium*) (Loves wet areas)

• Peppermint (*Mentha piperita*) (It spreads in all directions!)

- Sage (*Salvia officinalis*)
- Wild Indigo (*Baptisia tinctoria*)
- Wood Betony (*Stachys officinalis*)
- Yarrow (*Achillea millefolium*)

Plants that require a relatively large area to yield an adequate harvest

- Angelica (*Angelica archangelica*)
- Boneset (*Eupatorium perfoliatum*)
- Burdock (*Arctium lappa*)
- Chamomile (*Matricaria chamomilla*)
- Elecampane (*Inula helenium*)
- Fennel (*Foeniculum vulgare*)
- Globe Artichoke (*Cynara scolymus*)
- Joe-Pye (*Eupatorium purpureum*)
- Milk Thistle (*Silybum marianum*)
- Red Clover (*Trifolium pratense*)
- Scullcap (*Scutellaria spp.*)
- St. John's Wort (*Hypericum perforatum*)
- Stoneroot (*Collinsonia canadensis*)
- Vitex (*Vitex agnus-castus*)
- Wild Oat (*Avena fatua, A. sativa*)

Plants that do okay in pots and boxes

- Basil (*Ocimum basilicum*) (requires hot sun!)
- Calendula (*Calendula officinalis*)
- Feverfew (*Tanacetum parthenium*)
- Lavender (*Lavandula spp.*)
- Mints (*Mentha spp.*)
- Parsley (*Petroselinum spp.*)
- Rosemary (*Rosmarinus officinalis*)
- Sage (*Salvia spp.*)
- Thyme (*Thymus vulgaris*)

Wild plants to encourage in your garden and around the house

- Blackberry (*Rubus fructicosus*) (Keep an eye on this one and maintain control!)

- Black Cohosh (*Cimicifuga racemosa*)
- Bloodroot (*Sanguinaria canadensis*)
- Blue Cohosh (*Caulophyllum thalictroides*)
- Burdock (*Arctium lappa*)
- Chickweed (*Stellaria media*)
- Chicory (*Cichorium intybus*)
- Cleaver (*Galium aperine*)
- Coltsfoot (*Tussilago farfara*)
- Culver's Root (*Leptandra virginica*)
- Dandelion (*Taraxacum officinale*)
- Ginseng (*Panax quinquefolius*)
- Goldenrod (*Solidago virgaurea*)
- Goldenseal (*Hydrastis canadensis*)
- Joe-Pye (*Eupatorium purpureum*)
- Jewelweed (*Impatiens capensis*)
- Milkweed (*Asclepias spp.*)
- Passion Flower (*Passiflora incarnata*)
- Plantain (*Plantago lanceolata, P. major*)
- Slippery Elm (*Ulmus rubra*)
- Stoneroot (*Collinsonia canadensis*)
- Tansy (*Tanacetum vulgare*) (Takes hold and spreads!)
- Violet (*Viola spp.*)

Plants that require digging roots (although other parts of the plant are often used as well)

Divide the roots' crowns and replant whenever possible.

- Burdock (*Arctium lappa*)
- Dandelion (*Taraxacum officinale*)
- Echinacea (*Echinacea purpurea*)
- Elecampane (*Inula helenium*)
- Golden Seal (*Hydrastis canadensis*)
- Horseradish (*Cochlearia armoracia*)
- Poke (*Phytolacca decandra*)
- Valerian (*Valeriana officinalis*) (Likes it wet!)

Medicinal trees

- Black Haw (*Viburnum prunifolium*)
- Elder (*Sambucus spp.*)
- Ginkgo (*Ginkgo biloba*)
- Hawthorn (*Crataegus spp.*)
- Sassafras (*Sassafras albidum*)
- Slippery Elm (*Ulmus rubra*)
- Wild Cherry (*Prunus serotina*)
- Willow (*Salix alba*) (Likes a wet area!)

Plants for the medicine of their beauty

- Clary Sage (*Salvia sclarea*)
- Foxglove (*Digitalis purpurea*) (all parts are toxic taken *internally*—see Chapter Twenty-Four, "*Poultices*")
- Mullein (*Verbascum spp.*)
- Nasturtium (*Nasturtium officinale*)
- Poke (*Phytolacca decandra*) (toxic)
- Oriental Poppy (*Papaver spp.*)
- Sunflower (*Helianthus annuus*)

Fertilizer

- Aged animal manure
- Kitchen and garden compost
- Urine (diluted with water 1:5); do not put on leaves

Pest control

- Healthy plants
- Safer soap
- Garlic-Cayenne spray
- Beneficial insects (i.e., ladybug, praying mantis)
- Picking snails and slugs off plants every morning throughout the season. This will drastically reduce their population the following years.
- Gophers are highly territorial, so remove one and your garden is free until another moves in.
- Moles don't hurt anything; they merely plow the soil and eat creepy-crawlers, not plants.

• To discourage deer (glorified cows), hang from your plants nylon stocking bags full of smelly little motel soap bars.

Equipment

• Dehydrator

• Pruning shears (Good quality)

• Root-digging tool (Strong trowel or Japanese hori-hori)

• High-quality garden tools

• Gloves

APPENDIX C

Eight Principles of Excellent Medicine-Making

THE THREE ECONOMIC PRINCIPLES

Harvest only abundance

Harvest only in areas of plant abundance, leaving plant communities with no particularly noticeable physical evidence that you were there. Harvesting is not always the taking of plant parts, but often merely visiting their turf, observing, and harvesting feelings of connection, insight, and kinship with plant and animal companions (ally bonding).

Exchange energy

Leave an expendable but intimate part of yourself in exchange for your harvest: a power object that you previously found, a ritual, a prayer, a meditation, or some other personal, special expression of gratitude. Sanction the exchange with your gift, making the herbal harvest yours to transform into your potions and brews and dispense as you will.

Plant seeds

The wise carpenter and foresightful printer will honor and support the healthy life of forests and conserve their range of diversity. The bright plumber will assist in protecting water resources and esteem the Earth's bodies of water so people can continue to draw healthy fluid through their water pipes. The green herbalist will sow seeds throughout Gaia, participating in the circle of giving and the simple cycle of sow and reap. Every occupation draws its primary resources from Earth and can promote balance by contributing energy to conserving, recycling, and restoring, learning from Earth's intelligent technique for ensuring perpetual abundance.

THE INTUITIVE PRINCIPLE

Be intimately aware of the common life force in all things

Appreciate Unity. Experience, enjoy, and be nourished by your connection with all life. Recent evidence from several disciplines, including brain and consciousness research, anthropology, microbiology, neurophysiology, elemental physics, and mythology (and simple observation) reveals that body, mind, and consciousness are inseparable, an indivisible whole, a dynamic continuum. The universe too, so long thought to consist of innumerable separate parts, appears to be at its primary level an unbroken wholeness, a single dimension independent of time and space in which the seemingly separate parts are not in the least separated but are *all intimately connected.* All knowing is available to all beings.

THE TWO SPIRITUAL/SOCIAL PRINCIPLES

Have fun
When you are having fun, at that moment, you are experiencing most intimately and clearly who you truly are and what you enjoy doing. This self-knowledge can escort you to further creativity and joyful activity in your chosen work/play. Seek responsible instruction from an experienced teacher to build a foundation, but ultimately *make medicine in your own unique fashion.* This is self-fulfillment, self-nourishment, creativity, and independence. You are at your best when you're having fun with life; when you are joyful, you uplift others which is your most precious gift.

Hurt no one
Kindness is the foundation of peace and health. Honor and appreciate individuality as mutual appreciation begets mutual support. Protect the planetary rights of other persons and all species. Harming oneself and others is the fundamental basis of disease. Harvest from your heart; connect with the heart of the circle of giving. Base your herbal research on empirical investigation and scientific research that does not involve the confinement and ill-treatment of a member of any species.

THE TWO PRINCIPLES OF PERSONAL POWER

Come from the heart
Expressing our true feelings and intuition from the heart is how each of us measures up to all others and develops a sense of self-esteem, personal power, and fearlessness. Spontaneity lives.

Dance and sing
Herbal medicine-making is a Path of Passion. Cut loose and celebrate your life.

APPENDIX D

EXTRACT INFORMATION CHART

(As prepared for the California School of Herbal Studies)

Country name of herb: _____

Latin botanical name: _____

Method: Folk _____   Weight/Volume _____

W/V _____

    Total weight of herb used _____ Gm

    Total menstruum _____ ml

    Vol. 190-proof alcohol _____ ml

    Vol. distilled water _____ ml

    Vol. vegie glycerin _____ ml

    Other _____ ml

Batch # _____

Date prepared _____

Date pressed _____

    Yield 1st press _____ ml

    Weight wet marc _____ ml

    Weight dry marc _____ ml

    Final yield of filtered extract _____ ml

Source of herb _____

Quality: Primo ____ Excellent ____ Good ____

PROCEDURE NOTES: i.e., Methods of grinding used, what worked, what didn't; all idiosyncrasies of the herb being processed; how processing might be done better next time; performance of menstruum, suggested changes next time; alternate w/v, etc.

_____

_____

_____

EMPIRICAL NOTES: i.e., all feedback received about the use of this extract.

_____

_____

_____

APPENDIX E

HARVESTING INFORMATION CHART

(As prepared for the California School of Herbal Studies)

Herb gathered:

    Botanical name _____

    Common name(s) _____

    Batch # _____ Date collected _____ Time of day collected _____

Gathering site:

Private or public land; recently worked, farmed, or logged? Distance from nearest highway, power lines, or other manmade structures. Types of fertilizers used and when; any history of herbicides/pesticides used on this land.

_____

_____

_____

Weather conditions during harvest _____ Temperature _____

Handling methods:

Cleaning method (Shaking, peeling, washing, tools used, etc.) _____

_____

_____

Drying method (Hanging, racks, dehydrator, etc.) _____

_____

_____

Drying conditions (Light exposure, moisture, ventilation, temperature range, environmental factors such as dust, insects, and odors) _____

_____

_____

Fresh plant weight _____ Dried plant weight_____

The undersigned individual(s) guarantees that these herbs were harvested in ecologically sound areas with conscious care for the plant community and the natural environment in which they are growing.

Signature _____ Date _____

APPENDIX F

FIRST AID FOR POISONING BY ALKALOIDS

Plants ordinarily used by herbalists are not poisonous. Yet, as is well known, some plant components are extremely poisonous. As health allies and caretakers, it is practical to remember that in cases of alkaloid poisoning and other kinds of poisoning, the initial treatment consists in chemical *destruction* or *obstruction* and subsequent *evacuation* of the poison. While each alkaloid, when taken by mouth, will require its own special chemical antidote (see the Merck Index), if any is known, the following general procedure and drugs may be used:

GENERAL PROCEDURE

1. Remove noxious agent from contact with patient.

2. Keep patient warm and lying down. An unconscious or near-unconscious person should be placed on their abdomen, head turned to one side and tongue pulled forward.

3. Give 2–4 glasses of water immediately (milk can be substituted).

4. Induce vomiting immediately by giving 1–2 tablespoons of salt in a full glass of warm water, or a tablespoon of mustard in warm water, or have the patient place index finger far back on tongue and stroke from side to side. *Vomiting should also be induced after each dose of the antidote.* **Caution:** With strychnine, strongly caustic, or corrosive poison, *do not* induce vomiting.

5. Give patient the Universal Antidote (see below).

6. Get medical attention as soon as possible. Do not interrupt the above procedures.

UNIVERSAL ANTIDOTE

If the nature of the poison is unknown, give repeated doses of 1/2 ounce (15 Gm) of the following mixture or a like mixture, stirred in half a glass of warm water:

• **Pulverized, activated charcoal** (burnt toast as an alternative) — 2 parts

• **Tannic acid** (strong black tea as an alternative) — 1 part

• **Magnesium oxide** (milk of magnesia as an alternative) — 1 part

Never give oils, fats, or alcohol.

Tannin (tannic acid powder or common black tea) precipitates most alkaloids (as well as certain toxic glycosides and many metals). *But* remember that this precipitate *redissolves* in the *acidic* gastric juice, so it should be given with alkaline substances, such as sodium carbonate or bicarbonate, milk of magnesia, or the like, which neutralize acids, and then they should be removed by vomiting or with a stomach pump.

Iodine in the form of Tincture of Iodine diluted, or Lugol's Solution (iodine with potassium iodide) may be given as a general antidote. *But* this precipitate *redissolves* in the *alkaline* juices of the intestines, so it must be hurried through the bowels by means of a purgative if it is too late to remove it by vomiting or a stomach pump.

Activated animal charcoal (or vegetable charcoal as an alternative) absorbs and obstructs alkaloids. This may be used if quickly removed from the stomach before re-solution takes place.

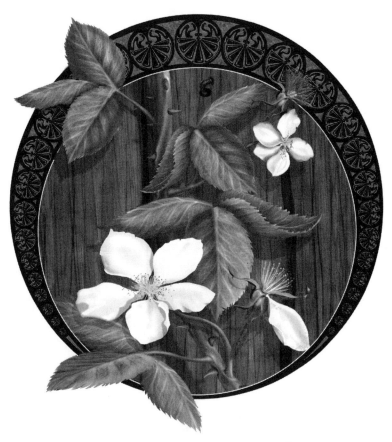

REFERENCE

All individuals have their distinctive way of doing things. Some folks put lids back on, some won't; some tuck their shirttails in, others don't; some do the dishes right after meals, while others let 'em soak. Medicine-making-wise the principles and instruction I have put forth in this handbook are pretty much how I do my thing. This how-to-herbal is a crystallization of what I have learned to date from sundry teachers, fused with the manifest magic of my salvaged blunders, and that which I have sensed or channeled, much of which popped into my head as a breezy "wow, that's a hell-of-an-idea." Certain folks may interpret some (maybe all) of what I have put forth in these pages as merely fond retrospection of brief psychotic episodes from which I have returned, or at least partially returned. Milking this compliment all I can, I will savor my particular madness by clarifying that my castles-in-the-air come fully endowed with lush gardens, talking plants, wizardly critters, and quaintly equipped kitchen-labs; the enchanting wonderment of all this invoking me to visit and water and attend to them regularly.

As to the pathway of my particular education and experiences in herbal medicine–making, it has been a winding road. At times I've jogged pointedly along its course, asking questions and making notes; and yet, often I've simply dilly dallied with Dandelions and watched the Mullein blossoms charm the bees. Any attempt to list in systematic fashion just who or what taught me this and that, would be very difficult indeed, for the evolution of my insights and methodologies progressed in a curlicue fashion rather than in any discernable linear sequence of research and events. Suffice to say the approaching list of highly talented, visionary beings touched, taught, and influenced me in one way or another, over and over again; and with warm heart, I give them my sincere appreciation and full credit for their profoundly creative work. At the same time, I probably should also ask their forgiveness if it appears that I have misinterpreted their teachings, or that I have gnarled the fiber of their clarity with the sometimes unyielding bent of my temperament. My grasp of these teachings intertwined with the passion of my personal direction is reflected to the reader by the substance of this manual. I hope this will inspire and serve you well, and any lucre that comes my way via your purchase of this compendium of herbal life force will be shared with hands-on educational centers that further assist anyone who wishes to become an informed and skilled herbalist.

So, companions, teachers, and esteemed peers, you, whose work has inspired and assisted me in this journey, as each of your names is read, wherever you are, will you please smile and nod to the reader and accept my deeply felt appreciation of your extraordinary Spirit.

LINA "CAROLYN" STAUB and FARA MARIE PEARSON, my herbalist soulmates, you beautify my life with your sweet hearts and artist touch

The PLANT SPIRITS forever dwelling in the CSHS herb garden and in the wild gardens that surround our home

NORMA MYERS, herbalist, wildwoman, and my first mentor

DR. JOHN CHRISTOPHER, herbalist and most jolly human being, my second teacher, author of *School of Natural Healing*

DR. EDWARD BACH, quiet master, floral medicineman, author of *Heal Thyself* and creator of the 38 original flower essence remedies

STUDENTS OF CSHS, your memory forever dwells in my heart; you are the green future

JAMES SNOW, most compassionate herbal therapist, my brother and teacher

MICHAEL MOORE, herbalist pioneer de magnificencia

ED SMITH, herbalist, storyteller, and medicine-maker extraordinaire

ROSEMARY GLADSTAR, my uncommon law sister, grand herbalist, visionary of United Plant Savers, and author of *Herbal Healing for Women*

7SONG, notorious herbalist, wildcrafter, and first-aid master

ROY UPTON, kindred spirit of many journeys, editor of *The American Herbal Phamacopoeia*

NAN KOEHLER, birth angel, author of *Artemis Speaks* and co-founder of Artemis College

JOSEPHINE GREEN, one of the bravest women I know, my role model for self-healing

AUTUMN SUMMERS, herbalist and teacher of green botany

LESLIE GARDNER, herbalist gardener and Deva whisperer

REBECCA MAXFIELD and JASON MILLER, nurturers of enchanting babies and the herb school campus

RUTH DREIER, herbalist, visionary, and health seer

KAREN MONDOUX, herbalist and seed gatherer

RICHO CECH, herbalist, medicine-maker, and medicineseedman

PAM MONTGOMERY, herbalist of the Green Nations, author of *Partner Earth*

SARA KATZ, most organized herbalist with a splendid eye for beauty

RICHARD LIEBMANN, N.D., Island captain of the good ship UpS

PAUL STRAUS, greenman forest healer

CHRISTOPHER HOBBS, herbalist, woodland dancer, teacher, and prolific author

BETH BAUGH, without whose brilliance many excellent herbals probably would have never been published

CHARMOON RICHARDSON, Shroomchef and mushroom master

DIANA DELUCA, who put delicious romance back into Western Herbalism by writing the *Botanica Erotica*

GREGORY TILFORD, herbalist, wildcrafter, and author of *The EcoHerbalist's Fieldbook*

RYAN DRUM, fearless wildcrafter of land and sea and herbal brewmaster

DAVID HOFFMANN, herbalist and phyto-bridge between the sciences, author of scads of herbals

PETER D'AMATO, caretaker of the carnivorous green and author of *The Savage Garden*

HILDA LEYEL and MRS. M. GRIEVE, authors of *A Modern Herbal*

WILLIAM H. COOK, M.D., wonderfully outspoken nineteenth century physio-medicalist

CASCADE ANDERSON-GELLER, wonderfully outspoken twenty-first century herbalist and wise woman

TIM BLAKLEY, herbalist gardener and co-author of *Medicinal Herbs in the Garden, Field, & Marketplace*

LESLEY TIERRA, herbalist and author of *The Herbs of Life*

CARLA EMERY, do-it yourself artist and pioneer, author of *The Encyclopedia of Country Living*

KATHI KEVILLE and MINDY GREEN, herbalists and aroma practitioners, authors of *Aromatherapy—A Complete Guide to the Healing Art*

DR. EDWARD SHOOK, N.D., D.C., author of *Advanced Treatise on Herbology*, your formula 57 made me a believer

JOHN URI LLOYD, the soulman of herbal pharmacy

D.C. JARVIS, M.D., author of *Folk Medicine*

JETHRO KLOSS, the Moses of Herbalism, author of *Back to Eden*

WILLIAM H. SHELDON, PH.D, M.D., author of *The Varieties of Temperament*

RUDOLF WEISS, M.D., doctor of herbal knowledge, author of *Herbal Medicine*

WILBUR SCOVILLE, PH.G., author of *The Art of Compounding*

CHARLES CASPARI, author of *A Treatise on Pharmacy*

JOSEPH P. REMINGTON, author of *The Practice of Pharmacy*

CLYDE M. SNOW, author of *Essentials of Pharmacy*

EDWARD PARRISH, author of *A Treatise on Pharmacy*

JOSEPH SPROWLS, Ph.D., editor of *American Pharmacy*

A.W. PRIEST and L.R. PRIEST, authors of *Herbal Medication*

J. H. KELLOGG, M.D., hydrotherapist, author of *Rational Hydrotherapy*; A. STILLE, M.D., and J. MAISCH, Phar.D., authors of *The National Dispensatory*; G. B. WOOD and F. BACHE, professors of materia medica, pharmacy and chemistry, authors of *The United States Dispensatory* (a very old edition)

WADE BOYLE, N.D., master of natural medicine, water therapist, and departed friend

FRANCIS JOHN FOX, who showed me that it's always best to laugh

ROBERT GREEN, who taught me the bitter, the sweet, and the sour of making a delicious medicine salad

BILL WATTERSON and GARY LARSON, you guys crack me up, your medicine is the best

and last, but certainly never least, joyful TIBET, mischievous little Shih-tzu Maltese cross, indomitable Spirit of the Little Folks.

I want to thank you...all.

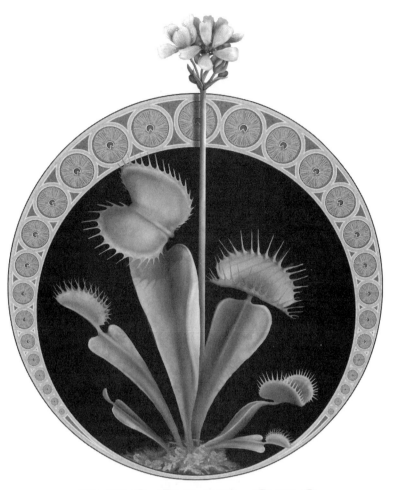

RESOURCES

The following compressed lists of resources will get you started and on your way. As like attracts like, each item you acquire will lead to another and your personal list of resources will take on a life of its own.

The herb books I recommend to you are all written by adept, hands-on herbalists. I am familiar with their work, and I trust the contents of their publications. They are good teachers and herbal craftsmen who love plants and draw from extensive experience.

BOOKS

Bach, Edward. *The Bach Flower Remedies*, Keats Publishing Connecticut, 1979. This is three books in one volume: *Heal Thyself*, by Edward Bach, *The Twelve Healers*, by Edward Bach, and *The Bach Remedies Repertory*, by F.J. Wheeler.

Batmanghelid, F., M.D. *Your Body's Many Cries for Water*, Globabl Health Solutions, Inc., P.O. Box 3189, Falls Church, VA 22043, 1995.

Black, Penny. *The Book of Pressed Flowers*, Simon & Schuster, New York.

Buhner, Stephen. *Sacred Plant Medicine*, Roberts Rinehart Pub., Boulder, Colorado, 1996.

Chancellor, Philip. *Handbook of the Bach Flower Remedies*, Keats Publishing, Connecticut, 1980.

Christopher, John R. *School of Natural Healing*, BiWorld, Orem, Utah, 1976.

Cech, Richo. *Making Plant Medicine*, Horizon Herbs Publication, Box 69, Williams, Oregon, 2000. This work is an excellent companion and reference for beginning and experienced herbal medicine-makers.

Cowan, Elliot. *Plant Spirit Medicine*, Wildflower Press, 1995.

D'Amato, Peter. *The Savage Garden: Cultivating Carnivorous Plants*, Ten Speed Press, Berkeley, California, 1998. Growing these captivating yet endangered wetland plants is a hobby of mine that I would like to turn you on to. This book is the very best in its field.

Emery, Carla. *The Encyclopedia of Country Living*, Sasquatch Books, Seattle, 1994. A magnificent resource for people who enjoy doing things for themselves in order to get high-quality products, includes an excellent chapter on making vinegar in the home.

Foster, Steven. *Herbal Bounty! The Gentle Art of Herb Culture*, Peregrine Smith Books, Utah, 1984.

Gladstar, Rosemary. *Herbal Healing for Women*, Simon & Schuster, New York, 1993.

Green, James. *The Herbal Medicine-Maker's Handbook*, 4th ed., (A compact, abbreviated version of this 5th ed.). James Green, Box 39, Forestville, CA 95436. $10 postage paid. Include your address.

Green, James. *The Male Herbal*, The Crossing Press, Freedom, California, 1991.

Grieve, Mrs. M. *A Modern Herbal*, Vols., I & II, Dover Publications, New York, 1971.

Griggs, Barbara. *Green Pharmacy*, Healing Arts Press, Rochester, Vermont, 1991. A history of grassroots herbal medicine and pharmacy.

Hobbs, Christopher. *Foundations of Health: The Liver and Digestive Herbal*, Botanica Press, Capitola, California, 1992. Christopher has written many other excellent herbals. Seek them out.

Hoffmann, David. *An Elder's Herbal,* Healing Arts Press, Vermont, 1993.

Hoffmann, David. *The New Holistic Herbal,* Element Books, Rockport, MA. 1996.

Jarvis, D.C. *Folk Medicine*, Crest Books, New York, 1962.

Keville, Kathi and Green, Mindy. *Aromatherapy: A Complete Guide to the Healing Art*, The Crossing Press, Freedom California, 1995.

Levy, Juliette de Bairacli. *Common Herbs for Natural Health*, Schocken Books, N.Y., 1974.

Levy, Juliette de Bairacli. *Traveler's Joy*, Keats Publishing, Inc., Connecticut, 1979. This is a gypsy's handbook to accompany your nomad travels.

McQuade Crawford, Amanda. *The Herbal Menopause Book*, The Crossing Press, Freedom, California, 1998.

Mills, Simon Y. *Out of the Earth*, Viking (Penguin Books), N.Y., 1991

Montgomery, Pam. *Partner Earth*, Destiny Books, Rochester, Vermont, 1997.

Moore, Michael. *Medicinal Plants of the Mountain West*, Museum of New Mexico Press, Santa Fe, 1979.

Moore, Michael. *Medicinal Plants of the Desert & Canyon West*, Museum of New Mexico Press, Santa Fe, 1989.

Moore, Michael. *Medicinal Plants of the Pacific West*, Red Crane Books, Santa Fe, 1993.

Poutinen, C.J. *The Encyclopedia of Natural Pet Care*, Keats Publishing, Connecticut, 1998.

Shook, Edward. *Elementary Treatise in Herbology*, Mokelumne Hill Press, Mokelumne Hill, CA, 1977.

Shook, Edward. *Advanced Treatise in Herbology*, Revisionist Press, New York, 1991.

Soule, Deb. *The Roots of Healing*, Citadel Press, New York, 1995.

St. Clare, Debra. *The Herbal Medicine Cabinet*, Celestial Arts, Berkeley, California, 1997.

Sturdivant, Lee & Blakley, Tim. *Medicinal Herbs in the Garden, Field & Marketplace*, San Juan Naturals, P.O. Box 642, Friday Harbor, WA 98250.

Tierra, Lesley. *The Herbs of Life*, The Crossing Press, Freedom, California, 1992.

Tierra, Michael. *The Way of Herbs*, Unity Press, Santa Cruz, 1980.

Tilford, Gregory. *The EcoHerbalist's Fieldbook*, Mountain Weed Pub., Montana, 1993. Mountain Weed Publishing, HC 33, Box 17, Conner, MT 59827.

Tompkins, P. and Bird, C. *The Secret Life of Plants*, Harper & Row, 1972. (A true fairytale)

Upton, Roy., ed. *American Herbal Pharmacopoeia* and *Therapeutic Compendium*, P.O. Box 5159, Santa Cruz, CA, 95063, 1999.

Vogel, A. *Swiss Nature Doctor*, Keats Publishing, Connecticut, 1990.

Weed, Susun. *Healing Wise*, Ash Tree Pub., Woodstock, NY, 1989.

Weiss, Rudolf. *Herbal Medicine*, Beaconsfield Pub. Ltd., Beaconsfield, England, 1988.

Willard, Terry. *Edible and Medicinal Plants of the Rocky Mountains and Neighboring Territories*, Wild Rose College of Natural Healing, Ltd., Calgary, Alberta Canada, 1992.

PLANT ID GUIDES

Find a plant identification guide whose drawings and photos appeal to you aesthetically and whose text speaks most clearly to you. A good series to begin with is *the Peterson Field Guide Series* (Houghton Mifflin Co.)—*A Field Guide to Wildflowers*. They offer a field guide for the Pacific States Wildflowers, the Rocky Mountain region, the Northeastern and North-central region of North America, and so forth. Obviously, any single volume that covers areas as large as these will identify only a small portion of the resident plant population. Other plant guides will zero in on specific areas. For example, I use one that focuses on *The Plants of the San Francisco Bay Region—Mendocino to Monterey* (Kozloff & Beidleman, Sagen Press, Pacific Grove, CA). With a little practice in the art and technique of using these guides, they become gratifying companions that can give you an introduction to the local flora by giving you the plant's family, common name(s), and its Latin binomial.

SCHOOLS, CORRESPONDENCE COURSES, AND OTHER EDUCATIONAL RESOURCES

Rather than present an exhaustive list of these resources and probably still leave out a number of excellent sources of herbal education, I will give you the address and phone number of the American Herbalists Guild. This organization has compiled a booklet, *The AHG Directory of Herbal Education*, which I regard as the finest listing of both residential and correspondence courses in Herbalism. This directory also includes many journals, newsletters, computerized databases, and Internet resources for the herbalist. It costs $10, which is a mere pittance for the amount of work that goes into compiling, updating, formatting, and printing the document. The AHG is a group of herbalists dedicated to the advancement of excellent herbal education, and with this booklet and other services provides a tremendous assistance to both serious and casual students of Herbalism; and the organization can use the funds to help continue its volunteer work.

The AHG Directory of Herbal Education,
American Herbalists Guild
P.O. Box 70
Roosevelt, Utah 84066
Phone (435) 722-8434 or Fax (435) 722-8452

A.H. Guild Directory
1931 Gaddis Rd.
Canton, GA 30115
(770) 751-6021
Fax (770) 751-7472

SUPPLIES

Alcohol

Aaper Alcohol
P.O. Box 339
Shelbyville, KY 40066
(800) 456-1017
Request 190-proof grain alcohol

Vie-Del Company
P.O. Box 2896
Fresno, CA 93745
(209) 834-2525
Request 169-proof un-aged brandy

Pure grain alcohol (190-proof, 95 percent) is available in liquor stores throughout the Western states except in California. *Everclear* is a well-known brand name. Pure grain alcohol can be bought in B.C., Canada, but only with a special use permit that can be applied for at a government liquor outlet. One can also bring a liter (1 per month legally and tax free) of pure grain alcohol over the Mexican border. It only costs about four or five dollars a liter. Possibly more than a liter can be brought over, but you will probably have to pay duty on this.

Glycerin (vegetable source)

Frontier Cooperative Herbs
P.O. Box 299
Norway, Iowa 52318
(800) 669-3275
Provides from 2-ounce to 32-ounce sizes to retail customers

Capsules (vegetable source)

Frontier Cooperative Herbs
P.O. Box 299
Norway, Iowa 52318
(800) 669-3275

EQUIPMENT

Vita-Mix blender

As suggested in the text of this manual, try to find a Vita-Mix blender that has the stainless steel container. The new version comes with a polycarbonate container which may (or may not, I've not used one) be damaged when used for powdering dense, dried herbal materials.

Vita-Mix Corporation
8615 Usher Road
Cleveland, OH 44138
(800) 848-2649 (1-800-VITAMIX)

A Press

The Mini-Jack Press—Horizon Herbs
Box 69, Williams
Oregon, 97544-0069
(541) 846-6704 or order on-line http://www.chatlink.com/~herbseed
Be sure to request their Growing Guide and Seed Catalog.

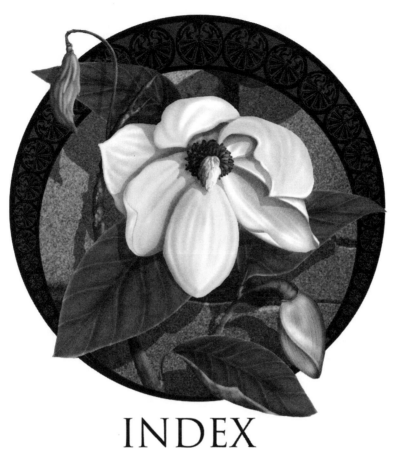

INDEX

Blakley, Tim, 23
Blender/juicer, recommendations for, 71-72
Bolus. *see also* Suppositories
defined, 220
Bottles. *see* Jars and bottles; Pharmacy equipment
Boyle, Wade, 250
Brandy. *see also* Alcohol
in syrups, 236
Bronchitis, remedies, 261, 262
Bulbs, 102
Bundling herbs. *see also* Drying herbs; Preparation
for drying, 59-61
Burdock (*Arctium lappa*)
actions and indications, 35-36
decoction, 115
extraction, 38, 76
glycerite, 192
Green's addendum to CSHS list, 24
infusion, 110, 200
percolation, 167
preparation, 55
salve, 208
tincture, 155
Bureau of Land Management (BLM), permit requirements, 53-54
Burns, Household Burn Center recipe, 282

C

Calculator, 70
Calendula (*Calendula officinales*)
actions and indications, 30
baths, 274
CSHS list, 23
drying, 58
extraction, 38, 313
harvesting, 56
infusion, 200, 211
poultice, 280
salve, 207, 208
tincture, 155
California School of Herbal Studies, list of 30 herbs, 23
Camphors, properties, 94
Capsules. *see also* Glycerin
capsule size, 294-295
circumstances modifying effect of medicine, 295-296
disadvantages, 294
dosage, 295
filling procedures, 295
in general, 293-294
herb preparation, 295
storage, 295
Castor bean, oil, 194
Castor Oil Fomentation, 287-289
Cataplasm. *see* Poultice
Catnip (*Nepeta cataria*), hydrosol, 119, 122
Cayenne (*Capsicum annum*)
actions and indications, 30
avoid during pregnancy, 37
baths, 274
CSHS list, 23
extraction, 38
infusion, 110, 200
percolation, 167

poultice, 284
salve, 208
tinctures, 148, 155
Centaury, flower essence, 133
Cerato, flower essence, 133
Chai syrup, 242
Chai tea, 166
Chamomile (*Matricaria recutita*)
actions and indications, 30
dosage, 297
extraction methods, 38
in general, 23
glycerite, 192
hydrosol, 122
infusion, 110
soil benefits, 17-18
Chaparral (*Larrea tridentata*)
extraction, 313
suppository, 221
tincture, 148
Cherry Plum, flower essence, 133
Chestnut Bud, flower essence, 134
Chickweed (*Stellaria media*), 57, 274
Chicory, flower essence, 134
Children. *see also* Warnings
baths for, 259-260
dosage recommendations, 86, 90, 297-298
formulation recommendations, 186, 187, 220-221, 242
Christopher, Dr. John, garlic oxymel recipe, 246
Cinnamon, extraction, 86
Cities, plants in, 44-45
Clark's Rule, dosage, 298
Clay, poultice, 284-285
Cleavers (*Galium aperine*)
actions and indications, 30-31
CSHS list, 23
extraction methods, 38
glycerite, 192
infusion, 110
succus, 314
tincture, 155
Clematis, flower essence, 134
Cocoa butter, in suppositories, 221
Collation. *see* Filtration
Comfrey (*Symphytum officanle*)
actions and indications, 31
avoid during pregnancy, 37
CSHS list, 23
decoction, 115
extraction, 38, 86
infusion, 110, 200, 211
lozenge, 302
mucilage, 86, 95
poultice, 280
salve, 208
suppository, 221
Commercial herbs. *see also* Herbs
evaluating, 16, 292
"commercial grade," 64
preparation, 66, 80, 171, 179, 298
purchasing, 63-64
Composting, 50, 58, 236
Compound formula, 26

Red Clover (*Trifilium pratense*)
  baths, 274
  drying, 57
Reishi (*Ganoderma lucidum*)
  actions and indications, 37
  decoction, 115
  extraction methods, 39
  Green's addendum to CSHS list, 24
Reproductive organs, remedies, 30
Resins, 96
Rheumatism remedies, 262
  Black Cohosh, 30
Ritual. *see also* Intention; Mindfulness
  of communion, 46-47
  in general, 44-45
  for harvest, 48
Rock Rose, flower essence, 138
Rock Water, flower essence, 139
Roots, 102
  evaluating commercial product, 16
  harvesting, 51-52, 54-55
  poultices, 284
  preparing, 55
Rose Electuary, 247
Rose oil, 96, 212
Rose water, 110, 122
Rosemary (*Rosemarinus* spp.)
  baths, 274
  harvesting, 56
  hydrosol, 122
  salve, 206
Rothman, Julie, 242
Royal jelly, 211

S
Sage, in honey, 244
St. John's Wort (*Hypericum perforatum*)
  actions and indications, 34
  CSHS list, 23
  extraction, 39, 148
  harvesting, 53
  infusion, 110, 200
  jello, 232
  mojo, 306
  properties, 95
  salve, 208
  threatened status, 52
  tincture, 155
Salicin, 95
Salves. *see also* Lotions; Skin
  dosage, 202
  Dried Herbs, Fixed Oil, Beeswax Salve, 203
  Ethyl-Oil Salve, 207
  from oil infusion, 204
  in general, 202
  general notes, 202-203
  Petroleum Jelly Aromatic Salve, 206
  preservation and storage, 202
  Vegetable Lard Vegan Salve, 205
Saponins, properties, 96-97
Saps, harvesting, 56
Saw Palmetto (*Serenoa serrulata*)
  actions and indications, 36

  dosage, 100
  extraction, 39
  Green's addendum to CSHS list, 24
  infusion, 110
  suppository, 221
  tincture, 156
Scales, 70
Scleranthus, flower essence, 139
Scullcap
  actions and indications, 34
  extraction, 39
  glycerite, 192
  infusion, 110
  tincture, 156
Seeds, 102. *see also* Fruits
  extracting, 76
  harvesting, 57
Sherry, 173. *see also* Wine
Siberian Ginseng (*Eleuthrococcus senticosus*)
  actions and indications, 36
  decoction, 115
  extraction, 39
  glycerite, 192
  Green's addendum to CSHS list, 24
  percolation, 167
  tincture, 156
Sieve, 310
Simple, defined, 293
Simpling, discussed, 293
Siphoning, 296
Skin. *see also* Baths; Hydrosols; Lotions; Salves
  effects of bath, 256
  liniments for, 301-302
  topical preparations, 101
Slippery Elm
  extraction, 86
  infusion, 110
  lozenge, 302
Solution, discussed, 312
Solvent exchange, procedure, 313
Solvents. *see also* Extraction
  alcohol, 81
    menstrua properties, 85-86
  in general, 80
  glycerin, 83
    menstrua properties, 89-90, 98
  maceration in, 75
  oil, 82
    menstrua properties, 91-92
  plant constituents and
    alkaloids, 93-94
    balsams, 94
    bitter compounds, 94
    camphors, 94
    enzymes, 94
    flavonoids, 95
    in general, 92-93
    glycosides, 95
    gums, 95
    mucilages, 95
    oils, 94, 96
    oleoresins, 96
    proteins, 96

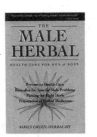